THE HEART OF COUPLE THERAPY

Other Guilford Books by Ellen F. Wachtel

Family Dynamics in Individual Psychotherapy:
A Guide to Clinical Strategies
Ellen F. Wachtel and Paul L. Wachtel

Treating Troubled Children and Their Families
Ellen F. Wachtel

The Heart of Couple Therapy

*Knowing What to Do
and How to Do It*

Ellen F. Wachtel

Epilogue by Paul L. Wachtel

THE GUILFORD PRESS
New York   London

The author has checked with sources believed to be reliable in her efforts to provide
information that is complete and generally in accord with the standards of practice that
are accepted at the time of publication. However, in view of the possibility of human
error or changes in behavioral, mental health, or medical sciences, neither the author, nor
the editor and publisher, nor any other party who has been involved in the preparation
or publication of this work warrants that the information contained herein is in every
respect accurate or complete, and they are not responsible for any errors or omissions or
the results obtained from the use of such information. Readers are encouraged to confirm
the information contained in this book with other sources.

Library of Congress Cataloging-in-Publication Data

Names: Wachtel, Ellen F., author.
Title: The heart of couple therapy : knowing what to do and how to do it /
  Ellen F. Wachtel.
Description: New York : The Guilford Press, [2017] | Includes bibliographical
  references and index.
Identifiers: LCCN 2016031560 | ISBN 9781462528172 (hardback : alk. paper)
Subjects: | MESH: Couples Therapy—methods
Classification: LCC RC488.5 | NLM WM 430.5.M3 | DDC 616.89/1562—dc23
LC record available at https://lccn.loc.gov/2016031560

To two very special couples:
Karen Wachtel and Sameer Parekh
Kenneth Wachtel and Margaret Noel

About the Author

Ellen F. Wachtel, PhD, JD, has a private practice in individual and couple therapy in New York City and is on the adjunct faculty of the Ackerman Institute for the Family. For many years Dr. Wachtel worked with Physicians for Human Rights and HealthRight International doing evaluations of people seeking political asylum, and she has mentored other psychologists volunteering with these organizations. Her books include *We Love Each Other, But . . . : Simple Secrets to Strengthen Your Relationship and Make Love Last*. She gives workshops on couples and families in the United States and internationally.

Acknowledgments

A big thank-you goes to Jim Nageotte, Senior Editor at The Guilford Press, for stimulating my thinking about what kind of book about doing couple therapy I wanted to write. Without his encouragement, this book would never have been written. Thanks too to Barbara Watkins at Guilford for her very helpful suggestions regarding the organization of the chapters.

The therapists who took the courses I've given at the Ackerman Institute for the Family also contributed valuably by challenging me with many thought-provoking questions, the answers to which form the foundation of this book.

Most of all, I want to thank my husband, Paul. Expressing my appreciation of him is a difficult task. Where do I start? When he helped me not be overwhelmed with anxiety as I started Harvard Law School? Or when he supported me in every possible way when I decided to give up the practice of law and become a psychologist? Or when he encouraged me to give talks and teach despite my fear of public speaking? Every step of the way he's been the voice of "Yes, you can." And so too with this book. He urged me to write it, wrote the epilogue himself, and spent much of a vacation reading a first draft and giving me exceedingly perceptive feedback. But in the end, my appreciation for Paul is not for the myriad ways he's helped me but for who he *is*—an incredibly warm, smart, supportive man who still, so often, makes me laugh out loud with his puns and quirky comments. So, thank you, Paul, for being the love of my life!

Contents

1

Introduction

Dilemmas and Choices in Couple Therapy

*D*oing couple therapy isn't easy. Even experienced couple therapists generally acknowledge that there are some couples with whom the work takes a serious toll emotionally; and even with less difficult couples, it's a not uncommon experience for therapists to feel at a loss and uncertain about whether anything they are doing is or ever will be helpful. Self-doubt often seems to come with the territory when it comes to doing couple therapy. So, when I sometimes say in conversations that I really *enjoy* working with even highly challenging couples, some of my colleagues look a bit surprised. I quickly clarify that it's not that I never have that stumped, "What do I do now?" feeling, but just that I've developed methods of working that generally seem to keep things moving in a positive direction.

The ideas in this book derive from numerous conversations with numerous people—students, friends, colleagues, my daughter (also a psychologist), and of course my husband, Paul Wachtel, himself a leading integrative therapist—who are curious about the specifics of what I actually do that might be similar or different from their own work. My aim in this book is to share with you in detail the methods that I have developed and my particular integration of theoretical perspectives that seems to make the therapy not only effective, but often actually quite enjoyable for both me and the couple.

I remember how hard doing couple therapy felt in the early years of my practice. To be in the presence of so much despair, frustration, anger, and contempt could leave me feeling as hopeless as the couple. Sometimes sessions seemed to go from bad to worse. After seeing some couples my head would be spinning and I'd wonder if I were really cut out for this work. It seemed so much harder than individual therapy and I'd feel so terrible when the tensions in the session hadn't been resolved and people left the office as upset as or perhaps even angrier than when they came in. Of course, this didn't happen with all the couples I saw or I would, in fact, have called it quits.

But after I had done couple therapy work for several years, I realized that I actually was finding this part of my practice more and more satisfying and that it was now quite rare for me to be so discouraged. In fact, I began to look forward to the sessions with the types of couples whom I had previously regarded as "difficult" because being able to help them turn the relationship around was so rewarding. Some of the change, I'm sure, came from simply having more experience. But I think a good deal of my increasing success in helping couples came from the fact that my work began to be more integrative, as did the work of many others in the couple and family therapy field (E. F. Wachtel, 1992, 2004; Sheinberg & Fraenkel, 2000; Fraenkel & Pinsof, 2001; Sheinberg & Brewster, 2014; Nielsen, 2016; Lebow, 1997; Pinsof, 1995; Gerson, 2009; Pitta, 2015; Feldman, 1992). Over time I gradually started to incorporate into my systemic orientation more cognitive, behavioral, and psychodynamic thinking and interventions. What I am presenting to you in this book is not a finished product. To this day, my work with couples continues to evolve as I incorporate experiential (Goldman & Greenberg, 2013; Greenberg & Goldman, 2008; Greenberg & Johnson, 1988; Wile, 2002) and attachment approaches (Johnson, 1996; Johnson, Makinen, & Millikin, 2001; Goldner, 2014), as well as information from neuroscience (Fishbane, 2013). My hope is that this book will be helpful to readers in their own efforts to meld new methods and perspectives into their work. It is meant to describe *one way* of working, my *particular* integration, and I by no means claim that this is the only way to be helpful to couples. There is increasing evidence that in couple therapy as in individual therapy, there are a number of "common factors" that cut across the party lines, so to speak, of the various schools of therapy that presently exist (Sprenkle, Davis, & Lebow, 2009). These include such elements as forming a strong therapeutic alliance (Norcross, 2002, 2010; Knobloch-Fedders, Pinsof, & Mann, 2007) and finding ways to motivate and instill hope (Howard, Moras, Brill, Martinovitch, & Lutz, 1996). Thus, many of the skills explicated in this book are essential regardless of the particular model from which one approaches the work. The reader doesn't need to adopt my approach in toto—rather, s/he can incorporate almost all the methods I describe into his or her own way of working with couples.

Clearly, interpersonal tensions are at the root of much of the distress that people feel, and a large proportion of people who seek therapy list problems with spouses or significant others as one of their primary complaints. The pros and cons, stresses and pleasures of a committed relationship are a topic of endless fascination both for the general public and for a variety of professional disciplines. There seems to be a voracious audience for the subject, and sociologists, psychologists, biologists, and even neuroscientists are weighing in on the topic and presenting their theories and findings to the general public. And, of course, in addition to the more academic findings, there are journalists, popularizing therapists, clergy, and self-proclaimed relationship experts giving advice on how to get and keep relationships, repair ones that are broken, rid oneself of ones that are destructive and addictive, or learn to enjoy being unattached. In the last year many thousands of books on relationships were published (Amazon had over 14,000 for sale) as well as articles and blogs too numerous to count.

It is thus not surprising that a growing number of therapists end up doing couple therapy, even though they may have very limited or sometimes no training in that modality. Many of the people who have taken my couple therapy courses feel that they *understand* what is going on with a couple but are often at a loss as to how to help the couple *break out* of destructive cycles, much less get what they crave from one another. Therapists who feel quite confident about the quality of their work with individuals can feel "lost" and insecure about their work with couples. This troubling feeling is quite understandable because many of the methods therapists use in working with individuals have to be significantly modified or even jettisoned when working with couples. For instance, psychotherapy outcome research has shown that a strong therapeutic alliance is a predictor of a positive therapy outcome. This is just as true for couple therapy as it is for individual therapy; but how the therapist forms a therapeutic alliance with the *couple* is quite different than forming an alliance with an individual (Pinsof, 1995; Pinsof & Catherall, 1986).

Becoming comfortable working with couples poses *particular* challenges for those therapists whose primary experience is in working with individuals in psychodynamically oriented therapy (E. F. Wachtel, 1979). In individual psychodynamic therapy, a strong transferential relationship forms between the therapist and the patient. Working with the nuances of that relationship is regarded by many psychodynamic therapists as a central therapeutic intervention. Therapists who work this way tend to like the intensity of the relationship they develop with the patient and may initially find the significantly different transferential configurations in the room in a couple session hard to adjust to. Though couple therapists too must foster a strong therapeutic alliance with the couple, it is nonetheless, in some way, a more distant, less intimate relationship.

Transference reactions toward the therapist do, of course, occur. But their intensity is less, both because of the methods used and because couples generally have strong transference reactions to *one another*. Although, as this book describes, couple therapists can have a great deal of influence on the emotional tone of the work, they do not have as much control over that as they do in individual therapy by virtue of the fact that the couple reacts to each other, not just to the therapist. One of the challenges for psychodynamically oriented individual therapists when they do couple therapy is that they see important unconscious issues that they would want to address with the person if in individual therapy, but which can be difficult to work on productively in the couple therapy modality. In the courses I taught at the Ackerman Institute, the psychoanalytically oriented therapists who were observing my work with a couple would often speculate about deeply buried intrapsychic conflicts that could be influencing the couple's interactions. Often the problem was not that these speculations were incorrect, but rather that issues of context, timing, the lack of a private relationship, and how the other partner would react to interpretations about unconscious motivations often pointed to the wisdom of foregoing that path of inquiry.

Carefully choosing what to attend to when faced with a myriad of choices is fundamental to good work with couples. At the heart of this book is a detailed examination of those choice points, and of the consequences of pursuing—or not pursuing—any particular line of inquiry. But the reader should rest assured that there *is* a way (and a time) in couple therapy to address many of these deeper issues and to help the partners mitigate the negative effect on the relationship of the issues they brought with them when they met. I will take up these matters periodically throughout the book and will go into detail about this issue in Chapter 8.

Another challenge for therapists originally trained in psychodynamic approaches is that they are often primarily trained to notice deficiencies, emotional damage, and impairment. Frequently these perceptions are accurate and important. But just how they are taken into account in the work—and how they are balanced with perceptions of the equally crucial strengths on which change can be (and must be) grounded—is the question that often is the critical difference between successful and unsuccessful couple therapy. All too often, being a smart, insightful therapist is understood to mean getting at the "underlying truth"—a truth that is almost never a flattering one, but rather one that exposes and uncovers the disavowed dark side of the patient (Havens, 1986; P. L. Wachtel, 2011a; Wile, 1981). One of the gratifying aspects of teaching has been helping students who have been trained in this way to be able to shift figure and ground. My hope is that this book will similarly help the reader learn to notice and work with strengths rather than responding first to deficits. Psychodynamic understanding is very much part of the integrative approach being described in this work, but, as is discussed further, it is used to understand longings and needs and not in the "gotcha" sense that characterizes so many interpretations (see, e.g., Orbach, 2004).

Focusing on, even seeing, the couple's strengths when they are in the throes of severe conflict is very difficult, probably considerably more difficult than diagnosing pathology. The latter shouts out to the therapist; the former whispers quietly and can easily be overlooked.

A key feature of this book is that it illustrates in great detail how this strengths-based approach is applied in difficult cases, cases where seeing strengths can, at first, seem at best a Pollyannish gloss on a raging tragedy. But my aim is to show the reader, case by case and example by example, just how this can be done—and how it can be done in a way that is precisely designed to *address* the very worst of what they are experiencing rather than to avoid it.

Those of you who have ever taken a fiction-writing class know the "show, don't tell" mantra of creative writing teachers. Though just *showing* what I do without explanation would not make sense, I am hoping that the book will, through numerous clinical examples, re-create the experience of my students who actually got to see me work with couples.

When I am learning a new approach that I want to integrate into my work, I find it useful to look at the exact wording of the therapist's interventions. To make it easier for the reader to do the same—and to enable the reader to easily see just what I actually said while also following the flow of the dialogue between me and the couple—I have *italicized* the therapist's statements throughout the book. I've tried to reproduce as accurately as possible the way I actually speak, and whenever what I wrote didn't sound like me, I rewrote it until I felt it rang true.

A different linguistic challenge arises in talking about what is going on in the session or for the couple. The challenge is actually twofold. First, as our understanding of the biases in our language has evolved, it has become clear that many sentences that use the generic "he" or "his" have a problematic gender bias. But sentences with lots of "he or she" and "his or her" become difficult to read, and although people are increasingly solving the problem in informal speech by using "they" or "their" essentially as nonsexist singular words, our written grammar has not yet adapted that convention, and so that solution still reads as ungrammatical. Further compounding the problem in writing about couple therapy in particular is that sentences like "The hurt partner may hide his feelings" or "The hurt partner may hide her feelings" may apply with one gender in one couple and the other in the next, so to make a general statement one can be caught in impossible-to-read sentences like "The hurt partner may hide his or her feelings when he or she finds that he or she is being treated in a way he or she feels evokes the old trauma." Reading such a sentence is itself a trauma, and one I don't want to inflict on the reader. Therefore, to make reading easier, I often will, in making general statements, alternate between "he" or "she" in different examples. Since the person who has an affair, the person who is preoccupied, the person who is uncommunicative, the person who brings excessive sensitivities from childhood, and so on, may be a man or a woman, this alternation also captures the reality that neither gender has exclusive possession of any of these traits or tendencies.

By addressing very specifically and in detail a range of difficulties that couple therapists commonly face, I am hoping that this book will be a little bit like supervision on your cases. In short, this book is intended to be *practical*, to give you the tools to do effective work with couples. What can look simply like good clinical intuition is actually based on principles and methods that enable the couple therapist to respond in ways that motivate and bring out the best in each person. At times what I will be describing may involve modifying or sometimes even completely giving up methods you are accustomed to using in working with individuals. But in my experience with students, when they try some of the methods I will suggest, they frequently see immediate benefits to this approach. For instance, almost every couple I see leaves a first session feeling a little more hopeful and eager to come back for another session. And if, as is often the case, one of the partners has acquiesced to the other and has come reluctantly, he usually feels, at a minimum, that it wasn't as bad as he expected! My aim too is that each individual not only feels heard but, if at all possible, receives some feedback about himself that is both positive and makes him feel known. Though a good first session doesn't necessarily mean that the rest of the work will go well or easily, it is of course an important first step and sets the tone for the work to come. Later in the book I discuss the structure I typically use for a first session and some of the variations on that format that arise from the variety of situations couples present.

Over the years many patients have commented that I'm an unusually positive person, and I respond to this comment by telling them that in my training I *learned* how to see what was going right as readily as to see what was causing problems. And one of my aims in this book is to help the reader learn to do that too. But, of course, the couple wouldn't be seeking help if everything was rosy, and great care must be taken to let the couple know that the fact that there are some, perhaps even many, positives by no means diminishes the seriousness of their unhappiness about what is missing or not going well in the relationship.

Though I try to make each session one in which the couple leaves feeling a little more hopeful than when they came in about ultimately working out their difficulties, this is not always possible. Later in the book I discuss the many reasons that sessions can, from the point of view of at least one of the partners in the relationship, be making things worse. Nonetheless, having the *intention* of facilitating some healing in each and every session is an important touchstone of my work. This may seem obvious, but unfortunately, all too often, therapists operate on the assumption that things need to get worse before they get better, and however relevant that idea may sometimes be for work with individuals (frankly, I'm skeptical!) it is almost certainly an impediment to good couple work. There is an urgency to couple work. Though couple therapy may at times be long term, couples need to feel that, even if slowly, they are fairly consistently making progress toward resolving the issues between them. Of course, even in individual therapy patients are evaluating the usefulness of the work and making judgments about whether or not to continue based on their assessment of how helpful the sessions seem. But in couple therapy, one person may be highly motivated to give therapy a try while the other is a reluctant or even hostile participant. This adds a level of complication to the evaluations each of them is making about the work. The person who has "dragged in" his or her spouse wants to show the other person that, in fact, talking about their difficulties with a therapist *is* helpful and thus is eager for some signs of progress. And the skeptical person, even if s/he has agreed to participate, needs, in a sense, to be "won over" fairly soon if the work is going to be productive. More so than in individual work, a few consecutive sessions that don't go well can lead to discouragement and withdrawal from therapy.

Keeping in mind that my job is to help *heal* often aids me when a session isn't going well. I ask myself what can I say or do that will calm things down, put the tension in perspective, and overcome feelings of discouragement. Subsequent chapters illustrate the kinds of things I say that bring me—as well as the couple—back to more productive work when, despite my best efforts, we've been going through a bad stretch. At the same time, it is also important to note at the outset that our job as couple therapists is *not* to try to keep together every couple who enters our office. In Chapter 10 of this book I discuss some of the ethical and therapeutic dilemmas of working with couples and will elaborate on the ways that my goal of having sessions be healing can encompass a variety of therapeutic goals and is not limited simply to saving the relationship.

Much of my work as a therapist, whether with individuals or with couples, is premised on the idea that understanding, both emotional and cognitive, must translate into change in how the person acts in the world. My task, then, is not only to facilitate new understandings and emotional experiences but to point the way toward new behaviors that follow from those insights. In writing this book, I have that same goal. That is, my intention is to help the reader go from understanding the general principles underlying my work to being able to employ various concrete interventions that derive from these basic tenets. Numerous case vignettes will demonstrate the points I am making. The cases are composites of the types of conflicts and personalities that I've encountered in the thousands of hours I've spent with distressed couples. I think you will experience the emotional truth of the situations I will be describing and that they will parallel closely what you encounter in your own work.

Many couple therapists, experienced as well as recently minted, feel swept along by the powerful force of the couple's emotions and can be as surprised as the couple about where they all land. We'll be looking later at some basic tenets about good relationships that enable us to have clear goals. But even when goals are clear, sessions can easily go awry. So, perhaps the most important skill of all in terms of being an effective couple therapist is to learn how to keep the session on course.

Taking charge of a session is not a matter of blowing a whistle like a phys ed teacher trying to get rowdy children to settle down and participate in the planned activity. Rather, it is done before there is even a perceived *need* to calm things down and in a manner that is subtle and often hardly noticed by the couple. This is because control and a clear sense of direction are the by-product of the many choices the therapist makes that affect how discussion of a particular topic will actually unfold. It is the accumulation of dozens of small, moment-to-moment choices about what to respond to and what to ignore that keeps the discussion moving in a useful direction and protects the couple from experiencing the session as out of control, hurtful, and little more than the mutual accusations that all too closely resemble what happens at home.

CHOICE POINTS

In order to utilize the suggestions that you will find in this book you first need to become very conscious of the choices you are making minute to minute in your sessions. Virtually everything said presents the therapist with numerous options regarding the direction of the work (Fraenkel, 2009). Even if we *think* we are just "following the couple's lead," how we respond to what is said reflects our assumptions about what we believe will be most helpful at that point in the therapy and contribute to the further direction a session will take. And, of course, what we *don't* respond to equally shapes and structures the course of the session. Implicit beliefs about what are the foundations and nature of a good relationship (see Chapter 2) and about what are the best methods for helping couples to achieve that status (see Chapter 3) underlie almost every word we utter in a session. One of the aims of this book is to heighten your awareness of the many choices you are making and to stimulate your thinking about *why* one would choose to go in one direction rather than another.

The following vignettes will give the reader a better understanding of what I mean by the moment-to-moment choice points that shape the session and the way they cumulatively effect the overall direction of the work.

Vignette 1: Francine and Mark

Francine and Mark had been separated for 2 months at the time they came to see me. After Mark discovered that he had herpes, he confessed to Francine that at the wedding of a high school classmate that he had attended without Francine, "I did something very stupid . . . I had a one-night stand with an old girlfriend." Within hours of hearing about this, Francine moved out of the apartment they had shared for the 8 years of their marriage. They had met when they were 20, and within months Francine had moved into Mark's apartment. They described being "soul mates" and Mark said that though there had been some ups and downs in the relationship they both had been ready to start a family until, as he put it, "I did this really stupid thing." Francine wondered whether the relationship had been "an illusion." She would never have imagined that Mark could do such a thing and felt that she didn't really know him. She questioned whether he really loved her. Recalling a few occasions when he had come home very late and hadn't called her, she wondered whether his tendency toward substance abuse—she knew that in his teens he had been to rehab—was kept in check by his marriage to her. "I think now that he never really loved me . . . I just served a function."

She was 95% certain that she wanted to end the marriage and had come to therapy only because it seemed like the responsible thing to do. She said, "I *believe* Mark that he was drunk and that this is the only time in the years we've been together that he did this. He thinks I'm overreacting, since it was just this one time, but I just don't think he gets it. How could he hurt me this way if he loved me? How could he put me at risk for herpes? And in the 6 weeks since he confessed, the only explanation he gives me is that he was drunk. He says the same things over and over again—it just happened, I don't know why, it has nothing to do with you, I was stupid." Francine was frustrated by the superficiality of what Mark was saying, and nothing he said could shake her belief that he didn't really love her.

In the third session, Mark said at one point. "I've been so depressed . . . I can hardly get out of bed. People at work have noticed. I even broke down crying once. My friends are worried about me." I asked Mark to tell me more about what he was feeling. *"What are you thinking about when you're depressed? What's going on inside you?"*

In response, he said the following: "I think about what a disaster of a person I am. How I messed up. How *ucked up I am . . . I'm always shooting myself in the foot. I have to start taking responsibility for my life. I probably should go to AA. I feel sick about how much I hurt Francine. And I miss her so much."

Here's the choice point I want to look at right now. When thinking about Mark's response to my question, I was aware of my brain sorting through a variety of responses and carefully deciding which I thought would be the most productive one at the moment in the work. Francine had been frustrated that his answers to *why* he had done what he did were not real answers. So, I could have asked him more about what he meant by "shooting himself in the foot" and have him discuss more his understanding of *why* he seemed to have done that to his marriage. But I had also been thinking that neither he nor Francine had been taking seriously enough his problem with drinking, so I could have asked him to elaborate more on his thinking about that. I could also have responded to his feeling "sick about how much I hurt Francine," because when he told Francine that she was making too much of this one betrayal, he clearly wasn't understanding and empathizing with her pain. All of these responses would have been fruitful, but I decided instead to ask him more about what he meant when he said he "missed" Francine. I did this because I thought the central impediment to Francine even considering trying to work on the relationship was her belief that Mark didn't really love her. So I asked Mark, *"What do you mean that you miss her? Could you tell me more about that?"* In response, Mark said, "I miss her when I come home. The house feels so empty. I miss her body next to me in bed. I miss calling her during the day . . . when something funny happens."

Again, there are numerous options in terms of my response. Missing her in bed or the house feeling empty could be "generic," so to speak, and could be incorporated into Francine's narrative that she was just a function. So I responded, *"Oh, you're missing calling her?"* "Yeah, I used to call her a couple of times a day . . . sometimes to tell her something that I knew she would get a laugh out of . . . sometimes to just check in to see how she was doing. She was my best friend . . . my soul mate. I can't imagine life without her."

Francine, who had been quite self-controlled up to then, teared up. His statement had broken through her defenses and it was difficult to just say, "He never loved me."

Let me make clear that there is no one right answer to deciding which fork in the road to take. My decision was guided by my goal of helping heal Francine's pain enough so that she was not making her decision to stay or to go reflexively, but instead would be open to examining in depth the nature of their relationship. The choice I made was my best guess about what would accomplish that goal at this moment in time. It is also possible that had I chosen another path, she would still have softened a bit. And the other potential topics I considered all represented topics that would eventually have to be addressed in our work together. My point in discussing this vignette and the others that follow is to heighten the reader's sense of how one's goals determine one's choices and thus shape the session.

Vignette 2: Luellen and Rosie

After living together for over 15 years, Luellen and Rosie had recently gotten married. They reported that they generally got along quite well—they both agreed that they were each other's best friend as well as spouse—but very occasionally they would have arguments that escalated to the point of viciousness. What concerned them both was that in the 6 months since they were *officially* married—they had considered themselves essentially "married" for many years—they'd been having explosive arguments once or twice a week. Rosie explained that when they argued Luellen would "hit below the belt" and say really hurtful things. Luellen didn't disagree. "I have a bad temper. I've talked about it with my own therapist. I think it's a fight-or-flight kind of thing—a survival mechanism—to deal with my overly controlling father who was a sergeant in the army and ran the house like we were the enlisted men under his command."

In the months that we had been working together, Luellen and Rosie came to understand why they had been arguing more frequently. Though in reality they interacted much the same way as they did prior to getting married—each had some separate friends whom they saw alone, each generally visited her elderly parents by herself—their *expectations* of one another since getting married had altered slightly. Rosie was more inclined to feel hurt when Luellen socialized without her. And Luellen was bothered by Rosie "becoming controlling" and "not letting me be my own person."

As their sensitivities became clearer and the pattern that led to escalations was identified, the arguments they had been having diminished greatly. Minor disagreements no longer escalated into emotional conflagrations. Rosie commented, however, that "Luellen still can be *mean* sometimes, but I try to let it go, and she cools off pretty quickly." Earlier in our work Rosie had alluded to, but didn't want to elaborate on "cruel things—things I can never get over—that have come out when Luellen's mad." But when I picked up on that comment, Rosie made clear that she didn't want to revisit what she referred to as "traumatic" memories for fear it would "set them back."

Rosie started the 10th session with the following statement:

> "I can't take Luellen's temper. I've really had it! We had one of those autonomy issue arguments, but this time it was like it was before we came here. Luellen screamed and cursed at me. Then she acted like nothing has happened. She went out for a walk and when she came back, she didn't want to talk about it. I'm sick of this! She thinks it's okay to say horrible things to me and then just because she said 'Sorry,

I didn't really mean what I said,' I'm supposed to forget about it. She's used to that approach. In her family you wouldn't dare talk about some horrible fight that had happened. Not that my family was so great, but at least they talked about things instead of sweeping them under the rug. Since that fight we've hardly spoken. I've really had it with all this."

First of all, I had to deal with my own personal reaction to what Rosie said. Though I "know" that couple therapy often has its setbacks, I nonetheless was aware of feeling disappointed. I thought I had been so helpful, and now this! Awareness of my feelings was very important, because it allowed me to not automatically follow my instinct and say *"Tell me what happened. What went on? How did this happen"* or *"It seems like a repetition of a familiar pattern . . . let's look at that again to see what happened."* Though of course it was important to know these things, it would not necessarily be the most productive direction to initially explore.

Knowing from prior sessions that Luellen felt terrible about what she called her "demonic temper," I thought that perhaps I should start by exploring with her such questions as *"How did she understand the loss of the self-control she had been working so hard to achieve?"* And though of course it is essential to eventually understand this issue, I decided not to ask that question at this point, because I felt that Rosie could experience that as yet another instance of "excusing" Luellen. I thought also of inquiring why Luellen didn't want to talk about the argument after it occurred, asking, for instance, such questions as *"What's your feeling after an argument? What's going on for you inside?"* Perhaps she felt ashamed of the things she had said, and a discussion of that would help heal the emotional wounds she had inflicted. But she could also not want to talk after an argument because she still felt angry about the dispute that had preceded the argument and was concerned that it would re-evoke her anger.

I could have chosen to focus on Rosie's statement that she "can't take it anymore" and ask her to explain more about what that means. I wondered to myself if she has been thinking of separating from Luellen. But since she had never expressed anything like that before, and they had only recently gotten married, I decided to leave that statement alone.

Though in prior sessions Rosie had explicitly said that she did not wanted to discuss the content of the hurtful things that Luellen had said in arguments in years past, I felt that she was making it clear now that she needed and wanted to talk more about how she had been hurt in this argument as well as in others. For this reason the choice I made was to respond to the part of her statement that indicated she'd been badly wounded by Luellen's words. I said, *"It sounds like you were very hurt by some of the things Luellen said and wanted to talk about it after the argument. Can we do that now?"* I asked Rosie to turn to Luellen and tell her about the things said that had pained her. After she had spoken directly to Luellen, I asked about how seriously she had taken Luellen's accusations. For instance: *"When Luellen said, 'You are a user—lazy—it's the "Latina" in you, just like your mother,' did it feel like Luellen's true feelings about you? Or that she really had prejudiced attitudes? Do you believe she really feels that way about you? About Puerto Ricans? Or did it feel like she didn't mean what she said and was just lashing out?"* Rosie responded that she had trouble believing that Luellen didn't actually feel that way about *her*, but didn't think Luellen was truly a bigoted racist. "She actually loves visiting my family and sometimes wishes she could be more 'Latina' herself." This led to a discussion of what in Luellen's history would make her prone to making that kind of accusation and what, if anything, would help Rosie believe Luellen's assertion that she actually didn't think Rosie was "a user" at all. The reader will see in Chapters 7 and 8 how to explore and work with the issues from each person's past that can so powerfully negatively affect relationships.

All of the discussion thus far did not address the differences in family background regarding talking about issues that Rosie had angrily highlighted in the beginning of the session. Thus, after we had discussed Rosie's feelings about the hurtful comments that had been hurled at her, I said, *"When you said earlier that you don't get over big arguments that quickly, I heard underneath that you had a wish to get over the hurt and that you know that if you talk more about it you'll be able to put this behind you."* I am attributing to Rosie *knowledge* about what will help her forgive Luellen. This is an example of an attributional statement, a method further discussed in Chapter 5. Because the session had focused on her hurt and Luellen's wish to repair the damage done, this statement resonated with how Rosie was currently feeling.

Vignette 3: Veronica and Tom

Veronica and Tom had been together on and off for 8 years. On numerous occasions they had broken up, but after a few months they missed one another and found themselves getting back together. They had great sexual chemistry and they both said they were "best friends." Around 6 months after getting back together, Veronica would feel that Tom was not as attentive or committed as he had been before. She would notice that he "checked out" other women—which he denied—and when she expressed her insecurity, Tom would at first be reassuring and then would start to feel annoyed by how "stifling" her insecurities were. When he responded with annoyance, she would become emotionally distant and this would in turn lead once again to their separating. They came to therapy to resolve their ambivalence once and for all. The therapy had been going well. Both of them felt that they were making progress and were not falling into the repetitive patterns that had previously led to their breaking up.

But one day Veronica called and asked if we could schedule an emergency sessions. Here's Veronica's account of what had led to their need for an earlier meeting:

> "I thought things were getting better between us. I really was beginning to trust him and thought I might even be ready to go ahead with the wedding plans that we had talked about. Ever since we started couple therapy, Tom was being so sweet and caring—acting the way I always wanted. I felt like these sessions really helped him understand my feelings and he wanted to make me feel secure. But yesterday he left his email open. I wasn't intending to snoop, but a familiar name caught my eye—an old girlfriend of his—and I found myself opening up the email. It was devastating.
>
> "They'd been communicating for months, and she sent pictures of herself practically naked. And the more I read, the worse I felt. In an email from 2 months ago, Tom told her we were in couple therapy and he might be available again soon. I just can't understand how he could do that. I feel so betrayed. To be fair, the last email I read was one where he was breaking it off. But still, for months he's been having an emotional affair."

Perhaps, at first glance, you will think that there aren't many choices here in terms of how to respond, because, of course, the topic is clear and Veronica's boyfriend needs to respond. But what I say next is important in shaping the direction of the session. There are again many options and subtle differences in wording that influence where the session will go. I could, for instance, ask Veronica more about the email that broke it off. *"What did he say in the email? How do you understand Tom's breaking it off?"* Inquiring about this last email starts with a question that has the potential to produce something positive to build on. Perhaps Veronica will say that he felt guilty, or didn't want to hurt her, or was feeling closer to her, or was ready to commit. But it won't necessarily go that way. For instance, Veronica *might* think that his cutting off the communication had nothing to do with their relationship. But by asking that question, there is a *chance* that some positive direction might emerge.

Or, I could pick up on her statement that she just doesn't understand, and say, *"You're so upset, but I sense that you really want to understand."* This is another example of an attributional statement. If I responded this way, it would be a decision to initially emphasize Veronica's wish to understand rather than her feelings of hurt and anger.

On the assumption Veronica needs to feel that Tom is truly remorseful, I could ask her to tell Tom how deeply hurt she feels. I'm less inclined to take this option because it seems too much like what they have done in the past—Veronica talking about her insecurity and Tom empathizing and then becoming tired of dealing with her feelings. Though the facts here are quite different than mere suspicions, I'm concerned that too much guilt and blame leads Tom to be defensive.

I decide to start by turning to Veronica, and reflect back that it was so devastating because things had been going so well. *"What do you mean that he was so sweet and caring? How? In what ways?"* I do this because it is a reminder of how good it can be between them and because it starts the conversation with Tom being appreciated rather than blamed. This, of course, is counterintuitive. I, like Veronica, am disappointed, and in a much more limited way feel that he has betrayed my trust too. Was his participation in therapy a charade? Was he just going through the motions? But, though I feel this way, I want to respond in a manner that will not make him feel attacked and will help him be as open and nondefensive as possible. After Veronica elaborates on how sweet he'd been, I turn to Tom and ask him to help Veronica understand what was going on for him.

I also highlight the point that Veronica had been developing trust, and ask her what she would need to develop that trust again. By this statement, I let her know that it *may* be possible to build trust again and that there are specific actions that can help that.

Of course I am concerned about what happened and wonder if Tom has not been forthright about his ambivalence or his "complaints" about Veronica. I scheduled a separate meeting with him to go into this concern in more depth.

In these three vignettes, we have looked at only a few of the possible responses to these statements. Many more paths could be taken. But I think the point is clear: the choices one makes initially and one's response to the comments that follow are what set the agenda for a session. Like driving a car, we are constantly making small adjustments or the car will swerve and possibly crash. Each sentence the therapist utters is a mini-intervention and it is the accumulation of these small decisions that keep the session on course.

The choice points I have been illustrating are not limited to couple therapy. The communication skills that are explicated and demonstrated in this book are as applicable to individual therapy as they are to couple work. Too often, in both individual and couple therapy, patients can feel that the therapist's goal is to get at deep, unconscious, or unacknowledged feelings that reveal something bad or weak about the person. What the therapist may think of as simply descriptive often has accusatory implications, and feeling "unmasked," the patient becomes defensive and resistant (P. L. Wachtel, 2011a; Wile, 1984). Throughout this book, the reader will be exposed to ways of saying things that get at underlying issues without inducing feelings of shame and the concomitant resistance that results from that feeling.

How one says things can make an enormous difference in the progress of the work. The numerous case vignettes you will find throughout the book highlight the wording that I think best invites the patient to give serious thought to the therapist's comments, interpretations, and suggestions (see also P. L. Wachtel, 2011a).

A LOOK AHEAD

The next two chapters present some basic assumptions and fundamental principles that underlie the chapters that follow. In Chapter 2, I present my own assumptions about the nature of a good relationship. These assumptions inform our decisions about what directions would be most fruitful to pursue. Equally important in our choices are some fundamental principles that underlie the work. Chapter 3 discusses some of these foundational principles regarding therapeutic method, procedure, and what I think is helpful overall and at different stages of the work. Chapter 4 describes my typical way of conducting a first couples session, including how I structure the session, assess the couple, and find strengths in the relationship. Most couples come to therapy with the goal of wanting their partners to change, but I start with the assumption that it is generally easier to change oneself than to get someone else to change. That's why in the first session I usually ask each person to think about "What makes you not the easiest person in the world to live with?" Chapter 5 discusses how to build on that question in Session 2 and the sessions that follow by using methods that foster self-reflection, humility, and the motivation to change oneself. Also in Session 2, the work of addressing the couple's difficulties begins. Chapter 6 overviews some of the issues that tend to underlie most relationship problems with suggestions for how they might be addressed. Then in Chapter 7, through case examples, I show how the methods covered in Chapters 5 and 6 can play out within the early sessions. The next two chapters discuss the influence on the couple of their families of origin and how to work with those issues. Chapter 8 describes how the process of doing genograms with the couple can itself be therapeutic, fostering empathy and elucidating aspects of each individual that the partner may not know. Given a more complete understanding of what each person carries into the relationship, Chapter 9 describes how to collaboratively move the couple from insight to action through new emotionally resonant experiences. Chapter 10 focuses on improving communication skills to work through a variety of issues and includes a section on the therapist's communication skills. Chapter 11 discusses how to handle seemingly intractable difficulties around affairs, emotional challenges faced by couple therapists, and knowing when it's time to end couple therapy.

SOME CLOSING COMMENTS

All couples need to find a balance between the "I" and the "we" (Lerner, 2012; Fishbane, 2001; Greenberg & Goldman, 2008). Maintaining one's individuality while being open to being influenced by one's partner is something that is not resolved once and for all by couples but rather is an ongoing challenge throughout the developmental stages of long-term relationships. Perhaps this issue is even more in the forefront when a couple's worklife overlaps, as it does for me and my husband, Paul, also a psychologist. Like all couples, we work to maintain our individuality while at the same time joining and intertwining our lives much of the time. Our thinking overlaps a good deal, though there are definite differences—for instance, he's a psychoanalyst and I am not—but one of the pleasures of a long marriage is to wonder whether we influenced one another or if we would have thought similarly regardless of how the other viewed things. The combination of similarities and differences to which I have just alluded is also what ultimately led me to ask him to write the Epilogue to this book.

2

⚭

What Is a Good Relationship?

*I*n this chapter we look at assumptions regarding what most couples need from one another in order to feel content with their relationship, and at what is required to repair the rifts that have occurred. The next chapter will discuss some of the foundational principles regarding therapeutic method and procedure upon which the remainder of this book is based. Much of what I have to say in these chapters about the foundations of good relationships and about how to proceed therapeutically will likely seem familiar to most couple therapists; but other aspects of what I offer here may be surprising or controversial. My aim in these chapters is to make clear to the reader the basic structure of how I think and work and why I believe this approach is especially helpful for couples.

You will likely have questions about some of what I say in these initial chapters. The principles described here have evolved over many years of trying to help very distressed couples and have been shaped by the direct experience of seeing relationships improve in dramatic ways. I begin with an overview of these principles in order to enable the reader to have a basic structure or map to understand just what I am up to in the more detailed descriptions of clinical exchanges from sessions that follow. But the map is not the territory. It will only be as you see these principles applied in the clinical accounts that are the heart of the book—including the ways that these principles must be modified as we hit the inevitable obstacles—that you will be in a real position to see which of these principles can serve as a useful guide for your own work.

This discussion is also intended to heighten your awareness of *your own* beliefs and practices. You may have some other assumptions that you would add to those explicated here. Or you may find that you disagree or at least have some reservations about what I have highlighted as primary. In these chapters, as well as in all those that follow, I encourage you to pick, choose, borrow, and incorporate what makes sense to *you*. My intention here is to stimulate you to think about and evaluate your own basic assumptions. You do not need to swallow whole my approach for it to be useful.

WE LOVE PEOPLE WHO MAKE US FEEL GOOD ABOUT OURSELVES

To my mind this simple statement captures much of what couple therapy is about. Generally, couples are so mired in their frustrations that they no longer give one another the good feedback that came naturally earlier in their relationship. Very often people get recognition and admiration everywhere *but* at home. This is not necessarily because the spouse just doesn't see anything positive anymore. Couples who are coming to therapy because they want to see if they can repair their relationship often *do* still see some or even many positive qualities in their partner. But by the time the couple seeks couple therapy, hurt, disappointment, and criticism have usually come to dominate their relationship. They are in no frame of mind to express admiration or to make the other feel good.

One of the challenges of couple therapy is to address dissatisfactions while simultaneously helping each person feel valued. If the relationship has some chance of being repaired, the therapist must facilitate the expression of positive perceptions of the spouse. In doing so, it can be helpful to point out that we don't have to be *completely* pleased with the person to give compliments, noting, for example, that most people continue to affirm their children's good traits even while they are less than delighted with certain aspects of their behavior or sometimes even their personality.

Many people feel that giving good feedback about *some* things undermines how seriously the complaints they do have will be taken. Saying something complimentary to their partner can feel like papering over legitimate concerns, and furthermore that doing so will decrease their partner's motivation to change. Paradoxically, just the opposite is usually true. The person who feels valued and loved is much more likely to respond nondefensively to the other's concerns and expressions of unhappiness. My belief in this principle affects my work in many ways. Couples are often quite taken aback by the statement, *"We love those who make us feel good about ourselves."* The startling obviousness of the comment can jolt the couple into seeing the ultimate destructiveness of the path they are on. I have found that saying this is more powerful than the corollary truth that *criticism erodes love*, which though equally true requires more explanation and frequently provokes debate.

Another way that this tenet about love informs my work is that I'm always alert for subtle signs of admiration that might otherwise go unremarked upon. Perhaps in an exchange in the session the husband says with annoyance something like, "Our house is constantly filled with people and it's too much. Sometimes I just want to come home and not have to interact with anyone. But Andrea [his wife] talks to someone for 2 minutes and they want to be her best friend, and before you know it, they're coming over for dinner. I've told her over and over again to consult with me before inviting people over, but she doesn't seem to care about what I want." As a 3-second aside, before addressing the main point of what he's saying, I might say to the husband, *"It sounds like even after all these years together, you're pretty amazed at the effect your wife has on people."* If the husband hears it as a momentary aside and not something that is detracting from his complaint, he might elaborate a bit more with something like "Yes, everyone loves her because she's so interested in them." And then, when we turn back to the more substantive issue, his wife is likely to be less defensive because a significant affirmation has just been highlighted.

Frequently one person in the couple feels hurt that the other doesn't express love verbally. "I know he loves me but he never says it and never compliments me." The partner hearing this remark may be puzzled by what feels like an inaccurate representation. He might say, "Didn't I tell you this morning that the dress was nice?" or "I do say I love you." What the wife is *really* asking for are statements that actually make her feel good about herself. If he had said, "You look great in that dress," rather than "The dress is nice," or "You have great taste," or "Everything looks good on you," it would be about *her*, not the dress. And similarly, it may be true that he says, "Yes, of course I love you" (not spontaneously, but when asked), but the whole exchange is not giving the wife the little ego boost that she is craving.

Sometimes my work with couples is frankly psychoeducational, and I'll explain to them how to make compliments more meaningful by being specific rather than general—for example, "You're good at lightening up a tense situation like you did the other night when Jim and Rould started to argue in front of us," or "You really have a way of getting Charlie [their 6-year-old] to give you details about school," or "You're good at thinking outside the box and coming up with solutions to things, like you did with Martha the other night." Often I'll give couples a copy of the self-help book I've written, *We Love Each Other, But . . .* (E. F. Wachtel, 2000) and suggest that they read the sections titled "Expressing Admiration Goes Beyond Saying I Love You" and "How to Convey Admiration Year after Year without Getting Repetitive."

The corollary of *we love people who make us feel good about ourself* is, as I noted earlier, *criticism erodes love*. Feeling constantly criticized and negatively evaluated is one of the most frequent complaints couples make about their spouse. Early in a romantic, intense relationship, couples can sometimes be open to critical input about themselves because it is experienced as deeply caring. As a new couple gets to know one another, they are interested in how the other sees them, and as part of that they often discuss aspects of each other's personality. For instance, a woman might point out to her new boyfriend that he seems to have difficulties with authority and that he acts in a too familiar, somewhat disrespectful, manner to her father. Or a man might tell his girlfriend that in her wish to show that she understands another person's feelings she too quickly turns the conversation around to something about herself. These are never pleasant things to hear, but in the context of new, intense love it is possible to hear this kind of input without feeling too hurt or defensive. But, in my experience, the willingness to be critiqued, particularly on big things like personality, social interactions, work habits, and the like rarely lasts very long. Frequently, one person in the couple will say, "I don't know why she wants to be with me. She criticizes me constantly. Nothing I do is right." Often I've heard one person say that "there's a knot in my stomach when I hear the key in the door because I'm on edge about the critique that's soon to follow."

Some people internalize their partner's criticism and feel inadequate and inept. Others are more apt to feel angry. But in either case, a fundamental bond in a relationship is frayed when one no longer believes that s/he makes the other feel happy. Frequently, a vicious circle can occur in which the criticized person withdraws, leading the other to be hurt and still more apt to point out the other's faults, and so on. Or the criticized person, out of anger, may consciously ignore his partner's complaints or, alternatively, may not realize that his "forgetting" is a passive–aggressive expression of his resentment at being criticized.

One of the most important things I learned early on in my training is that asking people to *stop* doing something is much more effective when it occurs in conjunction with focusing on and engaging some alternative behavior. It is far easier to *do something different* than to just *halt* habitual behavior. Thus, an important aspect of breaking the vicious circle of criticism and withdrawal is to heighten each person's awareness of the aspects of their spouse's personality that they feel positively about and to help them find comfortable ways to express whatever positives they find.

COUPLES NEED TO ENJOY ONE ANOTHER

Many couples coming to therapy have a "transactional" relationship. They interact almost exclusively around the *business*, so to speak, of family life.

Sometimes they spend almost no time alone, and when they do have time alone together, talk only about very practical things that they need to do and plan for. Often couples bicker or argue in the midst of these discussions, but even when they do not, this type of engagement, though of course necessary, is not experienced as something pleasurable.

It is important to be clear, however, that taking pleasure in one another's company does not *necessarily* mean spending time alone together. We must be careful not to impose our own personal or cultural preferences on the couples we work with. A couple may take pleasure in each other while entertaining together, or going out with other couples, or traveling with other families, or just being together as a family. The main issue is whether they feel that the other's presence enhances the enjoyment they are getting from the activity.

Here I want to distinguish *enjoyment* of one's spouse when in each other's company from *intimacy*. Having open and emotionally revealing conversations may, of course, be pleasurable (and much of my work does involve enhancing intimacy between the partners), but it is by no means the only way for couples to feel they are happy to be with one another.

The feeling that one's partner doesn't really have much desire to spend time with you is a source of serious hurt in relationships. Many couples don't put any effort into being appealing or interesting to their partner and the notion that one needs to consciously do so can come as somewhat of a surprise. To be sure, being natural and comfortable with one's spouse is a source of pleasure, and provides a respite from the public persona that one assumes in the world. Yet without some conscious effort to stay attractive, both physically and in many other ways, the relationship can easily become flat and dull.

To address this issue, it is commonplace for therapists to suggest that couples have a "date night." Occasionally this can be helpful but often it is not. Some couples, with a little push from the therapist, *can* enjoy time with one another away from the stresses and strains of parenting, and simply haven't made it a priority. But my experience is that often couples don't follow through on the "homework" to have a date because it feels like a pressured, forced interaction. And frequently, if they do follow through, the date turns out to be quite disappointing. Many couples report that they sit across from one another at a table and don't know what to talk about. The "date" feels strained and dull. Or worse, they may feel that the other isn't really *present*. Or the couple may not know how to have an engaging fresh conversation. Perhaps one or both of them "hold forth" on some topic and the conversation devolves into all-too-familiar positions that feel more like a debate than a real exchange. And worse yet, many a "date night" has turned into an opportunity for big arguments.

Emphasizing "enjoyment" in the relationship shifts the emphasis from what is *wrong* to what they can do to have more positive experiences. Sometimes this is as straightforward as asking couples to talk about some of the memories of fun they had together at one time and encouraging conversation about possibilities for new or similar experiences that they can incorporate into their current life patterns. Many couples do not have much desire to go out with one another primarily because their Saturday night date has turned into a predictable routine. Couples need to have enlivening experiences together, and sessions can be used to help the couple brainstorm in a productive way about ways to engage with one another in a less routinized manner.

Often, focusing on having a good time together involves looking at what goes awry when they try to do that. But the therapist can help to make an examination of what goes wrong an opening into how it can go better. For example, the therapist might ask about what happens when one person proposes some activity for them to do. Is the other "game" or does s/he go along with the suggestion in an obviously reluctant way. Or, in considering what happens when the couple goes out to dinner and the conversation falls flat, or becomes more of an argument then a conversation, a close examination of the communication style of one or both partners may point the way to small changes that can enliven the interaction.

COUPLES NEED TO BE "AGREEABLE" WITH ONE ANOTHER

It's been challenging to come up with the word that best describes the attitude that enables couples to get along well with each other despite the inevitable differences that two people have. I've settled upon the word "agreeable," though I know that it may have connotations for some readers of prefeminist subsuming of one's self to one's partner or a superficial adaptation that substitutes for real connection. But let me be clear, first of all, that a commitment to "being agreeable" must be made by *both* parties. I thought about simply saying that couples need to be more "easy-going" with one another. Being "easy-going" involves being relaxed about things and not being too demanding or critical. And though, of course, an easy-going attitude goes a long way toward making for a harmonious relationship, being "agreeable" involves *more* than letting a lot go. It is a *positive* attitudinal and behavioral stance rather than the mere absence of a negative one.

A shorthand way of describing this to couples is to say that it would be very helpful to their relationship if each of them were inclined to say *yes* and that *sure, yes, fine, okay* could be thought of as their default response. I sometimes lightheartedly suggest with some couples, who are aware that they are competitive with one another and tend to get into power struggles, that if they are going to compete with one another, perhaps they could compete around who can say *yes* more often. Though this is said in jest, there is a lot of truth to it, and the couple's laughter in response also entails their "getting" it.

Couples who get along well may find themselves in the situation where each is more than willing to defer to the other's preference, and occasionally, of course, this can lead to the humorous "Alphonse–Gaston" routine in which each one says, "No, it's up to you. . . . No you." But how much better a problem that is to have than the resentment which arises when a couple can't move forward because each is so dug into his or her own opinion and positions. If one person begins to feel that he is almost always the one who is going along with what the other wants, resentment will of course build up. *Each* person needs to be committed to an attitude of cooperativeness and a desire to make the other happy.

A further perspective on what I mean by being agreeable is to think of it as focusing less on the *I* and more on the *we*. It means that not every decision needs to be evaluated by assessing how *I* as an individual feel about it. Many of the difficulties that couples face have to do with negotiating the balance between being an individual and being a couple. Sometimes, to preserve one's sense of individuality, almost every decision becomes an opportunity to assert one's separateness and difference from the other, and when this happens effective couplehood is extremely difficult.

That is not to say that there aren't times when one person may need to stick with his or her individual preference. Each person needs to assess just how important what is at issue really is to him or her; it is not being wisely agreeable to go along with something that s/he will later feel unhappy about having agreed to. When two people really do differ on some issue that is genuinely meaningful to each, then "being agreeable" means that each person actively looks for a compromise or a third way, with the goal being to find something they can each truly feel comfortable with. Rather than there being a winner or a loser, each tries to find a solution that will make the other happy, but without making him- or herself miserable in the process. This is, of course, not always easy, but the very process of engaging in the effort is itself a strengthening of the relationship.

Preserving a sense of separateness and individuality undoubtedly is a key element in keeping relationships vital and interesting. Separate opinions, tastes, and pursuits can be stimulating and enhancing to the couple's interaction. Out of a legitimate concern for preserving a separate sense of self, one or both members of the couple may resist the "joining" that makes a couple feel closer and diminishes conflict. Autonomy and a separate sense of self are virtues that can also be overemphasized. Not only do some couples make every small choice an opportunity to highlight their differing individual preferences, and hence implicitly assert their individuality, but couples may also conform their *perceptions* to this aim, selectively attending to the numerous ways they *differ* rather than to the ways they may be similar. Most couples are together because they do share some fundamental values and assumptions despite differences in personalities and interests. Couple therapy can help them develop a "we" narrative by bringing to the foreground those similarities and consonances that they take so for granted that they are scarcely noticed, though they may be the very ground of the relationship. Perhaps they have similar sensibilities, humor, work ethics, attitudes toward creativity, or fundamental values, to name but a few of the characteristics that often go unnoticed in a couple's desire to define themselves through differences. Some couples, of course, have grown so far apart or have lost so much respect for one another that they just can't find a "we" identify. This state of affairs does not bode well for the longevity of their relationship and may at times be an indication of such extreme alienation from one another that couple therapy is unlikely to be effective.

COUPLES NEED TO EXPRESS LOVE AND AFFECTION PHYSICALLY

It is not uncommon for couples who seek therapy to barely touch one another. Often, they are quite physically affectionate with their children or a pet but not at all with one another. At times, the lack of physical demonstrativeness has come about because of tensions in the relationship. But often it seems to have just gradually happened as the couple shifts more and more into relating to one another as coparents rather than as romantic partners. Often, as this proceeds, there is an avoidance of all physical contact for fear that it will be misread as a sexual overture.

Sexual intimacy is both a *sign* of closeness and further *fosters* the emotional connection. It is now well known that when people have sexual contact, oxytocin is released and bonding is enhanced. But even apart from the explicitly sexual aspects of the relationship, closeness between couples is enhanced when affection is expressed physically. What I am referring to here are physical gestures of fondness and connection—for example, the spontaneous hug, the arm draped around the shoulders, the quick neck message as one walks past his spouse at her desk, the reaching for the other's hand in the movies or on the street. These warm gestures, though small and casual, mean a great deal to the recipient. And many people are particularly touched when physical affection of this sort takes place in front of friends or family because they are proud to have it known that they are close.

Frequently one person in the couple feels hurt that the other doesn't initiate any physical contact. Noticing the affection expressed by other couples, sometimes even one's grown children, stirs both longing and pain.

Even witnessing how warm and affectionate the spouse is with the children can highlight the absence of the same kind of affection between the couple. Each may feel wounded by the lack of demonstrativeness of the other. And often it has become a cyclical self-perpetuating interaction, in which each avoids possible rejection by not initiating contact and accommodating to a relationship where almost no touching occurs.

Therapists need to help couples break the ice with each other. Sometimes this happens naturally as the relationship improves; but frequently, even if the couple is now getting along well, the physical distance remains. This is even truer when it comes to sexual intimacy. A strong case can be made for addressing the lack of sexual relationship early in the treatment rather than waiting until other issues are resolved (Iasenza, 2010; Perel, 2010). When couples have a gratifying sex life together, all sorts of irritations may no longer seem as important. A remarkable number of couples almost never have sex. Sometimes they say that when they are sexually intimate it is actually very gratifying, but busy schedules and exhaustion make sexual contact a low priority. For others, sexual contact just hasn't been very gratifying. One or both may feel they don't have much of a sex drive or find masturbation, with or without pornography, a satisfactory outlet. Often couples do not raise the issue of the lack of sexuality in their relationship. When the therapist inquires about the topic, it can be a big relief because one or both have been very hesitant to bring it up.

To be sure, therapists need to be cautious when examining the couple's lack of sexual contact. There is a fine line between encouraging a discussion of the topic and pushing the couple to address something that they would rather leave alone. Frequently, however, one person is considerably more bothered about it than the other, and in that case, in particular, it is a topic that the therapist must find a way to address in therapy.

COUPLES NEED TO FEEL SECURE
ABOUT THEIR RELATIONSHIP

Of course, couples need to trust that each is faithful and is not having an affair of any sort: physical, emotional, or virtual. But even when that is not an issue, many partners do not feel emotionally safe with one another. They don't regard their spouse as someone whom they can reliably go to for comfort and support. Sometimes this is because there have been one or more serious attachment injuries from which the person has never fully recovered. And, of course, sometimes one or both parties have an insecure attachment style deriving from early childhood which gets reenacted in the relationship. It is one of the fundamental tenets of the work being described in this book that the effects of attachment injuries, as well as patterns that derive from attachment styles, can be greatly mitigated by changes in day-to-day interactions.

For big hurts and betrayals such as affairs, cathartic expressions of hurt may be an essential first step in healing the attachment rupture. But much of the time it is the mundane, quotidian alterations in how the couple interacts that results in the establishment of lasting emotionally security. One important premise is that the impact of the big hurt is often misunderstood because frequently what ultimately matters is not the hurt itself, but rather that it has led to a lifelong set of ongoing and repeated events that *maintain* the hurt (P. L. Wachtel, 2014a). But if new sequences are initiated in which day to day *a different* texture of experience is generated, then the big hurt from the past gradually dissolves. The ongoing, routine, predictable experience that my spouse is in *my* corner, rooting for me, defending me when need be and frankly, being biased in my favor can be one of the most powerful factors over time in generating a deeply felt sense of safety.

Many people are hesitant to confide their upsets to their partner because they want *support*, not an *objective evaluation* of the situation being described. Often the "objective" partner is not at all trying to be hurtful. He may be the type of person who, when asked, will convey to the therapist that he generally listens to almost *anything* he hears with unvoiced, silent skepticism. While that analytic, evaluative mind-set may serve the person well in his career it can be quite wounding when applied at home. Often a key component of couple therapy can involve coaching one or both partners about how to really listen, with the goal being to join, comfort, or offer support rather than to analyze.

Of course, honest feedback is extremely important too. One cannot be expected, nor would it be helpful, to blindly agree with everything one's spouse feels and thinks. But when people feel that their spouse is generally "on their side," receiving some objective critical input from time to time will be experienced differently than if it is a frequent occurrence.

It is a common complaint, from both men and women, that when they talk about a difficulty, their spouse responds with suggestions for how to solve the problem when really what's wanted is just a chance to verbalize one's upset. Though the problem-solving stance is often described as typically male, I have frequently heard men complain that if they tell their wife about some work-related issue, the wife immediately starts giving advice about a complex situation that would take a long time to explain. And, to make matters worse, often embedded in the solution being offered is some "constructive criticism." For instance, a spouse might respond to the partner's getting a smaller bonus than expected by saying, "I think you need to prove to your supervisor that you don't have to be so obsessive–compulsive about your work and can get the work in even before the deadline instead of perfectionistically refining it right up to the last minute." Though a statement like this might be intended to be helpful, it is likely to be experienced not as a constructive suggestion but simply as a covertly hostile criticism.

In loving relationships, being with your partner feels like a safe haven. This is not to say that one's partner should be blindly loyal; sometimes we really don't feel that our spouse is in the right. But I am talking here about having a *general inclination* toward seeing things from one's spouse's point of view. Women often express the wish for this attitude in terms of wanting to "feel protected." Men, in my experience, are likely to express their longing for something very similar via complaints that their opinions and input *are not valued* enough by their partner and that the judgments of friends or family are given more weight than theirs.

COUPLES NEED TO REMAIN ATTRACTIVE TO ONE ANOTHER

In a good relationship, couples feel very comfortable with one another. One of the pleasures of being in a relationship is that you can come home and shed your public persona. After work many people change out of their work clothes, perhaps vent a bit about the stresses of the day, and feel relief at being able to be their authentic self. But often this level of comfort goes hand-in-hand with an assumption that one shouldn't have to do anything to stay attractive to one's partner. I've heard many people say that they aren't interested in having sex because their spouse doesn't shower often enough, or has bad breath, or goes to sleep in a dirty, ripped t-shirt or sweat suit. But even when couples do make some effort to stay physically attractive to one another, they may make little effort to be attractive in other ways. Couples are often surprised by and may initially object to my suggestion that being attractive to one another needs to be a day-in and day-out undertaking for the rest of their life together and entails more than one's physical appearance. Frequently, couples relate to one another with little regard for politeness or manners.

By "politeness" I do not mean simply saying "thank you" and "please," though the value of these words and—especially—the attitude that goes with them should not be underestimated. A couple may be "natural" with one another, perhaps in the way they were with their siblings, and un-selfconsciously burp or pass gas because their partner is not thought of as someone with whom good manners are expected. Politeness also means making an effort to act with one's spouse the way one does toward a friend. This means taking responsibility for true dialogue and interesting conversation or being conscious of the effect of one's mood on the other person.

Of course, couples need to be able to vent, complain, obsess, or go into detail about something in ways that one just wouldn't do very often even with one's closest friends. But even in a marriage, this kind of behavior must be balanced with an awareness of the effect it has on one's partner and a commitment to trying to be a good companion. It is common in couple therapy for one person to complain that he is worn out by his partner talking endlessly about work and family stresses. The familiarity and comfort of long-term relationships can lead to boredom without some conscious effort to be interesting and engaging to one another.

At times the difficulty is that one person is suffering from anxiety or depression and is not getting the professional help s/he needs. Being a good companion is difficult when one isn't feeling well psychologically. Often it is only in couple therapy that an individual becomes fully aware of just how emotionally distressed he has been feeling. The spouse can provide critical information about the intensity of his or her partner's anxiety or depression that can enable the therapist to determine if the partner needs individual therapy and precisely what kind of help the person needs.

A DELICATE BALANCE

The basic principles just described are what couples need to aim for, but it is important to keep in mind that every relationship has areas of strength and weakness. While therapists need to help couples come nearer to reaching the goals described in this chapter, we must be careful not to unwittingly endorse perfectionism and striving after unrealistic, idealized images of good relationships. Much of the work of couple therapy helps to heal old wounds and prevent new ones from occurring by helping the couple interact differently. But equally important is helping the couple put the disappointments in the relationship into perspective. By the end of therapy, the couple should feel that generally (but not always) most (but not all) of their needs are met.

A similar tension occurs between conveying the belief that people can change and helping people accept one another for who they are (Jacobson & Christensen, 1996; Gottman, 1999). Though saying "This is the way I am" in response to one's partner's wish for change goes against the grain of therapists, there are times when that is essentially true. The therapeutic approach described in this book often results in couples being able to focus on what they can and do get from one another rather than what is missing in the relationship. Sometimes, of course "This is the way I am" just isn't acceptable, and one of the skills of a good therapist—whether individual or couple therapist—is to enable the person to begin to see that s/he can be different, and indeed sometimes *is* different.

The basic principles I have presented here are derived from my work with a very large number of couples. The reader will notice that there is a good deal of overlap with what other seasoned therapists have concluded about what makes a relationship work well. For instance, John Gottman has pointed out the importance of "fondness and admiration" and noted that "positive feelings that have long been buried can be exhumed" (Gottman & Silver, 1999, p. 67). Gottman's work on the importance of spouses responding positively to each other's "bids" for connection is part of what "being agreeable" means (Gottman & DeClaire, 2002). There is general agreement that couples need to feel emotionally secure with one another (Markman, 2001; Greenberg & Goldman, 2008; Johnson, 1996; Kaslow & Hammerschmidt, 1992), give more positive feedback, and be less critical (Gottman & Silver, 1999). And many couple therapists also emphasize the importance of couples having enjoyable experiences with one another (Doherty, 2001; Schwarz, 2011; Markman, 2001).

All couples will have conflicts, and learning how to resolve differences is an essential ingredient of harmonious relationships. But conflict resolution skills are a necessary but not sufficient component of gratifying relationships. Markman (2001) (see Parker-Pope, 2010) has said, "It turns out that the amount of fun couples have and the strength of their friendships are a strong predictor of their future" (p. 271). In this chapter we have looked at some of the elements of relationships that can transform a "good-enough" relationship into one that is both a safe haven—a place of comfort and security—and a source of joy and pleasure in each partner's life.

3

Principles and Methods

*T*he basic assumptions about good relationships discussed in the previous chapter help inform our decisions about what directions would be most fruitful to pursue. But equally important in our choices are some *fundamental principles* that underlie our work. Although there is some substantial overlap with individual therapy, there are also quite a few differences. Therapists who are new to couple therapy need to learn some new approaches as well as learn when to put aside their usual modus operandi.

FORMING A THERAPEUTIC ALLIANCE

Just as in individual therapy, so too in couple therapy: forming a strong alliance is an essential ingredient for therapeutic effectiveness (Norcross, 2002, 2010; Duncan, Miller, Wampold, & Hubble, 2010; Lambert & Barley, 2001; Pinsof, 1995; Pinsof & Catherall, 1986; Knobloch-Fedders, Pinsof, & Mann, 2007). But developing and maintaining the alliance in couple therapy can be a much more complicated and delicate process. In individual therapy, therapists help bond with the patient by showing empathy, initially seeing things from the patient's point of view before challenging his or her assumptions, offering support, and slowly building rapport. In couple therapy, these methods must be greatly modified. To begin with, there is often time pressure because one person in the couple may be a reluctant participant. Moreover, our usual ways of showing empathy when one person is expressing a lot of upset may make the other partner (often whom the first is upset *at* feel blamed). And finally, we cannot suspend disbelief in the way we do in individual therapy, initially seeing things completely from one person's perspective. Rather, we need to communicate that we are listening to one partner's version of the difficulties respectfully, but at the same time acknowledge that the other partner is likely to see things quite differently. In couple therapy a therapeutic alliance consists of creating three bonds, one with each individual and one with "the couple" (Pinsof & Catherall, 1986). To begin with, each person needs to feel that his or her point of view has been heard and understood. The therapist achieves this goal by being an active listener. He needs to summarize the core concerns expressed by each of the partners and then ask to be corrected if he doesn't have it quite right. For instance, I might say something like *"So what I'm understanding so far is that you feel that your wife is frequently, or maybe even constantly, critical of you and that it seems so unfair because you work so hard to support the family. Is that right or am I off a bit?"* He might then elaborate a little: "Well, yes, that's basically right, but the main point is that I'm sick of coming home to constant complaints!"

In addition to each person feeling that his or her point of view has been heard, understood, and respected, each also needs to feel *liked* by the therapist. Giving each person some personally affirming feedback as soon as possible begins the process of bonding. The input could be said almost as an aside (*"I see you have a good sense of humor"*) or it may relate to the content and process of the session. How and when to do this is discussed further below.

It is also helpful if the therapist finds a way to join with each spouse so that both the husband and the wife feel that you are similar to them in some way. I'm not talking here about major self-revelations, but simply some small gestures through which you bond. For instance, I always offer couples water or tea or what I describe as "my horrible instant coffee," and if someone actually said yes to the coffee, I might laughingly say, *"I like the stuff but I don't find too many other takers."* Or, if someone finds the couch too crowded with pillows and asks if he can remove them, I might say, *"I know what you mean. I'm always throwing pillows on the floor."* Or, more substantively, if someone says that he's a light sleeper and feels his wife is inconsiderate when she noisily comes in to bed, I might say, *"I know what you mean. I can wake up at the drop of a hat too, and that's a real problem for me and my husband."*

It is not uncommon for couples to feel embarrassment or even humiliation about the limitations of their relationship. How the couple looks to the world is often quite different from the way they behave with one another when they're alone. The therapist's ability to see some positives in their relationship helps mitigate the shame they may feel about how they act at home. A therapeutic alliance with the *couple* often begins by conveying respect for them as a "we." For instance, it may be that after hearing about what they were attracted to in one another (discussed further in Chapter 5), the therapist may comment on how substantial and meaningful their reasons for coming together were. Or, if the couple states that they have had a difficult relationship for many years and have seen other couple therapists, one might convey respect for their persistence in trying to find solutions.

Often, despite their marital problems, couples have been a successful team in some aspect of their life. They may, for instance, have cultivated a wide circle of friends, or run a business together, or have become close to each other's family, or cared for elderly parents together, or raised children who are doing well. By conveying respect for their ability to achieve these things and work together regardless of difficulties in their relationship, the therapist is bonding with them as a "we."

The most important factor in developing a strong therapeutic alliance with the couple is their sense of experiencing the therapist as skilled in making the sessions productive. Trust in the therapist and the process develops when the couple feels "safe" and sees that the sessions do not result in yet more conflict or the unraveling of the relationship. It is reassuring to couples when the therapist controls the emotional intensity of the session, follows up in detail on what was discussed in the prior meeting, carefully builds on aspects of their relationship that are still somewhat gratifying, and sums up at the end of the session what has been covered, especially any plans for trying new ways of interacting.

At the same time, although the therapist must convey that she is in charge, the alliance is strengthened by also conveying the message that the work is collaborative and that she does not have all the answers. While it is useful to "normalize" some of the difficulties the couple is having, the therapist needs to communicate that she is aware of the particularity and even uniqueness of *their* issues and that any problem-solving suggestions are derived from the specifics of their individual personalities and the particular characteristics of *their* relationship. Helping the couple to find their own solutions and giving them credit for the work *they* are doing with help from the therapist contributes greatly to a strong therapeutic alliance. And, of course, as in any relationship, admitting to mistakes you have made and apologizing when your error has done harm not only helps strengthen the bond but also serves as a useful model for the couple.

Perhaps most importantly, the working alliance is strengthened when blame, self-criticism, and shame diminish as the couple gains some perspective on how they are unwittingly caught in negative patterns of interaction. As the couple therapist helps them understand the role of family history, individual sensitivities, and different coping styles in the repetitive vicious circles that have developed—Wile (2013) describes this as constructing "a permanent platform or perch, above the fray" (p. 28)—they are more and more able to step outside of the impasse in which they find themselves and together observe the way "the pattern" is exerting its pull on them both. The objectification of "the pattern" as something separate and distinct from each of them as individuals helps them to join as allies against destructive habitual ways of interacting that their mature and healthier selves do not really want to engage in (Johnson et al., 2001; Scheinkman & Fishbane, 2004).

FOCUSING MORE ON LONGINGS AND VULNERABILITIES THAN ON COMPLAINTS

Whenever possible, I try to focus on what each person is longing for rather than on his or her complaints. Couples come to therapy because one or both of them is feeling quite unhappy in the relationship. Usually, they initially describe this unhappiness in general and mutual terms—"*We* argue all the time," "*We* live like roommates," "*We* don't have much in common any more"—but when asked to elaborate, the *we* often turns into complaints about the other: "*He's* too controlling," "*She* criticizes me constantly," "*She's* too sensitive and takes offense at everything," "*He* puts me down in front of the children," to name but a few of the dozens of critiques that couple therapists hear each day. Most couples think that couple therapy will be about venting their complaints and enlisting the therapist's help in getting the other to change. And though, of course, the therapy does need to focus on these dissatisfactions, the sadness, frustration, vulnerabilities, and implied *craving for something better* can all too easily get lost in the torrent of grievances (Scheinkman & Fishbane, 2004; Greenberg & Johnson, 1988; Greenberg & Goldman, 2008; Johnson, 1996). In the first session, I often state, *"Though our initial goal is to help you get along better and repair the hurts that have resulted in a frayed relationship, we could also aim higher, and see if perhaps you each can get more of what you may be longing for."* This is one of the reasons that in the initial session I usually spend considerable time hearing about the good feelings and experiences the couple may once have had with one another. Wishes, longings, and expressions of sadness about what used to be but is no more are much easier for the other to hear than criticism.

There are several components to what I mean by "shifting the focus" to what people are longing for. First, general statements need to be operationalized. By this I mean that all general statements must be grounded in day-to-day interactions. For instance, if the husband says, "I want to feel that I'm really important to her, that I come before work," I might ask, *"What would that look like? What would give you that feeling?"* Perhaps he would say that she'd call me during the day even if she was very busy, or that she'd invite me to business functions when bringing one's spouse was optional. I would also ask his wife if she has any ideas about the kinds of things she could do that would demonstrate her love for him. *"Nobody knows him as well as you do. What's your sense about what makes him feel important and loved? What do you think you could do that would make a difference?"*

The best way to convey to someone what you are wishing for is to give an example of when that person spontaneously did what you've been craving. Thus, in the example just given, I would also ask, *"Can you think of a time when your wife actually did something that made you feel you came first?"* Generally this question does elicit some instance of the longed-for feeling, but not always. For instance, he might say, "Yes, when she cancelled some appointments to accompany me to the cardiologist, but I don't want to have to be on the verge of a heart attack to know that I come first!" *"Of course not! Can you think of any other less dramatic times that you had that feeling? If not, why don't you give that some thought during the week? Maybe some instance will occur to you."*

By now his wife is probably jumping out of her skin with a desire to remind him of instances of devotion that have gone unnoticed. After she states some of the ways she believes she shows how important he is, I would ask the husband, *"Just give some thought to what your wife has said. Don't respond now, just think about it, and if you want to we can talk about it some other time."* I don't ask him to discuss how he feels about what she has just said *now*, because many people have difficulty retracting or changing their mind about a position they have just taken.

Even when dealing with the couple's statements about what the other is doing wrong, I look for a choice point to subtly shift from blame to longing. For instance, when Ginny stated that ever since coming back from their vacation, her husband had scheduled work engagements almost every night and he had completely forgotten about their regular date night, the therapist had many options for how to respond. One could focus on her hurt, or her anger, or ask him for his take on what she had just said. Though any of those responses might be productive, it is more likely that he will be defensive because he feels blamed and may countercritique his wife for exaggerating or being too needy. The response that most gets to desire and longing would be something like *"It sounds like you're really missing him after having spent so much time together when you were on vacation."* "Yes, that's it," said Ginny. "Really?" said her husband, Roberto. "I didn't realize that." Like Roberto, many people are quite surprised when they understand the positive feeling that lies beneath the surface of a criticism. Although Ginny may have to face the reality that, of course, her husband is simply not as available during their regular life as when they're on vacation, expressing her upset as longing rather than as criticism helps avoid the vicious circle that can develop as attack elicits defensiveness and countercriticisms. It is also possible that her expression of missing him will trigger his own feelings about the good time they had when they had an extended period of time together, and this in turn may enable him to better resist the pressures of work.

I am painting a rosy picture here. Perhaps he didn't enjoy their time together as much as she did, or sees her wish for him as controlling and excessively needy. But at a minimum, shifting from blame to wish opens up more possibility of something good happening in the session.

Here are a few more examples of how complaints can be turned into wishes. Austin angrily stated that "all I get from Serena is criticism. I don't have a minute to catch my breath all day and look forward to finally being able to relax. But the minute I walk through the door I face a barrage of my crimes and misdemeanors—how come you didn't empty the dishwasher before you left the house, or, you left the lights on again, or you didn't put away the stack of papers you left on the dining room table. I'm sick of it. You're obsessive–compulsive about the house and you do the same thing to our kids." Of course, there's more to this interaction than his complaints. Perhaps Austin's wife is so critical because she feels he's not engaged enough with her. Or perhaps she feels devalued in her role as homemaker and parent. Or perhaps she *is* too obsessive. There's much to be discussed. But again, in choosing a focus, it is useful to opt for one that concentrates on *wishes* rather than on anger.

Thus, the therapist could respond to Austin's angry outburst by following up on the part of the statement in which he refers to coming home and looking forward to relaxing. *"What would that look like, if you could come home and relax? How do you picture it?"* Or perhaps one could say, *"It sounds like you still think of home as a haven of sorts—can you remember times when it did feel like that?"* Of course, he might say, "No, never," or she might say, "His idea of relaxing when he gets home is to tune out and not relate to me at all."

One must not expect focusing on wishes to be a "magic bullet"; but it does at least open up the *possibility* of a discussion that is more than mutual accusations. But let me be clear: though my goal is to get the couple to shift from complaints to wishes, this task is often quite difficult to accomplish. People respond defensively even to the other person's wishes and often focus on the implied criticism in the other's statement. So, for instance, if a woman says that she would feel more loved if her husband spent more time with her, he might angrily respond that she just doesn't appreciate how demanding and stressful his work is and what *he* longs for is for her to be more appreciative of what he does for the family. In Chapter 4 we look at some methods for handling the common pattern of attack and counterattack in which many couples engage despite the therapist's attempts to get the couple to articulate longings rather than complaints.

Couples often reach a point in the work where they are getting along much better, yet they are still not feeling particularly close. They might report that "things are better, we haven't had any big arguments, and we're bickering a little less." At that point, if one of them hasn't already said it, I might respond with something like *"It sounds like you're relieved things have calmed down, but though it's better, it seems like it's just 'okay'—not bad, but not feeling particularly good."* Almost always, both partners will agree with that statement, and their response provides an opening to discuss what else they might want from the relationship now that they are getting along. I also explain that they are less likely to backslide the more they each feel fulfilled in the relationship. It's much easier to let a lot of the little annoyances go—to have a "don't sweat the small stuff" attitude—when important needs and wishes are being gratified.

I might at this point remind them of some of the things they said in the first session about what had drawn them to each other and made them want to stay together. These are usually things like long intimate conversations, intense sex, adventures, spontaneity, laughter, and the feeling, described in the prior chapter, that they are each other's biggest fan. I might say something like *"Of course, that was a different time in your life. You didn't have kids and the responsibilities you have now, but is there a way you can get some of that back?"*

Often couples are simultaneously intrigued and deeply skeptical about that possibility. Cory's statement about his wife is typical of this mix of feelings. "When we met, she was really adventuresome. But ever since we had kids, she's like a different person. I lost the wife I married. Of course, I miss that person, but I need to be realistic. I just don't think she wants those things anymore. She's become much more traditional." As often happens, the person in the couple who presumably has changed *also* misses his or her former self. When this occurs, the next step is fairly straightforward. The therapist helps them brainstorm about how to have experiences with one another that are somewhat similar to what they once had.

Sometimes the couple seems fairly satisfied with the improvements they have made and they come to sessions with not much to talk about. This may be an indication that it is time to wind down and set a date for termination. But often the therapist is aware from things said in earlier sessions that there are areas of their relationship that one or both feel are far from what they would ideally like. For instance, the couple may have no sex life or they may be living quite separate lives except for the time they spend together with their children, or one of them is extremely dependent on the other and knows almost nothing about their finances. Acceptance plays a big role in marital happiness (Jacobson & Christensen, 1996) and therapists need to take care not to destabilize a "good enough" relationship. It is all too easy, however, for *acceptance* to morph into resentful acquiescence. This is particularly true when what is missing is physical intimacy, and therapists, while respecting the couple's right to chart their own course, need to gently probe the parameters of what each partner is truly comfortable accepting.

Though the therapist does not want to stir up conflict, it is also important not to collude in pushing dissatisfactions under the rug. Topics that had been off the table may no longer seem so dangerous because the couple has experienced the therapist as building on their strengths and are no longer apprehensive that sessions will spiral downward into negativity and mutual accusations. But if the couple shuts the door on what the therapist has raised, it is extremely important not only to back off but also to help the couple feel good about all that they *have* accomplished—not bad about what they have chosen not to tackle. Feeling good about the work also makes it much more likely that they will come in again if what has been left unresolved becomes more of a problem.

LEARNING TO SEE POSITIVES

It takes practice to notice the subtly implicit positives in statements in which the main point is primarily a negative one involving emotions like shame, discouragement, hurt, and anger. Again, it's not that the therapist ignores the painful emotions. Not at all. Rather that he *also* notices and comments on an additional dimension that is readily overlooked. Therapists are accustomed to focusing on what is *wrong* in interactions in order to help fix the problems. It takes conscious effort to find the kernels of good interactions that one wants to reinforce and encourage. Further complicating this issue is that the "good" is *relative*, and may consist of the diminishment of negatives rather than actually being positive in itself. Just as I tell patients that they can *learn* to see the positive—that I was *taught* how to do so in my training—the reader too can become skilled at picking up the nugget of some strength or movement in the right direction (O'Hanlon & Weiner-Davis, 2002).

Below you will find two examples that illustrate the way therapists may be able to find some small things to build on even in a more generally negative account. Here's the first one:

"Al [her husband] again got into a screaming fight with Cole [their teenage son] and I was furious. Honestly, I thought they were going to reach a new low and actually come to blows—but thankfully, they didn't. I've been trying hard to stay out of it when it seems to me that they may be heading toward a fight. I know that my 'butting in' bothers Al a lot and just leads to the two of *us* having an argument. For a few days they actually did seem to be doing better with one another. I think maybe because you [looking toward her husband] tried harder to be understanding with him because you knew that I wasn't going to come in and calm Cole down. But you really blew it and acted as immaturely as he does! I know Cole can really be 'in your face' and he definitely was intent on pushing your buttons this time, but still, you're supposed to be the grownup!"

Here are some kernels of strengths that are embedded in this basically troubling statement:

- The wife had noticed that both she and her husband had been doing better at breaking the pattern of interaction they had in relation to their son. She didn't "butt in" and he was staying calmer in his interactions with Cole. Often people do not notice change, so it's to her credit that she was able to see that something good had been happening even if the change was quite short-lived.
- She was committed to trying to do something different because she knew it *bothered* her husband.
- By acknowledging how provocative Cole could be she was demonstrating some empathy for her husband's reaction.
- She had insight into the way her husband didn't have to try as hard because he knew he could rely on his wife to calm things down.

These points do not negate the fact that the husband had a serious lapse in self-control. But the fact that they were both able to do something differently can be used to combat the discouragement they both were feeling. It argues for trying once again to break the dysfunctional pattern, but this time with some plan for what each of them can do when their son is at his most provocative.

Here's another example:

"I tried to talk with her about what was going on at work. That's what she *says* she wants, right? But, just as I said last week, I don't believe Mary Sue really wants me to tell her what's going on in my life. But, I gave it a try . . . and just as I thought, within a couple of minutes there was a distracted look on her face—and she said—wait just 1 minute while I respond to my boss's email. I was really pissed off and needed to cool down so I walked out—actually—I slammed the door and said '*uck you' as I left. And instead of apologizing to me, she said I was making a big deal out of nothing and was furious that I cursed at her. I get it. She can't hear about anything that I'm upset about because she gets so anxious. I guess she thought when I told her my boss was hassling me that I was probably going to lose my job. I tried to tell her it wasn't anything serious so she wouldn't worry, but she gets so bent out of shape with anxiety that there's no point in talking to her. Later we had dinner and watched some TV together. She asked me about work again but I didn't want to talk about it. I'm not falling into that trap again. It's bullshit that she wants more openness. Well, maybe not *bullshit* because I think she believes that's what she wants. But really, I'm on my own when it comes to problems."

- The husband was aware of needing to cool off and though he remained angry, did get calm enough to reconnect with his wife in some way—dinner, watching TV.
- He tried to accurately report on the extent of his reaction—volunteering that he had slammed the door and cursed at his wife.
- He had insight into why she had trouble listening to him and retracted his use of the word "bullshit" to describe her state of mind.
- In the past when the husband had stormed out of a room, his wife would follow after him and insist on talking. This time she didn't do that and that helped prevent a further escalation of the argument.
- By asking him again what was going on at work, the wife was trying to undo the interaction that had led to the blowup. Implicitly, she was now communicating that she would try to listen despite her anxiety.
- Knowing that his wife was prone to getting anxious, the husband had tried to reassure her at the outset that the incident he was describing "wasn't anything serious."
- The husband was expressing some wish for connection. It was clear that he wasn't just trying to please his wife by trying to talk with her more intimately.
- By watching TV together they were trying to reconnect in some way.

Again, noticing these positives is not meant in any way to downplay the hurt, anger, or problematic behaviors that the couple is revealing and discussing. Rather, these are "asides" or short detours that plant a seed to encourage productive directions and thought processes even as the therapist also (as the couple requires) attends to the "main event" as the couple experienced it.

And finally, though the two examples demonstrate that there may be something good to build on even in accounts of troubling incidents, therapists should have realistic expectations in regard to noticing positives. Often it is simply not possible to find any without stretching the point in a way that feels unrealistic or insincere.

BEING GENEROUS AND SPECIFIC
IN THE USE OF POSITIVE FEEDBACK

Positive feedback, when sincere and specific, is an extremely effective method for getting the best out of people. I have already talked a bit about giving feedback that helps establish a therapeutic alliance with each individual as well as with the couple as a unit. Here I am talking about using feedback to encourage steps in the right direction. When faced with choices about what to respond to, underlining—and implicitly affirming—any bit of progress is uppermost in my mind. Here's an example: A couple states, "We lapsed back into our old pattern and had a terrible fight in front of the kids. We both felt terrible about them having seen us cursing and screaming at each other. Jimmy was being very provocative and I lost it." Though of course we need to examine how the argument started, why and if Jimmy was provocative, what they each could have done differently to prevent this kind of episode, and so on, it is useful to digress for a few moments to reinforce certain *positives* that the statement alludes to. In addition to reinforcing steps in the right direction, the brief focusing on something good—or more accurately, *relatively* good—helps establish an atmosphere that makes the discussion of what has gone wrong more productive; feeling acknowledged for some small bit of progress, the couple is likely to be less defensive.

Perhaps in the wife's opening statement we notice that she is acknowledging her part in bad fights more than she usually does. I might say something like *"Before we get into what happened, I just want to say that I'm struck by your openness in saying that you know that your 'losing it,' even though provoked, was part of what led to this bad scene in front of the children."*

Or if the couple rarely talks about feelings, or seldom acknowledges the other's feelings, my digression might focus on that aspect of what was said and I'd say something like *"I'm struck by your saying that you <u>both</u> felt bad about the argument. How did you know that Craig was upset about it?"* This might lead to a discussion of how they talked about it later, or how she had some empathy for him despite the fact that he'd been provocative.

When underlining what might seem like a mere footnote to the main point, it is crucial that the couple experience this as a brief detour, almost an *aside*, and not of equal importance to the central concern that was raised. If the therapist does not get back to the original topic, the couple may feel that he is too invested in seeing the couple as making progress and that he doesn't really *understand* the seriousness of their problems.

Even if the noticing of something affirming of the couple's attempts or success in interacting a bit differently has led to a productive discussion that the couple wants to continue, the therapist must make clear that we need at some point, if not today, to get back to the issue with which they started the session. If the therapist neglects to get back to what was originally presented, the couple can lose confidence in the therapist's ability to keep the sessions on focus. And even worse, the couple may see the therapist as sweeping problems under the rug or colluding with one or both of them in minimizing the gravity of their negative interactions.

UNDERLINING POSITIVES
THAT OCCUR IN THE SESSION

So far we have been looking at giving some affirming feedback about interactions that have happened outside the therapy office. Positive feedback is also extremely useful in helping couples make the best use of their time in the session. The old maxim—Catch people doing something right—is useful in getting the couple to have productive sessions. So, for instance, as the couple starts to talk about something difficult, I might stop them and say, *"I'm struck by the way you're talking about this sensitive topic—you raised it in a way your wife can hear and you're really listening nondefensively."* Or if a couple who have in the past been very adversarial with one another are doing better at listening to one another rather than each waiting his or her turn to rebut, the therapist can digress for a few seconds to note this change. Saying something like *"I know this is a difficult topic about which you clearly have a strong disagreement, but I'm really impressed by how hard each of you is trying today to really hear the other's point of view"* can be helpful. A statement like this encourages them to do this more, and the more they do this the better the session will go. Sometimes the comment is directed at just one person in the couple. For instance, if someone has described himself as not being good at talking about his feelings, noticing and pointing out those moments when he is expressing himself well encourages him to try harder and to begin to think of expressing himself as a less risky or failure-prone activity. Or perhaps someone who tends to be defensive is being at least somewhat more open. Attending to that increased openness will make it a little bit easier next time for him or her to again be less defensive. It's important, of course, to offer this type of praise without emphasizing that in the past s/he has been defensive because the compliment is then likely to be overshadowed by the implied criticism. Instead, one could say something like *"You're being so open today. I wonder what's enabling you to do that? Is your husband doing something differently so that it feels safer to be open to his criticisms?"*

Trying to be fair in one's description, seriously thinking about what your partner is saying, being open to the therapist's input, staying calm, not "indicting" your partner, listening with a mental set of wanting to understand and not just waiting to rebut, trying out new behaviors based on what has been discussed, moving toward one's spouse when s/he is upset, show-ing empathy, trying to put yourself in the other's shoes, breaking tension by reaching out physically to one's partner, listening attentively when one's spouse is talking about his or her family history—these are all qualities that if noticed and commented upon help the couple act in ways that make the therapy much more likely to be helpful.

One needs to be careful that saying something positive to one person in the session doesn't make the other person feel that s/he isn't doing well. Often it's possible to commend both partners. For instance, if one was to say to the husband, *"I'm really impressed by how open you are being about having a problem with your temper,"* you could turn to the wife and say something like *"I think your staying calm has really helped him experience his own contribution to the arguments,"* or *"You're nodding your head in agreement, and it's really helpful that you're able to recognize how hard he is trying."* One can't always find a parallel compliment, but if the therapist is generally attentive to steps in the right direction, both parties should be receiving approximately equal feedback. In Chapter 11 I discuss what to do when one person feels you see things more from the other's point of view.

Again, it is important to remember that the purpose of noting the small steps in the right direction is to encourage constructive changes in the way each person acts with the other at home as well as to "shape" behavior in the session so that the work is as productive as possible. By noticing some good moments *even while agreeing that the situation being described is indeed quite problematic*, the therapist communicates and perhaps models having a perspective that negative interactions do not entirely wipe out good ones, and that often negatives and positives can and do exist side by side.

KEEPING THE SESSION FOCUSED

Without clear direction from the therapist, a session with a couple can easily lose focus. When discussing one issue, couples often bring up many related concerns that if addressed at the time will lead to a feeling that many upsets have been voiced but little has been resolved. Often the larger the number of issues covered in a session the less the feeling of getting somewhere. At best the work will feel spread too thin and the couple will leave with the uncom-fortable feeling that the session didn't accomplish anything. At worst, it will feel like the session is spinning out of control, resulting in unresolved hurt feelings, anger, and defensiveness. Thus, the therapist needs to strike a bal-ance between letting and even encouraging the couple to voice pent-up feel-ings and frustrations and keeping a tight enough rein on the session so that it doesn't deteriorate into venting of mutual accusations. Borrowing images from both dance and jazz, one can think of the session as "choreographed," but at the same time improvisational. The therapist carefully moves the session along, one step at a time, leading to an organized pattern. But s/he is not following a rigid course that ignores the almost infinite number of ways that the couple introduces their own variations in whatever was planned or anticipated.

Of course, it is not realistic to expect that each session will result in some resolution. The problems couples discuss are often years in the making. It may take many sessions before the hurts, anger, and wishes behind the issues are sorted out. Often the difficulties need to be looked at from a number of different angles—both individual and systemic—before progress is made. Nonetheless, it's important that the couple leave the session with the experience that it had some coherence and direction.

The first step in keeping the sessions focused is to help the couple articulate clearly what issues they want to work on in the therapy *overall* and, again, in each session. Often couples feel a strong need to talk about an argument they have recently had even if it has been resolved. Paying attention to choice points can help the therapist use something that is said in describing the incident as a segue to focusing on a more general concern.

I try to start sessions by sharing my thoughts about what might be useful to discuss, for example, getting back to what was talked about last time, or getting back to what was put on hold, or getting to some new topic that was originally designated as a goal—and asking the couple what issue each of them had been thinking about raising. There is an important metamessage conveyed in starting a session this way. The couple will feel less anxious knowing that the therapist has a plan and is not as subject to the latest disturbance in the atmosphere as they are. Additionally, it communicates an expectation that the couple give some advance thought to the session and actively engage in choosing a focus rather than just respond to what happened to come up.

It is particularly important to communicate this expectation when one or both members of the couple have been in nondirective individual therapy, where spontaneously seeing what emerges is often the norm. Couples are usually pleased that the therapist has been giving thought to their situation. It's important, however, for the therapist to present his or her ideas for how to proceed and what to focus on not as an imperative, but merely as a suggestion, saying something like *"At some point, we do need to get back to what we put on hold last week. But we can get back to it next week if there is something else that seems more pressing or that you'd rather discuss."*

Even when there has been an agreement regarding the topic, it is natural for one thing to lead to another and for a myriad of issues to be raised. It is all too easy for the therapist as well as the couple to get sidetracked. Deciding together upon a focus at the beginning of the session provides some check against this drift from happening but often peripheral topics raised in the course of discussing an issue can be difficult to resist. There are, however, a number of ways for the therapist to nonetheless keep the session on track. Sometimes it's done by what the therapist chooses to focus on in response to statements: the session stays focused because the therapist responds to the aspect of what has just been said that furthers and deepens the topic at hand rather than diluting the focus through the exploration of some related but peripheral topic. At other times the therapist needs to more explicitly take control of the direction by saying something like *"I know that what you're raising is important but if you don't mind, I think it will be more productive if we put that concern on hold for a while and continue with this."*

Most couples are relieved to have the therapist step in and direct the session. But, of course, there are times when one partner (or both) has a lot of difficulty ceding control or when emotions are so intense that calming down and letting the therapist keep the work focused is very difficult. Chapter 7 describes in detail various methods for dealing with these kinds of couples. For now, suffice it to say that the therapist needs to express empathy for how difficult it may feel to let go of something that feels important to discuss and needs to assure the person that you, the therapist, will make sure that what s/he has raised will be revisited later in the session or in the next meeting. The therapist also needs to be clear and to explicitly acknowledge that it is ultimately up to the couple how they want to use the session. If they each agree that it would be best to change topics for now, then of course the therapist should go along with what they wish to do. This undercuts power struggles and gets the couple to reflect on whether or not they want to follow the path of whatever issue has momentarily most ignited their anger or outrage or rely on the therapist's best professional judgment.

Of course, there are the occasional times when an intense eruption of anger occurs and the couple is so aroused that the topic previously at hand seems far less relevant than what is going on in the room right now. If that occurs, the focus must shift to what is happening—what caused it, how they each can calm down, how to prevent this kind of interaction from occurring at home. The methods described in this chapter often prevent eruptions of this sort from happening, but sometimes, despite the therapist's best efforts to create a positive, problem-solving atmosphere, couples can become extremely angry with one another in the session and have little interest in the agenda the therapist thought would be most productive. Chapter 7 discusses how to calm down the couple in these circumstances and get them to step outside the situation and together analyze what triggered the explosive exchange.

It's not always easy to decide what is peripheral and what is germane to the topic at hand. Sometimes urgent issues raised by one or both partners seem clearly to be an avoidant response. At other times it is fairly clear that the new topic is raised because one person feels hurt and under attack and is responding defensively with a new, tit-for-tat complaint. But often what is raised is experienced by the couple as genuinely germane to what is being discussed, and yet to pursue this new example or event will lead to a confused tangle of topics.

For example, Sarah states that "I feel very lonely even when Charlie's at home. I know he works hard and needs to relax, but he spends all weekend plopped in front of the TV. He really doesn't want to spend time with me, much less have sex!"

In response, Charlie says, "Sarah has no idea how much stress I'm under during the week. She doesn't get it. I need to veg-out on weekends. If it were up to her, she'd schedule every minute with some chore or activity. It doesn't have to do with not wanting to be with her." He goes on to say, in a tone bordering between indifference and sarcasm, "If she wants us to be together, she should watch TV with me. But she'd never do that. She over-schedules everything and is constantly nagging. That's why Nickie [their 14-year-old son] is always fighting with her and spending as much time out of the house as he can. She never lets up on him. I've told her she should leave the kid alone, but she doesn't care about my opinion."

In response, Sarah states, "You always minimize things. Nickie is a kid who needs structure. His teachers notice it. They say he has to be reminded a lot or he'll just procrastinate. The guidance counselor told me to provide more structure for him."

"Well, I disagree," says Charlie. "They're probably picking up on your anxiety. He's doing fine. Sure—if you ask them what's wrong with Nickie, they'll tell you something! You always look for problems—look and you'll find them for sure!"

"If you spent more time with him, you'd see for yourself that he has to be reminded and watched carefully. He'd love to spend more time with you. You're just like your father. I know you love the kids but you barely make time for them. They never confide in you. You have no idea what's going on."

This is a very typical example of how therapists must make judgment calls in regard to what is on-topic and what is too far afield. Since the start of the discussion was the wife's wish for more closeness and time together, the anger Charlie is feeling toward his wife is clearly relevant. He is not simply "vegging out." In order to eventually help the couple become more intimate, they each need to give voice to the anger they are feeling. So, in this instance, the therapist would still be on focus if she were to follow up on Charlie's anger and irritation at his wife. But as described above, the quicker the focus on what is *bothering* someone can be redirected to what s/he is wishing for, the better it is. In this case, the husband's sarcastic comment about his wife joining in watching TV with him might contain a kernel of a wish both for her to join him more and to be more relaxed.

The topic of how each feels about the other's parenting is of course an important one. But to pursue that issue instead of the original topic raised seems too tangential and will likely lead to that "we didn't get anywhere" feeling. The therapist needs to acknowledge the importance of that topic while putting it on hold and bringing the couple back to the original topic of closeness. Again, everything is related to everything else but a line must be drawn somewhere. The therapist could say, *"I think the issues you have around parenting are clearly important and I'm going to make a note for us to get back to that in another session. But for now, I'd like to go back to what's getting in the way of your feeling good about spending time together and figuring out if there's something we can do about it. Is that okay with you?"*

There's rarely a clear answer to what is on-topic and what is not, but the therapist's attempt to keep the session focused provides an opportunity to step back, evaluate, and make collaborative decisions about what would be the most productive use of therapy time. This process is in itself therapeutic: it contributes to a thoughtful atmosphere and reminds the couple that though they both need to air their frustrations and will undoubtedly at times engage in mutual critiques and countercriticisms, ultimately our purpose is to find solutions.

In the remainder of the book, the reader will see how the methods described in this chapter are applied in dealing with the day-to-day clinical challenges that couple therapists encounter.

4

CR

The First Session

*I*n this chapter, and throughout this book, I'm going to describe my preferred and most typical way of working. But it is important to keep in mind that what I am describing are not hard-and-fast rules, but rather guidelines that I believe enhance the likeliness that couple therapy will be helpful. Good clinicians of any ilk are flexible and respond to the particularities of the situation and the culture of the individuals with whom they are working (Beutler, Consoli, & Lane, 2005; Brewster & Sheinberg, 2015). Nonetheless, it is important to have a structure from which you can then, in a sensitive and thoughtful manner, deviate.

GOALS

My goals for the first session are in one sense limited, and in another sense quite large. Limited, because we are not yet "officially" going to start working on the issues that made the couple seek help. Large, because I have numerous objectives that I am hoping to accomplish—not completely, but in a significant enough way that the couple leaves wanting to give couple therapy a try. To this end, my aims are as follows:

- To reduce the couple's anxiety about the process.
- To communicate something about the methods and "rules" to make the sessions a safe, controlled environment.

- To demonstrate the way in which I will be simultaneously in charge and collaborative.
- To stimulate thoughts and memories of any positives in their relationship.
- To instill some hope, if at all possible.
- To combat feelings of shame and demoralization.
- To address concerns they may have about the therapy.
- To give feedback as to how I see their difficulties.
- To assess whether or not one person has actually already firmly made up his or her mind that s/he wants to end the relationship.

When I go out to greet a couple for the first time, I'm aware that they are in a heightened state of emotion. One or both of them may actually be feeling dread. With that in mind, my first aim is to help them both have confidence that, at a minimum, I will do no harm. Being friendly, relaxed, and welcoming is of course important, but that in itself does little to reassure the couple that the session won't unravel an already fragile bond. Security begins to build when the couple feels that the therapist knows what s/he is doing and that there is a clear plan and structure to the session. From the moment the couple walks into my office, I am communicating to them that this will be a very different experience than what happens at home when they are trying to address their issues.

As I usher the couple into my office, I indicate that I'd like them both to sit on the couch. By doing that, I'm communicating that I have a customary way of doing things—that I'm going to be *directing* the session. Though I do lose some information by not letting them choose to sit far from one another if they like, by having them sit side by side I make it *possible* for them to be physically comforting if something transpires in the session that inclines them to do so. The other message conveyed by how they are seated is that they each will be conversing with me, not with one another. The issue of how much the couple should communicate directly to one another rather than through the therapist is a complex one and the various aspects of this topic are discussed later in this book.

Though I want to convey that I'm in charge, and thus they can relax a bit, I don't want to set off power struggles by their experiencing me as rigid or inflexible or authoritarian. Rather, I want them to experience me as an equal who is doing her job, and I invite them to call me by my first name. In the previous chapter, we looked at some of the ways I strengthen the therapeutic alliance by finding small ways to join with each individual. The therapeutic alliance is also strengthened by helping them feel that I will be taking care of them. Thus, after indicating where I want them to sit, I act like a host who, before we get started, wants to make sure her guests are comfortable. It's been one of my therapy traditions for many years that I ask if people would like some water or tea and I always have hot and cold water available. Of course, there are other ways to be gracious and solicitous as well—for example, "Would you like another pillow for your back?"; "Is the sun bothering you?"; "Is the office cool enough for you?" These caring gestures communicate that though you are in charge, it is in the service of helping them.

Generally, I've had a very brief telephone conversation with whomever made the appointment. If the caller wants to go into detail, I interrupt him or her by saying, *"I find it's best to get the information with both people present, just so we're all on an equal footing."* Usually this is readily accepted as sensible. At times someone is quite anxious about what the therapy will be like, and I do try as best I can to describe my approach. In order to avoid being inclined to see the issues from only one person's point of view, I usually also speak only briefly to the referring therapist (often the individual therapist of one of the partners) and defer getting more input until I've had a chance to form my own impressions.

I begin the session by summarizing the little bit I know about the couple's situation. I explain that I have purposely limited the prior information I receive because I want to hear about the issues with both of them present. And by including as much as I can about the phone conversation, I am letting the couple know also that I don't have secret or private conversations. This statement is of course reassuring to the person who may think he has already been indicted and is anticipating needing to defend himself or disprove my negative assumptions. But just as importantly, it communicates that I have a particular and thought-out way of doing things—and again, that in itself begins to instill some confidence.

Next, I tell the couple how I like to conduct a first meeting. I explain, *"I like to spend just a little bit of time hearing about the difficulties that have brought you here—10 or 15 minutes or so—but then I'd like to put the problems on the back burner for the remainder of the session and focus for today on what was once good between you. It's very easy for couple therapists to forget about the positives in a relationship, so it's important for me to get a really clear sense of whether any of those positive things are still there at all at this point in your relationship, before we actually start working on the problems."*

BRIEF DESCRIPTION OF PROBLEMS IN THE RELATIONSHIP

There is a decision to made right from the outset, about who will be *first* to describe the issues that brought the couple to my office. I turn to them and ask who would like to start. Just that question can at times lead to a struggle.

"You start."

"No, you start. It was your idea to come here."

"Yeah, but you're the one who's always mad—tell the doctor what you're mad about."

Here's a choice point. I can either look at what's going on right then or there, or stick to my original plan and get a statement from each of them about the nature of their difficulties. As discussed in the prior chapter, staying focused is of primary importance, and so, as tempting as it might be to discuss what is happening now, I generally step in and say to one of them, *"Why don't you start. Tell me very briefly how you see the difficulties the two of you are having."* But often, getting a couple to step back from this sort of skirmish is not possible. The couple may need to start the session by describing their feelings about being in my office and the power struggle that may have ensued before they made the appointment. Some couples simply find it too frustrating to follow my agenda without first airing their more immediate feelings. When that is the case, I hear them out and then ask if they are comfortable *"putting that issue on hold for now so I can get a more general sense of some of the issues that have brought you here."*

The couple therapist is often faced with the difficult task of interrupting someone who is going into too much detail. Therapists are trained to be attentive listeners and cutting people short can feel like you are being rude, disrespectful, or overly controlling. But interrupt we must. We need to ensure that each person has a chance to talk and that there is still sufficient time remaining for an examination of the strengths in their relationship. Not only is it uncomfortable to cut people short, but it can sometimes be quite difficult to get someone who wants to tell the whole story to summarize or more quickly get to the main point. When this occurs, I politely interrupt and mention again that for now I just want a sense of things—an overview. I explain that, of course, if we decide to proceed I'll need to get a much more detailed understanding of what goes on between them. If the person keeps going on with details, I'll again interrupt and say, *"I know this can be difficult and I want to apologize in advance, but the way I work often entails interrupting people and redirecting the conversation."* By doing this I am beginning to educate the couple about the way the therapy operates—not free-flowing, but directed. Also note that I don't assume that the couple will want to continue to work with me, and by saying *if we decide to proceed*, I am implicitly acknowledging that we are all trying to decide whether or not I can be helpful to them. This is another example of the perhaps paradoxical-seeming combination of structure and direction, on the one hand, and deep respect for the autonomy and choices of the couple, on the other. It is in the constructive tensions between these two characteristics that much of the therapeutic energy seems to lie.

Some couples make our work easier—when one person is talking the other listens intently. This is a relatively rare occurrence and when it does happen it's important to make note of it. I'll say something like *"I'm struck by how intently you were listening. You seemed like you really wanted to understand your wife's point of view."*

More often, one of the first challenges the couple therapist faces is how to intervene when the listener interrupts and they are both speaking at once, or even if quiet, indicates nonverbally that s/he is eagerly waiting for a chance to rebut what is being said. I use those occasions as an opportunity to convey to the couple the frame of mind that is essential for the success of couple therapy. So here's what I say: *"It's natural for couples when they're listening to one another, to want to correct, or clarify, or even debate what's being said. Almost everybody does it. But what can make the experience in this office unlike what you would do at home, and much more productive, is to listen in a different way. I'd like you to try to listen with the mind-set of noticing what part of what you are hearing is basically right, sort of right, even a tiny bit right. Try to listen for what you can agree with. Try not to get bogged down in details that might be incorrect, but ask yourself, can you see something 'right' in what's being said? Can you understand how your partner could see it that way? I know this will take effort, because that's just not how any of us usually listens, particularly when we feel we're being misrepresented or criticized. But if you could listen for what you can agree with rather than what's incorrect, you'll be taking an important first step in the work we are doing. This isn't easy to do, and I'll probably be reminding you of this many times when I see in your eyes that you're marshaling your arguments and waiting to have a chance to contradict. But with practice, you'll be able to do it and it will help enormously. People don't get close by debating one another. So, it's not just about not interrupting, which of course is important, but actually listening with a receptive, open state of mind."*

When each has had an opportunity to briefly describe the difficulties that have brought them to my office, I summarize what was said and ask if there's anything that has been left out. Often they each have presented the troubling aspects of their relationship in much the same way, and if that is the case, I would say, *"Clearly, things aren't going well between the two of you, but it was interesting how similarly you describe the problem. Probably you don't agree with 'why' these negative interactions happen—but you do seem to be able to come together quite well in terms of describing the problem."* This statement joins them for a moment and implies a respect for their ability as a couple to be on the same page, at least in that regard.

But not infrequently, the couple not only doesn't agree on the cause of the difficulties but also describe what happens between them quite differently. For instance, George stated that Phillip often screamed at him. Phillip forcefully disagreed, saying that he doesn't scream and it frustrated him that "whenever I get a little bit excited George says 'stop screaming at me'—he acts like the slightest raised voice is abusive." When couples have divergent views of what actually *happens*, I include in my end-of-session feedback that one of the issues between them is this difference in sensibilities and perception. Sorting that out would be one of the goals of therapy.

ASKING ABOUT THE COUPLE'S SEX LIFE

Couples often do not initially raise the issue of their sex life even though they may not have had sex for many months, or even years. Embarrassment, shame, not wanting to put their partner on the spot, and the belief by one or both of the partners that their sex life is suffering *because* of the other issues in their relationship which they *have* brought up are all factors contributing to their silence on this topic. Add to that the feeling that one or both may have that they're no longer, or perhaps never were, really attracted to the other, and one can easily see why there would be anxiety about opening up what might prove to be a can of worms.

With all this in mind, in the first session I ask about their sex life in a way that I hope will mitigate feelings of shame and also instill some hope that couple therapy can be of help. Thus I would say things like *"Many couples who come to see me because they haven't been getting along haven't had sex for a very long time, or if they do have sex, it's not very satisfying, and part of what we focus on is how they can get that going again or revitalize their sex life. Where are you on this? When you first were together was there a lot of chemistry or was it 'good enough' so to speak? There are a lot of things couples can do to make it more gratifying, and if it wasn't so great to begin with, it can sometimes be better than it's ever been."*

When I say this, often one person seems relieved that the topic has been raised while the other is more dismissive and says something like "He wants me to have sex and just forget about the things he says to me," or "I need to feel close before I can have sex," or "We're both so stressed and worn out . . . ," or "Sex isn't really the issue . . . We're not close or intimate at all . . . I don't think we like each other very much right now."

In response to these kinds of statements, I'll say something like *"Let's put this on hold for a few sessions while we get going on starting to resolve some of the more immediate issues that brought you here. But it is important that we not keep it on hold too long. When couples have a physically intimate relationship, it often helps them resolve some other issues too— they feel more connected and some of the tension between them eases."*

When I introduce the topic by saying we can focus on *how* they can get sex going again and things they can *do* to make it more gratifying, I am implicitly saying that it will not necessarily happen naturally if they get along better. By further saying that we should put this on hold for a few sessions until some of the issues are *starting* to get resolved, I'm communicat-

ing, that they do not need to be *fully* resolved before we can start to address
their sex life, and that my expectation is they will have made some progress
in a few sessions. By phrasing it this way, I get my point across without
directly contradicting the more reluctant partner and in fact, at the moment,
I am complying with what s/he would like by dropping the topic.

FINDING STRENGTHS IN THE RELATIONSHIP

I move on to the next phase of the first session by reminding the couple of
what I had said earlier, that *"now that I have at least an initial picture of
what's wrong, I want to get a solid sense of what was once good in your
relationship and what might be okay in your relationship right now, even
with all the problems you've just described."* The tone and exact wording
of this statement is important. I don't want to overplay the possibility of
positives in their current relationship, since that is not what the couple is
experiencing, and to overdo it might mobilize them to convince me of how
bad it actually is or convey to them that I don't "get it." Thus, I say might
be *okay*, rather than what might be *good*.

To avoid any conflict (e.g., "You go first"; "No, I want to hear your
account") at a point when I'm hoping to generate at least some warm feelings, *I* make the decision as to who will speak first. Most people are used to
telling the story of how they met, but my aim here is to shift the focus from
the *factual* account of their meeting to what it was about the other that drew
them in emotionally. So, for instance, when James told the story of how he
and his wife had been in elementary school together until the third grade
when his family moved, and that, amazingly, his wife recognized him when
they ended up in the same college, I asked him, *"So, how did it progress
from that first excitement and hanging out with one another, to a committed relationship? What was it about her that made you get more deeply
involved? What did you see in her—what qualities—that made you want
to be together and that made you feel you could spend your life with her?"*

I follow up with questions that encourage the person to elaborate and
that give me a sense of what their relationship was like in the past. So, for
instance, if John says, "She was really supportive and caring. And very loyal
to friends," I would ask him what he noticed that made him see her that
way? Does he remember any specific incidents that he noticed? I ask too if
he remembers what it was like when things were good between them and
they were falling in love. Are there any memories of times when he felt particularly close to her?

When one person is talking about his or her experiences, the other
is usually listening with rapt attention. Often it's been years since they've
heard their partner speak so positively. And sometimes they have actually

never heard their partner articulate what traits were noticed and deeply valued. It's not uncommon for the couple to be tremendously touched by what the other has said. This exchange is usually an emotionally meaningful experience for both the speaker and the receiver—for a few moments, they have been able to access loving feelings that may have been deeply buried for quite some time.

To build on this exchange, I next ask if they ever still see, from time to time, any of the traits that they just described. And frequently, despite the fact that earlier in the session the couple described one another very negatively, they respond with an almost incredulous tone that I could possibly think otherwise—"Yes, of course, I still think he's very funny" or "Yes, she's still incredibly loyal to her friends." Or even, "Yes, we can still go out and have a really good time together—we like a lot of the same things and I still think he's one of the smartest people I ever met." Later in the session I will come back to this when I give them feedback, but at that moment I would usually make a little positive aside, like *"That's great—you both have the ability to put the bad feelings aside and have some fun."*

Troubleshooting

It is important to be clear that trying to elicit warm feelings from the past does not always go well. Here are some of the difficulties that you could encounter:

1. One person in the couple is hard-pressed to remember anything positive. Instead s/he talks about how there were problems right from the start or perhaps even that they broke up with one another several times. In response to this kind of reply I might say something like *"I'm not sure if the negative feelings you've been having for such a long time are making it hard to remember what once went well between you, or if, even though you did end up together, the good feelings most people have in the beginning just weren't there for you."* This statement respects what the person is feeling and doesn't pressure him or her to say something that isn't authentic.

In the situation just described, the listening partner will likely have some strong feelings about the partner's inability to say anything positive and may need room to express what may be considerable distress arising from what the partner said. The reactions can range from hurt to anger or even skepticism, though sometimes it may be an angry (or forlorn) statement that "Yes, this comes as no surprise to me. I've had that sense for years." Some partners may see the spouse as not being candid and just withholding anything positive in order to be hurtful or punishing. Sometimes people are so hurt or angry, if this "nothing" response occurs, that they feel it's not even worth trying to work things out. Whether to be encouraging or not about continuing to work on the relationship depends on the therapist's assessment of whether the person who can remember nothing positive has actually already made up his or her mind that the relationship needs to end.

If it seems like that person actually does want to find a way to make the marriage work, I would say something like *"So our problem here is different from those couples where the aim is to recover something lost from the past. Here the question we will be exploring together is whether—and how—the two of you can build—build now—the kind of relationship that will be meaningful and gratifying to both of you. Not every successful relationship begins with people being really in love from the beginning. It's well documented that in cultures where marriages are arranged, many couples come over time to love one another deeply, even though the marriage did not start out with the Western expectation of romance. So the question we need to pursue is do you see qualities in each other now that could make you happy if the problem in the relationship could be worked out?"* This type of statement takes some of the sting out of what the other has said, enabling his or her partner to hear it in a way that doesn't preclude a meaningful loving relationship from developing. The fact that both people want to work out the relationship, usually indicates that implicitly they *do* see characteristics in the other now that they feel positively about and that, in fact, there may still be something to build upon.

2. Sometimes even when both partners are able to convey something positive, one person's positive statements are much more richly evocative than the other's. When someone gives a description in very general terms ("She was fun," "She was nice," etc.), the therapist needs to try to get the person to elaborate. Often the difficulty is in *articulating* feelings rather than that the feelings themselves are shallow. I usually start by asking the person to give me an example of *how*, for instance, she was "fun" or "nice." I prompt the person to see if he can remember any *particular moments* when he noticed how "nice" she was. Maybe he'll recall some specific event, like "When my brother-in-law was in an accident and she brought food over to their house." But there are times when a person really seems unable to elaborate, and in response to my asking for an example, just repeats, "Nice, you know what I mean, just nice." There's a fine line between trying to help the person give a richer description and being too persistent, and thus making the person feel inadequate.

3. Sometimes a spouse focuses almost entirely on situational factors to explain why the couple got together, and there is often an implication in that description that the person wasn't really special, but simply fit the bill at the time. So, for instance, a woman might say, "All my friends were getting married, and I was tired of being a bridesmaid and never a bride."

Or "My wife had died suddenly, leaving me with two small kids to raise, and it was a relief to have someone who was willing to take that on." Or "We were seeing each other very casually—I'm not even sure if I should even say 'seeing each other,' since we were seeing other people too. I got pregnant accidentally and thought about possibly getting an abortion, but I knew that I just couldn't do it. But I hated the idea of being a single mom, so I decided to go ahead and marry him." Or "I was in college and a mess. I had been suspended and was back again but barely getting by. I needed someone to really be on my case and to kind of hold my hand while I tried to study. Maybe because he's a little older and has a much younger sister who he dotes on, he made me his 'project' and got me through." This type of description can be painful for the spouse to hear. S/he may feel devalued and denigrated by the fact that his or her only attractive qualities were in relation to what s/he could *do* for the other.

Before accepting this narrative at face value, I try to see if with a little prodding the person is able to convey anything special about the spouse's qualities that also entered into the decision. Again, note in terms of choice points and staying on focus, that I do not *immediately* change the focus to the listener's feelings, but rather *first* see if I can elicit anything positive or more specific that may mitigate the hurt. Thus, with the woman who was eager to finally get married, I might say, *"So, you were eager to get married, and what was it about Joe that made you feel okay about marrying him?"* Notice, that by saying "okay about marrying him," I am accepting her assumption that she wasn't that picky, but at the same time I'm trying to get something more positive and personal. Or, with the man who needed someone to take his wife's place, I might say, *"So, she was ready to take on that role. What made you think she'd be good at it—good with the kids, a good substitute mom?"*

Rather than ask more questions, I will sometimes extrapolate from what the person has said to certain *implied* positive characteristics about the spouse, with the hope that the speaker will then be able to join in and elaborate. For instance, in the case of the woman who needed someone to "hold her hand" in college, I would try to get more depth by saying something like *"It sounds like you saw him as unusually mature and supportive and someone who you could really count on."* I am choosing to highlight the kernels of a more meaningful emotional connection rather than what is lacking in the statement.

Sometimes what I get when I push for more is still quite minimal. If it is truly the case that the spouse was simply a means to an end, then this is important information and it will be tactfully incorporated into the feedback that I give at the end of the session. If I continue to work with the couple, then what was missing right from the start will need to be examined with the hope that they will be able to create something new together.

4. A related "situational" problem is when each person in the couple basically says that they married *because* they'd been together for years. Of course, this is not really an explanation, since the real question is why *were* they together for so long. Some couples describe having, and continuing to have, extreme ambivalence about one another, and they may have attempted to break up many times. The therapist in these kinds of cases needs as best she can to get a clear sense of what the "glue" is that has bound them. How do they each understand what kept drawing them back to one another?

To get a sense of what they saw in one another that led them to commit despite the emotional ups and downs, I might say something like *"So, what was it about John that made you feel, even despite all the difficulties and uncertainties that you could make a life together . . . that you could cast your lot with his . . . that you could face all the challenges in life better with him as your partner?"* Or, if the couple are intending to have children, one could say, *"What made you feel that he was someone you could go ahead and have children with?"*

These questions *may* elicit something positive, but not necessarily. Many people, when looking back on what kept them together, feel that in retrospect their motives were not psychologically healthy ones. They know that they were attracted to each other for wrong or superficial reasons. A man may realize that he liked being with a dependent, much younger woman who would allow him to run the show. Or a woman may realize that she always was attracted to "bad boys" and difficult-to-pin-down men. Similarly, it is not uncommon for couples to realize that they bonded when they were both heavily into drinking and drugs. The excitement and connection they felt with one another could not be sustained when one or both of them changed their lifestyle.

The point here is that the therapist must be flexible, and though my aim is to focus in a first session on past and present positives, there are times when that is just not possible. Instead, one may need to shift to what didn't go well right from the start and how those issues continued or changed over the years.

THINKING ABOUT THE SESSION: KEY QUESTIONS

As I listen to the couple I am pulling together my thoughts in preparation for the feedback I will be giving them at the end of the meeting. It is important to note that I, of course, do not share all my hypothesis and observations with the couple. Later in this chapter I'll be discussing the types of feedback that I may give and how to present my initial ideas in a way that can be most useful. But for now, here are the questions I am asking myself.

1. How strong was the foundation of their relationship? By this I mean, did the couple become deeply attached to one another? Did they have shared values and a genuine respect for the other's character and personality? I think about the basis of the initial bond. Sometimes, the foundation of the relationship was a strong sexual attraction but not much else. Or the couple may have come together when they were both doing a lot of "partying" or "bar hopping" or were both abusing drugs. I ask myself if the couple was excited about having found one another or if it was more of a "good enough" feeling and they perhaps were motivated by prior feelings of failure in relationships or feeling that it was time to settle down, or the ticking of a woman's biological clock.

2. How deeply ingrained are the negative cycles and problematic interactions? Did the couple engage in these patterns early on in their relationship, or are they of more recent origin? Not infrequently, there are life stresses (illness, aging parents, finances, careers, parenting) that have altered the way the couple interacts and that play a large role in the negative cycles that have brought the couple to therapy.

3. Are there still warm, loving feelings left, or has hurt, anger, disappointment, and criticism severely eroded the good feelings that once existed? So, for instance, do they sometimes, despite their difficulties, give each other good feedback and thus enhance each other's self-esteem? Are they still able to enjoy one another? Are they still attractive to one another in some way? Is there a physical aspect to their relationship?

Sometimes a couple will want to work on a relationship and yet one or both of them may speak about the other in ways that are so contemptuous and disparaging that, even if they assert that they still love one another, it is hard to know what that actually means.

4. Throughout the first meeting, I am also getting a beginning sense of each person's individual issues and personality characteristics that play an important role in determining how to work with the couple. Does one person find it aversive to talk about their difficulties? Is one person inclined to minimize the other's concerns, seeing them as unwarranted complaints? Does one person respond very intensely to any discussion of negatives and quickly get angry, despairing, or defensive? Is it difficult to engage one of the partners? Do I feel like I am pulling teeth and can't get any traction? How defensive are they? How blaming? Are they spontaneously reflective about themselves, or the relationship? Are they forthright? Evasive? Guarded? Are they suspicious of the other's motives? Are they suspicious of the therapist? Are they inclined to get into power struggles with their partner? With the therapist?

5. Is couple therapy appropriate for this couple? There are a number of considerations that may lead the therapist to conclude that couple counseling is an inappropriate modality at the present time. If there is current or recent physical abuse the therapist must assess whether it is safe to proceed with therapy (Stith, McCollum, & Rosen, 2011; Goldner, 1998). How committed are they to doing what it takes to never let arguments escalate to the point of physical encounters? One or both members of the couple may treat too lightly his or her loss of self-control and may think that the occasional pushing, shoving, restraining the other, blocking the partner's way, scratching, or the like is not "abuse," and thus is not serious. Couple therapy can only be effective if there is no fear that there will be violent repercussions from what is discussed.

One or both partners may need to be in his or her own therapy concurrent with, but possibly *prior* to doing couple therapy. Drinking heavily is an aspect of everyday life for many couples, and even where it contributes to some of their problems, is not necessarily a central defining feature of their difficulties. But for other couples substance abuse is so critical an issue—whether the couple think of it as so or not—that doing couple therapy without specific and intensive work on the substance problem may be close to futile.

6. Lastly, I'm trying to assess whether or not both partners actually want to work on the relationship. The question I'm asking myself is *Are both parties hoping that they could find a way to stay together, or is one or both really wanting to move toward separation?* This is a complicated question. Sometimes one person is clear that s/he regards couple therapy as essentially a final, last ditch try before they separate. S/he is skeptical that the relationship could improve enough to reverse the course that seems at this point in time almost inevitable. Perhaps that person has already announced the wish to divorce and may have agreed to see a couple therapist largely to appease the spouse. That partner may be cooperative in the session, but basically is participating reluctantly.

Of course, my answers to all these questions are in no way set in stone, since my assessment is based on only having seen the couple for one highly structured session. When I share some of my observations with the couple, I will make clear that what I am saying is tentative and will assuredly be subject to much revision if we work together.

SUMMARIZING AND GIVING FEEDBACK

I close the session by first summarizing what each person has said about what is bothering him or her, and then, once I know that I have understood each of them correctly, sharing with them some of my preliminary thoughts and observations about their relationship. For instance, I might say something like *"For now, here's how I understand why you are here.* [*turning to the wife*] *You want more out of the relationship, you feel lonely, you don't feel important, you feel that he's not really interested in spending time with you and that when he does he's checking things off his to-do list. When you talk about it, it leads to a fight, and you think maybe you should separate now that the twins are almost ready for college. You're feeling very worried about having these feelings and thinking of separating. You always thought you'd be together forever."*

And, in similar fashion, to the husband: *"You're upset that your wife could even think of separating. To you, the problem seems like she's going through some kind of a midlife crisis—maybe because the boys don't need her as much now that they are older. You feel that you haven't changed. You describe yourself as always having been a type-A person who devoted a lot of time to work. As I understand it, you don't really have many complaints about the relationship. Maybe you'd like sex more often, but basically you feel things are okay. You're here because your wife is unhappy and your home life isn't what you'd like it to be—you're arguing a lot—but from your point of view, that's because your wife isn't herself."*

I conclude by saying something like *"I know this is a very quick summary and of course we will need to delve much deeper. And also, you probably omitted a number of things that are concerning you because I only wanted you to focus on your difficulties for a brief part of the session. If we continue to meet, we'll of course go into these issues in depth. But did what I describe seem basically accurate? Did I miss something important or did I not quite get something?"* At this point the couple may want to modify or elaborate on something that I didn't get quite right. We'll spend a few minutes on this, but I keep it short because I want to share with them my impressions, and answer any questions or concerns they may have.

When describing how I understand each person's concerns I use language that makes clear that I am aware that the description is from that person's perspective, and thus by implication is not an "objective" account. So, for instance, I'll use phrases like *"You feel," "From your point of view," "You describe yourself as. . . . "* It's also important to use each person's exact words whenever possible, since it's another way to help underline that you are just *restating* what was said and not assuming that what was said was factually true. Thus, for instance, in the above example when I say *"lonely," "midlife crisis," "to-do list,"* it is because those were the exact words that had been used. And I even refer to the couple's children as "the twins" when summarizing the wife's statement, and "the boys" when reiterating the husband's statement. Not only does this again make clear that I am only restating what I have heard, but it also helps each of them to feel that I am listening empathically and trying to understand them in their own terms.

Couples are often very discouraged and not at all sure that their relationship is worth trying to salvage, much less whether it would be possible to repair it even if they wanted to. They may previously have had unsuccessful couple therapy, and though they've come for a consultation, they aren't sure that trying counseling again makes sense. Thus, the feedback the therapist gives regarding their relationship and what would be required to change it is an important part of the initial session and should be taken very seriously by the therapist. The aim is not to persuade the couple to pursue therapy but to enable them, using the therapist's observations and expertise, to make the best decision *for them* as to whether to proceed. And if they do continue, the careful and specific feedback the therapist provides will be of great benefit in getting the work started on the right foundation.

Starting with the Positive If Possible

If at all possible—and sometimes it just isn't—I start by giving the couple some positive feedback. It is essential, of course, that the feedback be authentic. If the feedback feels superficial, forced, or like a Pollyannish "feel-good" message, it is scarcely likely to be useful. But as discussed in the previous chapter, the therapist can *learn* to notice strengths that often get overshadowed by the anger, upset, and serious difficulties that the couple present and when these *genuine* strengths are noticed, the work is placed on a more effective and comprehensive foundation. In order for the positive feedback to feel right to both the couple and the therapist, it must be presented in a manner that in no way diminishes the seriousness of the problems that have brought the couple into treatment. Thus, I might say to a couple who were considering separating, *"I know that you've been having serious problems in your relationship for a long time and that you're not at all sure that you should be together, which made it all the more striking to me that somehow [to the husband] you were able to make a joke, and [to the wife] you still could laugh. You seem to have retained pleasure in each other's humor despite the fact that you have really intense arguments."* Or, to a couple who was listening to each other nondefensively, *"I know that you really see things very differently and, as you both described, if she says black, you say white. Yet it was interesting to me how readily you were able to shift gears and do what I suggested you try—to listen for what was basically right."*

Sometimes the positive feedback is directed toward one individual, but as discussed in the previous chapter, it's always important that *both* members of the couple feel acknowledged. For example, the therapist might say to a husband who reached for his wife's hand when she cried in the session, *"Even though you've been terribly hurt and quite angry at your wife for her betrayal, it's impressive that you have not closed off to her emotionally and reached out to her when she was so upset."* The positive feedback to the spouse can be related to what was just said, but can also be something completely different. The therapist might say to the wife in the above example, *"I was impressed by your ability to acknowledge how defensive you often are—you were really forthcoming about the role of your own tendency to deflect criticism in what happened between the two of you."*

Some of the positive feedback may be about ways of interacting that the couple take for granted but that are actually characteristics that distinguish them from couples whose "prognosis," so to speak, is not as good. For instance, the couple may speak to each other respectfully and, even when very angry, take care to not say anything truly hurtful or mean. Or the therapist might note that the couple was already inclined to try to understand the other's point of view and that she didn't have to give her "speech" about listening for what you could agree with because the couple was doing that naturally. Or perhaps in describing their difficulties, they each spontaneously acknowledged that their spouse saw it differently, and they spoke about their feelings in a way that was not an indictment of the other. The therapist might thus note that the couple is *not* interacting in some problematic ways that he frequently encounters, saying for instance, that *"often couples who come to see me are very guarded with one another. They find it difficult to be open to what the other person is saying and I need to remind them periodically to try to listen nondefensively and without marshaling their arguments for when they have a chance to rebut."* Or nothing that *"many couples who come to see me are so hurt and angry that they can barely look at one another, much less laugh at the other's joke."* Or *"You take for granted a respectful way of interacting that many couples find difficult to do."* Or *"Many people when they first come to see me seem to really want to hurt the other. . . . They can be sarcastic and very wounding to one another. . . . Sometimes there's still a lot of caring underneath but it isn't always as easy to see as it is with the two of you."*

For younger therapists who do not have the credibility that comes with the couple knowing that there's years of experience behind these statements, citing research can lend weight to the feedback. The therapist might say "highly regarded research [Gottman, 1994] has shown that when couples disagree in a way that's contemptuous, they are more at risk of eventually separating—and that's why it's noteworthy that the two of you generally speak to each other in a respectful way even when clearly very angry." And, of course, similar statements could be made about defensiveness, stonewalling, and excessive criticism. The point is that the therapist wants to make clear that the interaction s/he is noting is of significance, and not something that all couples are able to do.

It is important, of course, that the positive feedback the therapist offers not be experienced by the couple as superficial "feel good" bromides. Here the emphasis on *specificity* I have highlighted throughout is particularly important. The feedback must point to very specific features of the couple's behavior that they can recognize instantly is accurate about them. Relatedly, the therapist must also be clear that she knows that they probably are not as respectful with one another at home as they were in the office today, and that all couples will, from time to time, want to hurt one another, be defensive, stonewall, and so on. In fact, that is what makes the observation she just offered so noteworthy. Bridging the therapist's attention to the couple's still evident strengths and her very strong commitment to a clear-eyed appreciation of the reality and substance of their difficulties, she might say something like *"I'm sure you're not always as nice with one another as you were today, and if we work together I hope you'll let me see some of the not so pretty behavior that you each engage in."*

Giving Difficult Feedback Regarding the Nature and Severity of the Couple's Difficulties

After sharing with the couple whatever positives I may have noticed, I sum up some of the impressions I have about the nature and severity of their difficulties. If there is still good feeling between the partners, or the difficulties are clearly connected to some stressors they are encountering in their life, or they are strongly committed to one another, the feedback is direct and easy. I can assure them that couple therapy is likely to be quite beneficial and may even be fairly brief. Couples are often surprised by this assessment because they do not have a basis of comparison and, despite the good feelings that they share, feel very "stuck" in their inability to resolve certain issues.

Often, however, the feedback one must give is not as wholeheartedly positive. If the couple's problems are quite long-standing and not related to recent stressors, I might say something like *"Despite the fact that you both report being 'crazy about one another' from almost the moment you met, it seems that you have each had difficulty with certain aspects of the other's personality from very early on in your relationship. You have deeply ingrained ways of interacting that don't work well. I'm sensing that at this point a lot of the warmth and positive feeling that had been there for a long time has eroded, and you both seem quite discouraged about your relationship. I do want to assure you that it is possible in couple therapy to recover a lot of the good feelings, but you both would need to put a lot of effort into changing the ways you interact with one another."*

If I had noticed some of the positive ways of interacting that I described in the previous section, I might reiterate them at this point as part of explaining why I think there's a real possibility that therapy could help them turn around their long-standing problems. I might highlight that there was a strong foundation of shared values and sensibilities, and that although they have had a rocky history with one another, they still do see the other as possessing the traits that attracted them in the first place. If, on the other hand, the couple *did not* have a strong foundation, I might say something like *"You connected with one another at a time when you were both very young and didn't know yourself or the other that well. You had fun with each other . . . there was a lot of drinking and great sex. So, a big part of the work in couple therapy will be to see if you can enjoy one another and be close in <u>new</u> ways that fit better with your current stage of life and who you each are now."*

If in my preliminary assessment I noticed a predominance of some of the negatives discussed above—for example, defensiveness, blaming, expressions of contempt, inability to enjoy one another—I might say something like *"You are each so hurt and angry that you talk to each other with a kind of hostility that makes you each even more defensive and blaming. That's where my job comes in—the first thing I would need to help you with is how to talk to one another in a way that the other could actually hear and understand. I would also need to help each of you be less blaming and look at your own role in what's going wrong."* Or I might say something like *"Right now, you both seem cutoff from caring, loving, tender feelings toward the other. But you both say that you do want to make the relationship work. If we do work together, my goal would be not only to help you avoid the terrible arguments that brought you here, but to see if together we can figure out a way to soften the hard-edge way you relate to one another so that warmth has a chance to develop."*

Sometimes the feedback has to do with how they interacted with me, and whether or not my approach will work for them. So, for instance, if I had a lot of trouble taking charge of the session, I might say something like *"I could see that you were having a bit of a hard time with the way I work— my saying things like, okay now you talk, now you, let's move on—a bit like a traffic cop. I can really understand your having trouble with that—it can feel pretty awkward at first—and by the way, it's <u>my</u> least favorite part of my work—but unfortunately necessary. You are used to going with your gut feelings, and both of you can be highly reactive and emotional. But as I said earlier, I believe that the only way couple therapy can be of help is for you to have an experience with one another that is quite different than what happens at home. In order for that to happen, I need to intervene in these ways. This type of therapy is very difficult for some people. My experience is that generally couples get comfortable with this and learn how to listen to the other in the way I described. Of course, I would help you with figuring out how to control the impulse to interrupt, defend yourself, and so on. I think you might want to give it a try and see if you can adjust to my directing things. But I'd like you to think about and consider whether my way of working is what you want."*

The reader should note the phrasing of the feedback. By saying, *"That's where my job comes in—the first thing I would need to help you with is how to talk to one another,"* I am conveying both my expertise and my assumption that these ways of interacting can be taught and learned. This mitigates feelings of blame, humiliation, and failure that can arise from telling the couple about their "hard edge." Similarly, when I tell a couple that they need to be able to control themselves in the sessions but I can help them learn to do that, I am conveying that my comment is not about "character" or fixed traits, but rather is about a skill that can be developed.

ADDITIONAL CONCERNS AND COMPLICATIONS ABOUT FIRST SESSIONS

Thus far this chapter has provided the reader with some general guidelines for conducting a first meeting with a couple. But guidelines are just that, not hard-and-fast rules. In addition to altering the format of a first session when infidelity is the reason for the consultation—I will be discussing that in detail, shortly—there are many other circumstances that also call for modification of the standard approach described earlier in this chapter. Couples may be facing time-sensitive situations of all sorts. One person may have been offered a very desirable job in another city and the other may be reluctant to move. Or a couple may need to make a decision about an unplanned pregnancy. Or one person in a soon-to-be-married couple may be seriously thinking of breaking off the engagement. Regardless of whether or not there is some *actual* time pressure, some couples are so upset about what is going on between them that they really feel they *must* talk in detail about their difficulties right away and the quick overview of difficulties with a shift to positives approach has to be jettisoned.

And even when there isn't a crisis, there are situations that couple therapists encounter that may make following the structure I've just described not so straightforward. All good clinicians need to be "quick on their feet," so to speak. We need to be attuned to our patients, and often that means being willing to change course when our usual approach isn't a good fit for a particular couple.

One Person Wants to Meet Individually before Meeting as a Couple

Sometimes the person who has made the initial call wants to first meet with me individually to assess whether or not I'm the right person for them to work with. That person's partner may have very reluctantly agreed to couple therapy, and the one advocating for it is understandably concerned that if his or her partner has a negative experience, the door will be shut and the partner won't try someone else. In this type of situation, I generally agree to a first meeting with that person, but explain that if we were to go ahead with couple therapy, I would also want to have an individual meeting with the partner so that s/he can feel that I have had a chance to hear his or her experience and point of view just as fully. I also make clear that I can't work with a couple if in the individual meeting secrets are revealed that could not be shared with the partner.

Not infrequently people ask if we could start by working individually and then after a while bring in the partner. I explain that in my experience a prior relationship with one person hampers the effectiveness of couple therapy and that if I work individually with one of them I would refer them to someone else for couple therapy. Although I know that many therapists do make that shift, or even see one person for individual therapy while simultaneously doing couple therapy, it is not a way of working that I have found helpful. When we work with an individual, we tend to see things very much from his or her point of view (E. F. & P. L. Wachtel, 1986; Leone, 2013; Gerson, 2013) and it is challenging to maintain the systemic perspective so necessary to couple work.

As with every general rule, there are exceptions. For instance, a particularly fragile individual therapy patient may *only* be able to tolerate couple therapy when the couple therapist is also his or her individual therapist. The trust that developed in the course of the individual therapy may enable such patients to tolerate feedback in couple therapy that would otherwise be experienced as devastating criticism. But even if there are times when playing a dual role *can* help, I am not inclined to begin by first working with one person individually. Having a dual relationship is fraught with unpredictable pitfalls even when both parties are initially enthusiastic about it. This issue is further discussed in Chapter 10.

One Person Wants the Other to Commit to the Relationship before Couple Therapy Begins

Essentially, that person is saying, I can only work on the relationship in the context of knowing that you (the spouse) want to be with me. The frame of mind is something like this—I want you to affirm that you are committed to staying together regardless of the problems and only *then* am I willing to work on the difficulties in couple therapy. That person doesn't want to feel as if s/he is being evaluated, and experiences the other's ambivalence as a sword over his or her head.

In these situations, the therapist needs to empathize and help each elaborate more on what they are feeling. But ultimately, the spouse who wants commitment prior to therapy will need to accept the reality that one can't actually *demand* that the other feel what s/he doesn't feel. The fact is that one's spouse may believe that to make a commitment *before* seeing if therapy results in greater satisfaction would entail a sacrifice of happiness that s/he is unwilling to make. Many people voluntarily do make the choice to honor their previous commitments or marriage vows, despite having an unsatisfactory relationship. But making it a precondition to therapy can feel coercive, and the resentment that it stirs is counterproductive to the aims of therapy. The therapist can often help resolve this stalemate by making it clear that if they did decide to do couple therapy, it would be about *both* people acting differently in a variety of ways and would not feel like the "change or else" scenario that a sword over the head implies.

At times, a person who is insisting on commitment finds the ambiguity so intolerable that s/he would actually rather end the relationship than risk further hurt and disappointment. Or perhaps, by making a demand that is unlikely to be acceded to, the person is indirectly expressing his or her *own* ambivalence about working on the relationship. With this in mind, the therapist needs to explore the complexity of feelings that underlie such a demand and the choices and options that *both* partners have.

Often this impasse can be resolved by the uncommitted spouse agreeing to put the "stay or leave" decision on hold for a set number of months. This can feel like a great relief to the person who is uncertain about what s/he wants to do. Deciding on a specific date on which one will take stock can relieve the ambivalent or uncommitted spouse of incessant rumination, which is not only highly taxing emotionally, but in itself is a severe impediment to making progress on the relationship. If instead, the uncommitted spouse can give his or her *all* to working on the relationship for a set number of months, they'll both be in a better position to make a decision about whether they want to stay together or separate. It is helpful to actually mark the "take-stock-of-relationship" date on the calendar. Note, that the agreement is not to make a final decision on a specific date (which the person at that point may or may not be ready to do), but rather is a way of putting on hold one person's reoccupation with whether or not to end the relationship so s/he can move fully engage in couple therapy. It is important to be realistic, and to acknowledge that despite the designated date, they are likely to have times when one or both of them find themselves seriously contemplating the issue anyway. Perhaps they will have had a fight, or some progress that they seem to have made is followed by a step backward, and all the old obsessing about staying or leaving is evoked anew. By having a specific date in mind, however, they are more likely to be able to again put the decision on hold while they continue to work on their relationship. But here again, this is more likely to be helpful if the therapist makes it really clear that s/he is not *presuming* that they will or should stay together, but only that both will feel better if they know that they have given it their all.

When one person is ambivalent about working on the relationship, I ask whether or not there is another person in the picture or someone whom s/he *might* be interested in if they were separated. I will also state that *"to see if couple therapy can really make a difference, it's important to put a lot of time and effort into the relationship, and that it's best to avoid or step back from even <u>potentially</u> romantic relationships or friendships while trying to decide on the viability of the marriage."* I explain that when one satisfies the need for intimacy outside the relationship, even if not having an affair, couple therapy is much less likely to be effective.

One Person Wants to Work on the Relationship and the Other Is Reluctant to Do So

Very frequently one person is more committed than the other to trying to make the relationship work. Although this is usually not news to the couple, it is important to include it in the feedback at the end of the session. The more reluctant partner needs to know that you, the therapist, *get it* and that you are not assuming that s/he is committed to the relationship even if s/he is agreeing to continue in therapy. That person is much more likely to give couple therapy a try if s/he knows that you respect, and accept, his or her ambivalent feelings. So it can be useful to say something like *"I understand that your wife was so upset about your wanting to separate that you said you'd come to couple therapy. But it's important for us all to acknowledge that you are quite doubtful that this could really help and are here mostly because your wife wants to see if the relationship can be salvaged."* At the same time, it can also be helpful to state that *"couple therapy can result in people changing quite a bit, and that since you have already invested so many years in the relationship, why not invest a little bit more time to see if things change enough that you really feel differently."*

THE FIRST SESSION IN THE AFTERMATH OF AN AFFAIR

When a couple has come in because of the discovery of an affair, the standard first session described above does not apply. Instead, the therapist must immediately deal with the situation at hand. The couple is usually extremely distressed. The person who has been betrayed is often experiencing intense emotional pain. She[1] may be profoundly hurt and may be in the throes of an

---

[1]As discussed in Chapter 1, for the sake of avoiding convoluted sentences with multiple "s/he" and "his or her" constructions, I will here simplify, by randomly using just "he" or "she." The reader should bear in mind in every one of these instances that the sentences could have been written with the opposite gender.

almost primal sense of abandonment. She may be unable to eat or sleep. He may be overcome with grief or rage. Side by side with the pain is the almost unfathomable, dizzying challenge to sense of reality. What was accepted on face value—business trips, staying late to work, needing to go into the office on the weekend—was actually part of a plan to deceive. Many people who have been betrayed are shaken to the core. They may feel that they do not know who their partner *is* or *was* throughout their relationship. It is common for the one who has been hurt to become obsessed with uncovering every possible deception. They search for evidence from years back and become preoccupied with the quest to uncover the truth. They are tortured by the doubt and suspicion that consumes them. The tectonic plates of the earth have shifted and there is no longer a solid foundation upon which their relationship is built.

The partner who has been unfaithful is often also extremely upset. He may be surprised by, and profoundly disturbed by the depth of the pain his actions have caused. The betraying spouse probably never expected his spouse to find out about the affair, and may have had no intention or desire to break up the relationship. He may never have questioned his love for his spouse and sees the affair as something apart and separate, having nothing to do with how he feels about his partner. Suddenly, the betraying spouse may find that his life is collapsing around him and he may desperately want things to get back to normal. He may be overwhelmed by the roller-coaster ups and downs of the spouse's emotions. At times the hurt partner's love seems to still be there, and she seems to want to find a way to reconcile. At other times she may be engulfed by anger and seems only to want to hurt and even destroy the spouse who has inflicted such pain. She may threaten to humiliate the spouse in front of family, friends, or business associates. In some cases, the betrayed one may have already done some of these things before they arrive in the therapist's office. Even if the betraying spouse feels great remorse, she may simultaneously be appalled by the vengeful and mortifying actions in which the spouse has engaged.

The disloyal spouse also often feels dizzying, fluctuating emotions. At times feelings of empathy and remorse are overshadowed by a loss of patience with his or her partner's suspiciousness, and what can feel like endless interrogations and recriminations. Complicating the situation further, betraying partners may greatly resent that their spouse has invaded their privacy by reading their emails and texts, getting their phone records, or even perhaps hiring a detective. In their view, their actions do not justify or excuse the moral transgressions committed by their spouse even if it was in reaction to betrayal. Will this ever end? Can we get back to normal? Will I always have to account for every minute? Will she always hold this over me? Will I forever be regarded as an immoral untrustworthy miscreant? Will I ever be respected and held in high esteem again?

Furthermore, though the unfaithful spouse may be certain that she wants to remain with her spouse, she may, nonetheless, have a deep emotional connection to another person and may be finding it quite difficult to give up that relationship. Or he may feel a good deal of guilt about hurting and possibly having misled the person with whom he had the affair. And even when all ties have been severed, the betraying spouse may still miss and long for the person whom she has given up.

The goal of a first session—which if you know you are going to be dealing with the aftermath of an affair should be a longer one than usual—is to help the couple become a little calmer and to slow down the emotional whirlwind that has engulfed them. Often, the first issue that has to be addressed is the hurt spouse's feelings of humiliation about even *considering* staying in the relationship. Perhaps that person had always thought that she would not tolerate any betrayal and would end the relationship immediately if that were to happen. So, finding herself in a couple therapist's office adds insult to injury, so to speak. The therapist's first task, then, is to help the "betrayed" person feel that it is not a sign of weakness to seek counseling before making such a momentous decision. It is helpful to normalize and reassure the person that *"many, probably most, people who believed that they would immediately end the relationship if betrayed, when faced with the decision, realize that things are often not as clear-cut as they may seem when it's just a theoretical discussion. Relationships are complicated. And, at a minimum, most people want to understand more about what happened before deciding to leave."*

Another consideration that sometimes weighs heavily on the shoulders of the spouse who has been betrayed is that family and friends may be urging him to leave the partner. Again, normalizing this phenomenon can be helpful. Saying something like *"Though this advice is undoubtedly coming out of deeply caring for you and wanting to protect you from further hurt, it's almost impossible for anyone but the person actually in the relationship to understand the complex feelings both about being betrayed and about the potential loss of a future with one's spouse."* It is important to emphasize that a decision to do couple therapy is by no means a decision to stay in the relationship, but merely a chance to take a closer look at what happened, why, and *whether or not* the relationship can be repaired, *even if* the betrayed one is willing to work on the repair.

One of the most pressing issues when the couple comes in soon after an affair has been discovered is how much information the hurt one wants to receive, the nature of that information, whether or not getting that information will do more harm than good, and whether, painful as it might be, it is a necessary first step toward the possible restoration of trust. There is not one standard answer to these questions. People differ in what they need and how much ambiguity they can tolerate. In the first session the therapist explores these questions with the couple and helps them come up with some preliminary ground rules that are agreeable to both. Often, the plan needs to be very concrete—for example, should the hurt one have all passwords and free access to information that was once considered private? Can he talk to other people about what happened? When asking questions of the betraying partner, are there questions on topics that should be considered off-limits? It is important to emphasize the provisional nature of the plan and that together we will revisit the issue to see whether or not what has been agreed upon is actually working in practice or whether it needs to be revised.

The first session in such cases also needs to address the couples' concern that trust and a normal relationship may forever be out of reach. Often the one who has been hurt is tremendously distressed by how suspicious she has become. She may be horrified at the thought of having to live in a chronic state of mistrust. Will she ever not worry when the spouse is presumably on a business trip, or staying late at the office? And conversely, her partner worries that he will always be seen as the wrongdoer and will never get out from under this burden.

The anxieties of each partner must be both validated and, at the same time, put into a larger perspective. Thus, I might say something like *"Yes, it's probably true that something permanent has changed. You never thought it possible that your wife could do. . . . "* And to the unfaithful one, *"You never understood how deeply he loved you, how primal the trust was, how deeply hurt he would be. . . . It will take a long time—but for many couples who have been just as deeply shaken as you have been, gradually, what happened recedes, as months and years of a gratifying relationship overshadow the trauma of what has happened. It may never be quite the same as before—you can't erase the past—but assuming that there are no more deceptions—even small, seemingly inconsequential ones—you are likely to once again feel secure that what seems to be true and real actually is."*

I follow this advice by explaining that a big factor in the development of trust is the couple having a clear understanding of what factors led to the affair and the concomitant ability to both prevent the buildup of destructive patterns and to develop other ways of handling personal and relationship stress when it does occur. Together, the couple needs to make sense of what happened. The individual who was disloyal needs to understand what was going on for him or her as an individual, not just as a member of the couple. By this I mean that sometimes the motivation behind an affair has little to do with problems or dissatisfactions in the relationship. I've seen couples where the person who had the affair was using it almost like a drug that gave temporary relief from depression or feelings of low self-esteem. For some people it is a reaction to aging and reflects more a longing for youth than any serious unhappiness in the marriage. Or perhaps it is an enactment of attachment issues—a fear of emotional reliance on just one person.

Far more often, however, there are issues in the relationship that contributed to a spouse becoming emotionally involved with another person. One of the goals of a first session is to help the injured spouse be open to examining some of the problems in the relationship that were the backdrop for what happened. It can feel to the betrayed party that examining what wasn't working well exonerates the "guilty" spouse or "blames the victim." The therapist needs to help the couple shift focus to what was missing in the relationship and what *each* of them might have been craving without in any way condoning the spouse's seeking an affair as a *solution* to their marital difficulties.

Even with a lengthy session, the goals described above are not easy to achieve. The therapist needs to convey the message that recovering from an affair is often a slow process, and the spouse who has been unfaithful cannot expect the partner to quickly shift from anger and blame to a willingness to examine aspects of the relationship that may have played a role in setting the stage for the transgression. It may take many sessions before the actual work of "unpacking" what happened can begin.

Although a first session when the discovery of an affair is the issue is quite different than the standard first session I have outlined, the therapist should still look for any strengths that can be highlighted and reinforced. It may be a particular challenge for the therapist to find any positives to note in first encountering a couple in this kind of crisis. And while it may be especially valuable to do so where the sky looks so grey, it is important not to overreach here. Clinical sensitivity and skillfulness are especially important in these instances. If either party feels you are ignoring or overriding the seriousness of their pain or despair, the work will be severely impacted.

As described earlier, strengths can be underlined in two spheres: the way the couple relates to one another and the way each of them acts in the therapy session and with the therapist. In a first session after one person has discovered the other's infidelity, the therapist might notice such things as *"You are very angry, but you're not just indicting her—you seem to truly want to understand what happened."* Or *"I'm struck by your willingness to look at what was going on in your relationship despite your concern that he might think that doing so means you are excusing what he did."* Or *"You are tremendously hurt but you seem to know that you have an inner strength that will allow you in time to recover."* Or *"You seem at times— though it is hard to hold on to this—to be able to see this as something he's going through and not a reflection on you or a measure of his love for you."* The therapist can also give some positive feedback to the "betrayer" without in any way condoning his actions. For example, a therapist might say, *"I noticed that you are taking the <u>initiative</u> in doing concrete things to* *make your wife feel more secure—not just doing what she explicitly asks you to do."* Or *"You seem to be genuinely trying to understand how you could have acted in a way that fell so short of your ideals."* Or *"You are trying hard to understand your husband's feelings even though to you, the relationship you had with your coworker wasn't really an affair."*

Often the hurt partner is crushed for the very reason that in so many ways the relationship seemed *good*. Perhaps they enjoy each other's company when out with friends. Or perhaps they do a good job parenting together. Or they still can joke around with one another. It's particularly important to make note of these positives when the injured person feels humiliated by the fact that he is in a therapist's office rather than responding to the violation of trust by immediately ending the relationship. Furthermore, often the betrayed party questions whether *anything* she thought was good in the relationship actually was or whether the whole thing was a sham. If the unfaithful partner confirms that the good things *were* real, the therapist can help the hurt spouse understand that the betrayal does not actually negate the positive experiences that they had as a couple. Understanding how a spouse who still claims to have always loved you could have simultaneously been emotionally involved with someone else is perhaps the most difficult hurdle to overcome in getting past the affair. The therapist's input about the caring, or empathic, or simply open and undefensive features of one or both spouses' behavior in the office, as well as some of the genuinely good aspects of their relationship as reported by both partners, can be enormously helpful to the hurt partner who is trying to grasp what seems emotionally incomprehensible.

OKAY, NOW WHAT?

Often, as the first session draws to a close, whether it has been the standard one, or one in which because of a crisis we immediately start working on the couple's problems, the couple usually is feeling more hopeful about the prospect of therapy actually being able to help them. Fears that the session would devolve into heated accusations and counterattacks have been allayed. They have experienced the therapist as having a plan for how to proceed and as capable of containing the often overwhelming anger, hurt, and sadness that the couple brings to the session. And, for some couples, the therapist's ability to see some positives buried in the myriad of complaints and dissatisfactions has helped lessen the shame that they may feel about being in a highly dysfunctional or seemingly loveless relationship. But, as discussed above, the feedback the couple gets is by no means only positive. They will have received input about the strengths *and* the weaknesses in their relationship, and, by the conclusion of the first session, the couple should have a realistic sense of the difficulty (or in some cases, *ease*) of making the kinds of changes that could result in a more gratifying relationship.

The session has also provided them with an experience of how couple therapy works. If one or both of them has been in individual therapy, they may have assumed that the session would be a venue where they could vent their concerns and frustrations with minimal control or direction by the therapist. Despite the session being different from what they expected, most couples are satisfied with what the session has accomplished. If, however, the therapist senses that one, or both, aren't sure about whether or not they want to proceed, it is important to suggest that they take some time to think about what they want to do next. They should be encouraged to voice concerns and questions they may have. As discussed earlier, no matter how good the session was, it is not uncommon for one person in the couple to remain uncertain about whether or not s/he wants to embark on an attempt to repair what seems to be a severely damaged relationship. When this is the case, it can be helpful to suggest an individual meeting to talk through his or her concerns, with the proviso, however, that the therapist can't work with them as a couple if in that session the therapist is made privy to information that could not be shared with the other person in the couple. It's important to make clear that, if after a meeting with the ambivalent spouse, if s/he decides to give couple therapy a try, then an individual session with their partner will also be scheduled.

Before concluding the session, I give the couple information about what to expect in the next meeting. If, as in most cases, they have put on hold a full discussion of their difficulties, the therapist needs to reiterate that in the *next* meeting we will begin to go into more depth, both about what is wrong and about what they are longing for. With this in mind, I tell couples that when we meet again I'm going to ask them to tell me about a recent example of when things went wrong between them. *"I want the kind of detail that will let me see, almost as if I were there, what happens between the two of you. It doesn't need to be anything big—it could just be when you're getting that here we go again feeling. For the first couple of meetings, I like to go into this kind of detail about arguments or bad feeling so I get a really good sense of the patterns that have developed. After that, we won't be using sessions to hash out arguments—not only because I think that you will find that they diminish significantly as we begin to work on the issues, but because I'd like to help you talk to one another about what you long for and crave—not just the elimination of negatives—but what you'd love to get from one another."*

And lastly, in further preparation for the next session, I give the couple some "homework." I ask them each to *"think about what you know about yourself that makes you not the easiest person in the world to live with. From listening to you today, I have a sense that you each know a great deal* *about yourself, and in addition to talking in depth about your relationship, I'd like to hear your thoughts on this topic. We all bring particular sensitivities, and some not-so-great habits and characteristics to relationships, and it would be helpful for me to understand what you each know you bring to the interactions between you. The kind of things I'm talking about, for instance, are having a quick temper, or having a particular reactivity to being told what to do, or closing off when worried about something, or being a little obsessive–compulsive about neatness, or being moody, or being sensitive to criticism, and so on. These, of course, are just <u>examples</u> of the kinds of personality traits people have—but of course there are dozens of other things too. The point here is that I'm not talking about things that your spouse might have said about you, or even that other people have said. I'm really interested in what <u>you</u> actually know about yourself."*

The challenge of the second session is to get more clarity on the difficulties and to "dig in" in a way that while focusing on their serious problematic interactions manages to instill and maintain hope, a crucial ingredient for therapeutic effectiveness (Frank & Frank, 1991; Wampold, 2001).

5
ೞ

The Individual in the System
A Critical Pathway to Change

*C*hange in a couple's way of interacting very largely comes down to
each *individual* being willing and able to expand his or her sense
of self and to behave in previously uncharacteristic ways. In this chapter we
look at some methods that facilitate each person having an expanded view
of who s/he is and how s/he is capable of being.

SELF-REFLECTION AND HUMILITY

Most couples come to therapy with the goal of wanting their partner to
change. Often for years one or both of them has been pointing out the other's flaws and failings, and they come to therapy frustrated that they can't
seem to get through to their partner. Frequently, one person critiques a good
deal more than the other, and it is that person's dissatisfaction that results
in their coming for counseling. The partner who is being critiqued is usually
quite pessimistic about how helpful couple therapy could be and comes in
with the expectation that the therapy will be more of the same: a focus on
all the things about him or her that makes the partner unhappy.

It can be tempting to therapists to right this imbalance by probing for
things that the less critical spouse is actually unhappy about but doesn't
voice. At times this is a useful intervention, but it can also be the therapeutic equivalent of "two wrongs don't make a right." As I have previously

discussed, shifting the orientation to *wishes* rather than what is lacking is likely to be much more effective than mutual critiquing. But another conceptual shift can also help create the opportunity for a new approach to the couple's difficulties—fostering self-reflection, humility, and the motivation to change oneself. I start with the assumption that it is generally easier to change something about *oneself* or the way one interacts than to get *someone else* to change. If one person changes, the other inevitably will change too—since, as I discussed in Chapter 2, the ways we act—and even feel—are contextual: different aspects of our behavioral and experiential repertoires are activated in different contexts, and since each member of the couple is a context for the other, changing ourselves almost inevitably leads to change in the other. Of course, if only one partner is working hard to change, there will likely be resentment, and additionally, with only one pulling on the rope, the load will feel heavier and movement will be slower. When both take responsibility for generating change, movement is much easier.

This orientation is introduced early in the work and continues throughout the sessions. As I have described in the previous chapter, toward the end of the first session I ask them each to *"think about what you know about yourself that makes you not the easiest person in the world to live with."* Often one or both of them immediately volunteers something and I respond by acknowledging, and thus implicitly praising, his or her ability to be open. Even if they've answered right away, I encourage them to give more thought to this question since it's quite likely that other ideas about this will occur during the week.

In fostering an attitude of self-reflection and commitment to working on one's own contribution to the difficulties, it is important for therapists to be alert to even a small increase in self-awareness or a less blaming perspective on the problem. Consider, for example, how one might respond if the husband angrily said, "She just doesn't listen to me, she never takes no for an answer. I *know* I shouldn't start screaming—it makes *me* look like a real jerk—but sometimes I just can't see any other way to get through to her, and I get crazy and blow my top!" In response to this, the therapist could say, *"I'm understanding from what you're saying just how angry you get and how when you get so angry it makes things worse, but I'm also struck by how aware you are that this isn't a good way to respond and how you are struggling with the knowledge that despite your intentions to stay calm, you end up losing control. I hear you saying that even if you're provoked, you really don't feel good about responding this way."* The patient may well respond to this kind of statement with a "Yes, but . . . " statement and go back to focusing on how provocative his wife was being. If this happens, the therapist could then say, *"Yes, we do have to figure out together how to change this pattern that makes you both so unhappy, but it sounds to me that you'd like to figure out not only how to get through to Emma [his wife], but how to stay calm no matter how she's acting."*

An important route to helping each person in the couple acknowledge his or her own role in negative interactions is to explore family history. An understanding of the way one's family background gets played out in the current relationship can make it easier to acknowledge and then work on one's own contribution. Just as we need to accept that we, like everyone else, are inevitably flawed, we also need to accept that, like it or not, our family background has had an impact on who we are and how we act. This does not mean that we will inevitably act like our parents. In fact, often it is a determination *not* to repeat patterns we grew up with that have a greater influence on our behavior. For instance, Robert regarded his father as completely "henpecked" and acquiescent to his wife and her domineering family. In contrast, Robert would all too easily get into power struggles with his wife. He so feared losing his sense of self that he had difficulty "joining," and almost reflexively asserted his separateness and individuality even when his position and his wife's were not so far apart.

When someone is having difficulty seeing his or her role in negative interactions, it can be helpful to normalize problematic reactions by talking about what other couples experience. I might remark on how frequently I see a particular couple dynamic in my work. For example, if a woman is bringing to the relationship a level of irritability that she can't acknowledge and believes that she is *only* responding to her husband's actions, I might comment empathically that *"so many of the women I see are terribly stressed by juggling the demands of work and parenting that they feel burdened by their husband also wanting their attention—lots of things bother them that might not matter nearly as much if they didn't feel pulled in so many directions."* The hope is that a comment of this sort will help the woman be more comfortable in seeing her own stress level and reactivity as part of the problem rather than simply pointing the finger of blame at her husband.

Or when a man feels very annoyed with his wife for repeatedly asking him for help with common computer problems, but can't see that his annoyance is more complexly motivated, I might say something like *"It's strange how many highly competent women repeatedly turn to their husbands for tech support. But for some men it's just a minor irritation, whereas other men, like you, react to it very strongly. Sometimes the strong reaction is related to the man having a particular issue with highly dependent women— and even if his wife isn't very dependent in other ways this triggers feelings about too much neediness. Or sometimes the man feels that his wife only needs him for practical things and isn't interested in sexual intimacy, and thus he reacts strongly to what otherwise would go in the 'not a big deal' category. Do you think any of these feelings might be going on for you too?"*

Statements of this sort give the nonintrospective person food for thought as well as provide a model for how one's reaction to something may be influenced by feelings that have not been consciously articulated. Additionally, referring to what *other people* say about their experience provides a tactful way of pointing out that the person may be overreacting and that these same events could be regarded as little more than the normal irritations of married life.

Personal anecdotes can go a long way in conveying an attitude of humility about one's own shortcomings. It is helpful to realize before pointing the finger of blame at our partners that we are far from perfect ourselves and that a "live and let live" attitude is essential to long and happy relationships. I sometimes tell couples that I personally know how easy it is to overlook our own faults and focus on our spouse's failings. There are many times when I come home to a messy kitchen and, ready to pounce, I keep myself in check by reminding myself that I'm far from perfect in the neatness arena and ask myself if I really want to make my husband feel bad or start a fight. Or I might say that I, like many people, have an instinctive blaming reflex and when something is missing from my study, my first feeling is that my husband must have taken it, even though it is much more likely that I myself misplaced the lost object. Or when I'm busy getting ready for guests and start to get steamed up about the fact that I've been in the kitchen all afternoon and generally do the lions's share of shopping and cooking, I need to remind myself of a number of onerous responsibilities that are almost completely in his domain, not mine. These anecdotes normalize our baser impulses and model both the need to "talk oneself down" from the feelings and the awareness that we are all far from perfect.

BRINGING OUT EACH PERSON'S
BEST AND COMPLEX SELF

A fundamental assumption underlying my work is that people can and do continue to change throughout life. This may seem obvious, but too often therapists as well as patients unwittingly endorse a view of personality as fixed and immutable. Side by side with the fact that we do, of course, have many enduring traits is the familiar phenomenon that who we are interacting with has an impact on which of the many facets of our personality are activated. For example, with some people we may find ourselves being able to joke around in a way that is unusual for us. And with others we may get in touch with a more spiritual or philosophical aspect of our self.

It is common for couples to feel hurt when their partner is not seeing them in the positive ways that they are seen by others outside the home. For instance, a man who is seen by his wife as not showing sufficient empathy may be regarded by his colleagues as a particularly sympathetic and caring manager. Or a woman who seems to her spouse irritable and controlling may be regarded by her friends as easy-going and quick to laugh. Thus one of the goals of my work with couples is to help them each develop or express aspects of his or her self that are not regularly actualized in the relationship.

Elsewhere (E. F. Wachtel, 2000) I have talked about the wish to be seen in these positive ways as part of what propels some people to have affairs. Often the new person brings out traits that one no longer exhibits with one's spouse.

There are numerous intersecting influences that frequently result in rigidified roles in relationships. One person's behavior triggers a particular response in the other, and then that *response* in turn is reacted to in a way that highlights only one particular aspect of the partner. For example, when Lucinda is hurt because she feels Frank isn't attuned to her and sensitive to what she feels and doesn't value her opinion, she expresses her hurt through anger and criticism. Frank, in turn, responds to her criticism with anger and defensiveness and this further confirms Lucinda's belief that he isn't a nurturing person who will respond with empathy to her emotional pain. After years of similar interactions, Frank has been "pegged" as "not very empathic" and his hurt about being perceived this way by his wife is expressed in angry withdrawal and distance, further confirming Lucinda's perception that "Frank just isn't a warm, compassionate person." One's reputation in the couple is further reinforced because we all tend to see what we are expecting to see, and thus new and varied ways of behaving are often not noticed or responded to positively. Additionally, people in couples can feel threatened by the other changing. Often when one person goes into individual therapy and gets in touch with unfulfilled or unactualized parts of his- or herself, the other feels anxiety about how this new self-awareness will affect their relationship. The person worries about whether "He will be dissatisfied with who I am or the life we have together" or "Whether she will still need or love me?" Even when the spouse has actively encouraged his or her partner to go into individual therapy with the hope that s/he will change in some ways that will make their relationship better, there is often anxiety about the insights and self-exploration that is occurring. There is some comfort in what is predictable and familiar even if it has been one source of the couple's difficulties.

Even though partners are often troubled that they are perceived differently by their spouse than they are by other people with whom they interact, by and large couples tend to define themselves in relation to their spouse's characteristics. For instance, one might say, "I'm the social one, he's more of a loner"; or "I'm the tough one, and she's the pushover"; or "I'm emotional and he's all logic." It may be that people feel that their "real" self is the one that is manifested in their most intimate relationships. It is interesting to note that the couple may disagree about many things but rarely do they quibble with each other about these types of characterizations. Couple therapy provides an opportunity to examine these reified, rigid beliefs about the self and the other so that both have an opportunity to expand their self-narratives in a way that is more complex and less self-limiting (Freedman & Combs, 1996; White & Epston, 1990).

NOTICING "OUT-OF-CHARACTER" MOMENTS

In a previous chapter I discussed the role of positive feedback and the importance of noticing small steps in the right direction in helping couples change long-standing negative interactions. This approach is also quite helpful in expanding an individual's beliefs about himself. For instance, if the husband in a couple states that he's not good at expressing feelings, the therapist needs to be attentive to any moments in the session when he actually *is* expressing his feelings. Men who say this are usually comparing themselves to a highly verbal, articulate wife who can describe the subtle nuances of her emotional life. A man may feel inadequate in comparison to his wife and as a consequence not put into the "expressing feelings" category various statements he makes that *do* in fact capture what is going on for him emotionally. The therapist's noticing and highlighting of these moments challenges a reified definition of himself as "not good at feelings," and by so doing increases the likelihood that there will be more frequent instances of his taking a chance and trying out what he thinks he isn't good at. At some point in the session, for example, he might say, "I didn't want to come today. It's Cecile's [his wife] birthday tomorrow and I'd hate to say something today that upsets her. I want her to have a good time at the party tomorrow—she's been so down lately." In response to this, the therapist might say something like *"I know you say you're not good at expressing feelings and maybe there are a lot of times when that's true, but just now, your feelings came through really clearly and poignantly."* And to the wife, *"Did you notice that too? Did you hear how strongly he felt about wanting you to enjoy your birthday?"*

Often a spouse will respond by noting that in the sessions their partner does open up in a way that doesn't happen at home. At this choice point, the therapist could say, *"Let's put our heads together and figure out how we can enable that to happen more at home too."* It may be that it does happen at home, but isn't noticed because it doesn't fit with the wife's conception of talking about feelings. Or, if the husband actually doesn't express himself at home, it may be because his wife usually presses him to elaborate and he doesn't feel able to expand on what he's already said.

NOTICING COMPLEXITY AND NUANCE

When people make global statements about themselves, it is useful to help them notice the nuances that add complexity to their self-described personality. For instance, when Rachel says that she is indecisive and unsure of her opinions, this is likely to be accurate in some instances but not in others. She may be the one in the couple who has strong and clear opinions about child-rearing issues, for example. Or perhaps she's the one who has more definite opinions about restaurants, who she wants to socialize with, or where she wants to live. Most people are intrigued by feedback that they are more complicated than they thought. The point of underlining the exceptions to the rule that both she and her spouse may not have noticed is not to say, "It's not as bad as you think," but rather to inspire and give hope to the person about being the way s/he already *is*, but to do so in more situations.

NOTICING WHEN PEOPLE ARE "BECOMING"

Another way therapists can help couples expand their beliefs about themselves is to give feedback about how they are changing and *becoming*. This is different from acknowledging new ways of acting. Rather, it is noticing and underlining changes in what had been thought of as fixed aspects of one's personality. For example, Lara would often describe feeling very overwhelmed by the responsibility of caring for her elderly father, as well as the demands of juggling a job and children. She thought of herself as someone who "can't take a lot of stress" and who "breaks down when I'm pulled in too many directions." The therapist noticed that in the last several sessions Lara seemed calmer. This was attributed in part to the improvement in the couple's relationship but also to the fact that she had resumed taking yoga classes and was arranging to see friends more often. Lara had mentioned several times in the past weeks that she wished she could get a handle on her anxiety. When she reported that she was feeling a little better, the therapist said that he thought Lara was *"becoming someone who takes stock of herself and figures out what to do when she's feeling overwhelmed."* A statement like this not only acknowledges change but reinforces the message that who we are is not fixed in stone but rather constantly evolving. Similarly, when John, who described himself as someone who doesn't like change and prefers the comforts of home to "running all over the place looking for excitement," admitted that he was enjoying some of the outings he had agreed to do in order to please his wife, the therapist could say something like *"You seem like you're the kind of person who really gets into things even though it isn't necessarily what you would have chosen to do. Is this new for you? Are you becoming more that way lately?"*

By inviting the spouse to join in observing how his or her partner is "becoming," the therapist models giving a type of feedback that is usually responded to very positively. Most people are pleased and touched when a person who knows them intimately notices change and says things like *"You seem to be becoming more confident about doing presentations"*; or *"You're becoming more relaxed around your family"*; or *"You've become able to be yourself at parties."* Instead of being locked into roles that may no longer fit comfortably, the spouse is being seen anew and feels known.

When couples begin to notice and give positive feedback about *change,* the partner is experienced as a facilitator of growth and potential and the emotional bond between the spouses is strengthened.

ASSUMING THE BEST IN PEOPLE— AND FINDING IT

A key goal for the couple therapist is to encourage couples to try new ways of being with one another. When behavioral change feels like a natural manifestation of evolving feelings rather than something that the couple has *contracted* to do differently, the new ways of interacting are more likely to be sustained. They will feel like authentic expressions of feelings that were already present but not displayed because the couple had gotten into negative cycles of interaction.

There are two ways that therapists can help facilitate these seemingly spontaneous enactments of new behaviors. The first way is simply by assuming the best of people. If we respect someone, it is human nature to want to live up to that person's good opinion of us. Earlier I discussed the importance of developing a strong therapeutic alliance with both individuals in the couple. When people feel liked, known, and respected by the therapist, they naturally want to live up to the therapist's positive expectations. So, in a situation where the wife has been feeling neglected and wishes her husband would set more boundaries about work, the therapist could say to the husband, *"I'm sure you'll figure out a way to do this because you are so clearly someone who takes a lot of pleasure in being a caring man who looks after people, and this is what your wife is needing at this point in her life."* Or, when a man wishes that his postmenopausal wife would make more of an effort to reignite her dormant interest in sex, the therapist could say to the wife, *"I know from the things you've told me about yourself that you are the kind of person who persists until you figure out how to do something— like when you continued your Photo-Shop class even though you felt overwhelmed at first, or when you managed to put together the 100-piece Ikea entertainment centerpiece instead of sending it back. It seems that you always want to grow and have new experiences and that's why I have a sense that you'll figure out this sexual drive thing too—which of course I'll help you with. You're not the type of person to succumb to a 'this is just the way it is' attitude about the loss of yourself as a sexual person."*

Another method of helping people expand their sense of self is for the therapist to pick up on minute indications of feelings that the person has not yet reported having or consciously articulated. This involves noticing and highlighting slight indications of emotions, intentions, or wishes that lay beneath the surface of the overt content of what the person is saying.

For instance, when Walt expressed strong indignation at his wife, Meredith's, mother for complaining bitterly about Meredith's father, the therapist picks up on the empathy for his wife that was the source of his anger at his mother-in-law. The therapist could make an attributional statement, such as *"I get a sense that when you express anger at Meredith's mother, you are wanting to let Meredith know how much empathy you have for the pain her parent's marital problems are causing her."* Or, in another example, the therapist could say, in response to a wife's statement that "in my family we believed in being honest and had a 'no holds-barred' attitude toward expressing what we really felt," that *"it sounds like you are beginning to feel that you're not so comfortable anymore with the damage that full expression of anger can do."*

Attributional statements have an element of suggestion in them. But the suggestion only takes hold if there actually is at least a kernel of truth to the feedback the therapist is giving. In the first example, the therapist is in a sense suggesting to Walt that he is feeling empathy, but the seed of that feeling must actually be there for the empathy to grow and be directly expressed. And in the second example, the woman must actually have some real ambivalence about being "authentic" at any cost, in order for the idea that she's rethinking the wisdom of that approach to actually influence her.

THE BEHAVIORAL IMPLICATIONS OF NEW UNDERSTANDINGS

Couple therapists need to help couples *use* the insights they have gained about themselves, their spouse, and the patterns of interaction between them. Thus, a thread that runs through every session is the implicit (and often explicit) question, *"What are some of the possible actions and new ways of behaving that flow from what we have been talking about?"* This question applies equally to both big and small insights, to expanded understanding of one's self and one's spouse, and, of course, to the new appreciation of how the couple falls into routinized patterns of interactions that lead to hurt and anger. Even when couples have had a new and deeply meaningful understanding of one another in the session and have felt that they really *get* how they each have been responding to one another in a way that leads to vicious circles, it can be difficult to avoid falling into familiar patterns of behavior. It helps to think of these patterns as automatic, habitual reactions that are, in a sense, the default position to which they each return unless they make a very conscious choice to do something different. For this reason, it is important to help the couple spell out in detail both how they plan to interact differently and what provocations and pitfalls they can anticipate that could reflexively lead to their customary, unwanted behavior.

So, for example, Mark and Carly had come to understand the pattern that had led them to become increasingly alienated from one another. Mark would withdraw because he often felt that his wife "has no use for my opinions," and she, feeling his aloofness, would respond by "doing my own thing" and hoping his bad mood would eventually pass. In a particularly open and heartfelt session, they each expressed regret for wounding the other. They both understood that the hurt they each experience is only made worse by their habitual way of handling the feeling. In order to help this insight "stick," the therapist needs to ask them what they will each do differently when they feel ignored or unimportant. Based on what they had come to understand, both said they would try to say something to the other about how they were feeling instead of just withdrawing. But this is easier said than done, and by asking specific *questions* about the "doing it differently," the therapist can boost the odds that they will have some success in resisting the old way and trying something new. For example, the therapist could say, *"Let's put our heads together and think about what could make you go back to the old way even though you get it and really don't want to do that."* The husband might say that if he tells his wife he felt ignored, "it may just make her angry." Or she might say that if she were to ask her husband what's going on instead of her usual pattern of just doing her own thing until his mood passed, he's likely to say, "It's nothing" or "It's not important." The couple, with the therapist's help, can plan for how to prevent these reactions from occurring. It is also important to have a plan for what to do if, despite their best intentions, the cycle does get the best of them. *"How could you cut the cycle short? Can you do something different if you do withdraw? How can you remind yourself that you are caught in the habitual vicious circle? Can you put a cartoon on your computer that will help you keep perspective? Is there a friend you've confided in who could help you get back on track?"* The therapist can lightheartedly challenge the couple with hypothetical "worst-case scenarios" with the purpose of bolstering their resolve and helping them recognize potential glitches and pitfalls—I'm a big fan of the "I'll Never Be Jealous Again" song from the musical *The Pajama Game*, in which a character who promises to trust his girlfriend and not be jealous anymore is presented with challenging hypotheticals to test his determination. Along these lines, I might ask the husband something like, *"How would you handle it if you tell Cyd [his wife] that you are upset about something and her first response is 'Oh, you're being ridiculous!'?"* Or, to the wife, *"What if you text Charlie that you really need to speak to him about something and he never responds to your text, and then says he doesn't have a free minute at work? What then—how will you respond?"*

Even when a couple reports that they successfully avoided the repetition of a recurrent pattern, it is important to ask *how* they managed to do that and what each did differently. A detailed analysis of their triumph over destructive negative cycles of interaction not only positively reinforces their accomplishment, but also helps them articulate exactly what each *did* to make the new way of engaging with each other possible. It can also be helpful to ask if there were any moments when one or the other felt the "here we go again" feeling and, if so, how did they avoid letting the missteps escalate?

It is important for this action orientation to permeate all aspects of one's work with couples. Thus, it applies not just to insights about the couple's interactions, but to individual insights as well. For example, Melissa recognized that she would get so angry sometimes that she split off from consciousness the awareness that the man on whom she was showering venomous insults was the same person she genuinely felt she loved. The therapist explored with her *how* she could counteract that tendency when angry to dissociate the loving part of herself. It is not realistic for her to just resolve that she will no longer let herself express anger in a "go for the jugular" way. Rather, she needs some methods that will help her live up to her intentions and that will take into account the psychological process that allowed her to be so unrestrained. She might, for instance, commit to practicing visualizing her husband doing something that she associates with her tender feelings toward him—for example, hugging her, playing with the children, cooking pancakes—and then when starting to get angry close her eyes for a moment and go to that image. Or she might learn some relaxation methods that can be used when she is feeling highly agitated (Wilson, 1995), which will allow her to calm down and be her whole self. Though each individual must take responsibility for his or her own emotions, we can also ask if there is any way the spouse might help. Perhaps, for instance, a one-word signal from her husband that serves as a reminder of the good feelings that are often there could be incorporated into the plan. Or perhaps her husband could gently touch her for a few seconds to help bring back her awareness that he is her loved one, not her enemy.

Many individual issues have a large impact on the spouse even though they are not directly related to the relationship or the couple's interactions. And, as discussed in the previous chapter, sometimes a referral for individual therapy is clearly what is needed. But even if one person is in his or her own therapy, the couple therapist needs to include in the work some brainstorming about what the individual can *do* to deal with these issues, both for the person's own happiness and for the purpose of mitigating the effect on the couple. Thus, for instance, Leonard described himself as having an "obsessive" personality. He checked his email incessantly and if he didn't respond right away he couldn't relax. On weekends he couldn't "not notice" all the things that needed to be done around the house and even when trying to "hang out" with his wife and children, he found himself preoccupied and waiting for the moment when he could sneak off and get to work on the things that he felt needed to be organized or repaired. He agreed with his wife that he was compulsive about completing tasks and was often irritable by the end of the day because he was disappointed that he had not accomplished as much as he had hoped.

To make matters worse, Liz, his wife, felt that he held her to the same standard and would frequently "nag" her about tasks she needed to attend to. Even if she resisted the pressure he put on her to do chores that were not time-sensitive, she felt tense and guilty when, after a hard week's work, she wanted to use time on the weekend to relax. Understanding the effects of Leonard's obsessiveness on the relationship, as well as coming up with a plan for how the couple could handle it differently, was a central part of my work.

In working with couples like that, the couple therapist should pair expressions of empathy with questions about what the person is trying to *do* about the problem. So, for instance, the therapist might say, *"This obsessive tendency is really hard on you—and of course it affects your wife too. I hear in how you talk about it that you wish you could let more things go—it's really making you pretty miserable to be controlled by these feelings. How have you tried to handle this problem? Do you have any sense of what has worked for you in the past?"* Often, the spouse, as someone who has observed his or her partner closely, may have a sense of what approach might be beneficial, and that input can be quite useful in devising therapeutic strategies. For instance, the spouse might have noticed that this is much less of a problem when they are out of the house or on vacation. Or, perhaps he has noticed that she can resist the temptation to be compulsive when she has gotten a good night's sleep or has remembered to meditate. Sometimes the spouse wishes the partner would consider medication because they've observed, for instance, that "when he was on Prozac he could let a lot more go." But, realistically, as any therapist knows, there is no easy answer for how to get out from under the grip of obsessive or compulsive tendencies, and much of the couple work will consist of coming up with ways to not let it lead to negative interactions between the partners.

Similarly, it's not easy for people to change many other aspects of their behavior despite good intentions about doing so. A frequent occurrence in couple therapy is that one or both partners don't follow through on things they ostensibly *want* to do. Their difficulty in changing their behavior may be due to feelings and intentions that are out of the person's awareness, leading them to be a good deal more ambivalent about doing the things they've committed to than they realize. In working on this ambivalence, it is important to first take the person's frustration with him- or herself at face value. She may feel baffled and frustrated by her own "stuckness" because she genuinely does *want* to do the things that would make her partner happy. When the therapist tries to explore any possible ambivalence, the person may strongly assert, "No, I really *do* want to be more romantic . . . but I'm not good at that, I never have been," or "I understand why she's upset that I forget to ask her about her doctor's appointment or other stuff that's important to her. . . . I don't know why, but I just don't remember these things," or "I know he wants me to hug him more and give physical affection but that just doesn't come naturally to me. I'm just not that way."

When people don't live up to what they intend to do, they usually approach their "failure" with a renewed determination to try harder. But without a plan for *how* to overcome one's habitual mental states (e.g., forgetting, single-minded focus on a task to the exclusion of all else, self-absorption, inhibition) the person is unlikely to succeed, and, discouraged, may retreat into a "This is just the way I am" stance. An action orientation actually starts with helping the couple accept that they each do have some ingrained traits that are hard to overcome and that they can't expect new behaviors to come easily or naturally. If each can understand the other's behavior as something about the way that person *is* and not as a reflection of how much they care, they can brainstorm together about realistic ways they can each stretch to meet the other's needs.

The first step is for the couple to agree that the new behaviors *do not have to come naturally* to be a meaningful expression of love. So, for instance, rather than berating himself for his failure to remember to ask about events that are important to his wife, the husband could accept that he is likely to forget unless he puts daily reminders on his calendar. Or, similarly, the woman who does not show physical affection spontaneously could come up with a plan, for instance, that she will give her husband a hug and a kiss every time they say hello, goodbye, or goodnight. Helping the spouse accept that the show of affection is *real*, even though the person is doing what he *should* do, is an essential part of encouraging action strategies. If the spouse dismisses the gesture because it feels contrived, the person who is making these efforts is in a no-win situation.

Everything discussed thus far is based on the idea that changed behavior will not necessarily happen even when the couple therapy has led to greater closeness and understanding. This is particularly true when it comes to resuming or reinvigorating the couple's sexual relationship. Chapter 10 discusses methods for helping the couple bridge the chasm between emotional closeness and physical intimacy.

But no matter where and when action strategies are used, it is an essential part of the work to convey that all plans are "trial-and-error" experiments that may or may not be useful and will almost certainly need to be fine-tuned. Though any *particular* plan of action may not work, the solution-oriented stance described above makes it much more likely that the gains seen in the sessions will actually be enacted at home.

6

Common Underlying Relationship Issues and How to Address Them

*T*hough I've seen hundreds of couples in the course of my career, I still have a little knot in my stomach when I anticipate the second meeting with a couple. We've had a successful first "date" and the couple is definitely interested in seeing where things will go. But I feel concerned about whether or not the second time we get together will be as good, or whether instead the romance will fizzle out. Of course, I'm stretching this metaphor a bit—but just by a little. Usually the end of the first session has left the couple feeling hopeful and more positive about one another. But now it's time to get to the nitty-gritty of the difficulties and begin to work on their issues.

The challenge is not only to understand more of what is problematic in the relationship, but also to give the couple some sense of how their difficulties can, with the help of couple therapy be resolved. This chapter examines some of the issues that often underlie problematic interaction patterns. I also discuss ways to keep the couple hopeful, even while deeply exploring the hurts, angers, and disappointments that have led the couple to seek therapy. In the next chapter clinical vignettes will show how the methods described in Chapter 3 and Chapter 5 and the therapeutic formulations discussed in this chapter are utilized in a variety of therapeutic situations.

I approach each case as unique. I do not have an overriding theory about the etiology for most relationship difficulties. I don't assume almost all problems couples present have to do with attachment injuries, or autonomy conflicts, or power struggles, or conflicts between individuation and merger. It's not that I don't think these theoretical perspectives are useful—they are *very* useful—but rather that preconceived categories can lead therapists to overlook the *particularity* of the dynamic that exists in the relationship one is seeing before one's eyes right now.

Of course, after years of working with couples, I've accumulated a good deal of information about the types of issues that underlie relationship difficulties. Although I try to approach each couple with as much of a fresh sense of discovery as I can, I am also inevitably listening to and evaluating their difficulties on the basis of what I've observed in working with other couples. Below I describe some of the more commonly occurring concerns that couples have. But the reader should keep in mind that there are always a *number* of issues at play. In categorizing, we are painting a picture with broad brush strokes while the uniqueness of each couple's distress exists in the fine details. The reader should keep in mind that the common issues described below are meant to be used as an organizational framework to help extract some themes from the often overwhelming amount of material that couples present. But hypotheses are no more than that, and we must treat them not as definitive, but merely as *ideas* that we will use at choice points to help us determine what we think would be the most productive areas on which to focus. We must not be wedded to our initial formulations, nor fit new data into preconceived ideas. A willingness to change course and understand a couple's issues with more specificity engenders confidence and is the hallmark of a skilled clinician. Additionally, in order to build on strengths, we must pay as much attention to the *exceptions* to the problematic rule. With the above provisos in mind, the issues described below are ones that, to my mind, often underlie relationship problems.

CONFLICTING EXPECTATIONS REGARDING RELATIONSHIPS

Each person in a relationship has assumptions about what being a "couple" means. These expectations are often unarticulated, both to oneself and to the other. In the early stage of a relationship, it is common for dissimilarities to be obscured by the heightened sense of romance, in which couples who are falling in love naturally notice the ways they are similar, not different. And if they *do* notice disparities in what they each assume is basic to a committed love relationship, they may override concerns and disappointments because they so want the relationship to work out. But as the couple transitions into day-to-day *couplehood*, tensions may arise as these differences come to the fore. The topics about which significant differences can emerge range from what might seem relatively limited—for example, cuddle and sleep in on Sunday mornings versus one of them getting up and out early to jog with a friend—to issues of more obvious import—for example, how much and what type of *arguing* is "normal"; how much *critiquing* is acceptable; and what it means to be "loyal." If one person's behavior does not comport with the other's assumptions about how love is shown, the other's feelings of hurt and disappointment can lead to spiraling negative cycles of blame, withdrawal, and defensiveness.

In the first few sessions, I am listening for some of the underlying (if often unarticulated) suppositions each partner has about love and closeness: not infrequently, these unexamined premises play an important role in the tensions the couple is experiencing. Often these disparities can become more clearly apparent when one looks closely at each partner's family history. For example, if a woman comes from a family where there is a great deal of *togetherness*, such that on vacations they tend to all do things as a group, she may feel hurt by her husband's wish to pursue separate activities. Interestingly, even if the woman has come to feel her family is too "joined at the hip," she may nonetheless feel hurt by her husband's wish to do things separately. Her conscious view notwithstanding, she has been schooled from childhood in a definition of love that assumes togetherness. A man who consciously wanted to be with a woman who was independent and had her own life may nonetheless feel hurt that his wife rarely shows love as his mother did, by cooking his favorite meals.

The point here is that the emotional significance people attach to particular behaviors as signs of love, or lack of love, often have roots that are deep and not always conscious, and these powerfully emotional assumptions are not easily overwritten. Similarly, each person has deeply held feelings about what constitutes *unloving* behavior. Many people express dismay about what their spouse says in anger and feel that the spouse must not *really* love him or her if those words could be said. Or some people feel that a spouse's turning to someone other than themselves for advice and support when faced with an important decision indicates lack of trust and love. These are but a few examples of the many ways the couple can differ in their basis assumptions about how love is expressed or shown. Couple therapists need to look for the ways these divergent assumptions are enacted and negotiated as well as at the way the *meaning* attached to these differences is a source of the couple's difficulties. Does the husband who accommodates to his wife's wish for closeness by joining in her activities—for example, a trip to the farmers' market—feel resentful or overly compliant? Does the wife emotionally withdraw when hurt by his reluctance to be a couple in the way *she* defines it? How does he understand her motivation? Does he see her behavior as too controlling? As insecure? Does she express her disappointment as a critique of him? As a condemnation of his character? Together we work to articulate the ways in which the couple's differing assumptions have led to negative patterns of interaction that widen the already preexisting gulf in expectations.

ISSUES AROUND LOSS OF AUTONOMY
AND INDIVIDUAL ISSUES

Some couples' tensions are rooted in difficulty finding the right balance between being an *I* and being a *we*. One or both members of the couple may find negotiating this issue quite a challenge. Perhaps he comes from an enmeshed family in which achieving separateness and autonomy involved a hard-fought battle. This is not just a practical logistical issue but rather one that touches upon people's core sense of self and identity. Sometimes one fears one's own tendency to become too needy or dependent, and in reaction to this anxiety has a heightened need for independence. Many arguments that couples have are at bottom an enactment of *I–we* dynamics.

Couples who dig in to their position may be doing so because they experience compromise as a loss of a separate sense of self. People who have a sensitivity to the loss of individuality may find it difficult to see a middle ground as a satisfying outcome. "But what about what *I* want" is a frequent refrain of someone who feels that his *individual* needs are not being met. And if the couple's underlying assumptions differ about the amount of separateness that is consistent with love, the effect on the relationship is further exacerbated. One person may feel that the other is too focused on his or her personal preferences rather than making choices, or even sacrifices, for the good of the family. The anger and hurt generated by a difference of opinion about how *selfless* one should be can lead to bitterness and a feeling of betrayal.

Differences in regard to this issue may have been there right from the start of the relationship, or may have intensified by situational changes in the couple's life that stirred anxiety about loss of identity. Moving in together, having a child, becoming empty-nesters, unemployment or retirement, or, conversely, new career opportunities are all events that may stimulate and magnify anxieties about losing one's identity. A balance between the *I* and the *we* that worked for a long time may thus need to be renegotiated in response to changes in the couple's life cycle.

Often issues of *individuality* versus *joining* are not presented as such but may nonetheless underlie some of what the couple presents as a problem. For instance, when a couple says they argue over many things, or when one states that s/he feels lonely, or they both feel that they have few interests or even friends in common, or one is frustrated that the other seems not to be influenced by his or her opinion, it is helpful to explore whether or not issues of autonomy and the balance between the *I* and *we* are part of the underlying problem.

People are often unaware that a change in life circumstance has stirred up anxiety about the loss of identity or individual selfhood. With one couple, for example, it became clear that the husband's rejection of his wife's friends as "too bookish" was a result of his not-fully-conscious fear that with the upcoming arrival of their first child, his identity as a "free-spirited wild man" was soon to be forever lost, and that he was dealing with that anxiety by more sharply differentiating himself from his more "conventional" wife. Similarly, with another couple, exploration revealed that the underlying reason for an affair the wife had within months of the couple moving to the suburbs was that she mourned what she believed to be the loss of her identity as a sophisticated urbanite.

ISSUES AROUND FEELING LOVED AND VALUED

A common issue that brings couples to therapy is their concerns around attachment and love. Affairs, jealousies, ambivalence about moving in together or getting married, as well as painful thoughts about whether or not to break up, are all issues where concerns about love and emotional security can play a central role. And not infrequently, even when there is no particular crisis or decision to be made, one person will bring up in therapy that s/he doesn't feel loved, has felt abandoned or betrayed, or feels that his or her spouse's love can't be counted upon.

And even when couples are coming to therapy for reasons that on the surface have nothing to do with questions of love and attachment, these concerns may be embedded in other dissatisfactions and disappointments. For example, if a woman is unhappy that her spouse is a "workaholic" and never comes home until quite late, it might mean he is insecure about his value to his clients, or that showing how many hours he can work is a form of *machismo*, or that he is addicted to the praise he gets from his boss. But it is important to be alert to the ways his prioritizing work concerns over time with the family is an indication to her that he doesn't *care* deeply, or even love her very much.

In a different dynamic involving work, a woman who is upset with her husband for not taking a job that he thinks he's overqualified for may contrast him with her father, who "would do anything for his family and gave up being a teacher in Haiti to work as a street cleaner in New York so his kids could have a better life." She takes her spouse's behavior to mean he doesn't love her and the family strongly enough. Or when the couple is seeking couple therapy because they argue a lot, one person may say, "Everything I do seems to bother her, I don't know why she wants to stay with me or what she means when she says she loves me."

When expressions of concern about love and attachment are *not* the explicit and focal issue bringing the couple to therapy but rather are mentioned in the context of other topics, the couple therapist needs to carefully assess just how much weight to give to the matter. Not infrequently, a statement questioning the other's love is made out of anger and hurt but does not actually reflect the person's deepest feelings. Although attachment anxieties and injuries are undoubtedly a central issue for some couples, there are many couples who deep down do feel loved by the other but who nonetheless have serious frustrations and concerns about the marriage. Underestimating the health and strength of a couple's love and attachment is as serious a therapeutic problem as failing to notice the attachment injuries that underlie the marital difficulties. Even when one partner is upset about the lack of overt expressions of affection in the relationship—physical and/or verbal—this may not necessarily be experienced as a fundamental lack of love or caring but instead as something akin to carelessness or being taken for granted. Similarly, a wish for one's spouse to be more *present* and less preoccupied with work or other interests is a common complaint, but it is often experienced as something "annoying" about the other and not as a sign of a lack of love. On occasion, even an affair doesn't lead to fundamental insecurities about the spouse's love. S/he may be terribly hurt and angry, yet see the affair as the product of an "identity crisis" or avoidance of dealing with tensions in the marriage, rather than as something that calls into question the spouse's love.

ISSUES REVOLVING AROUND POWER, CONTROL, AND FAIRNESS

Underlying many of the arguments and frustrations that bring a couple to therapy is one person's belief that there is an imbalance in the relationship that she feels is unfair. The perceived inequities may have to do with finances, household responsibilities, child care, freedom to come and go, decision making, and even the right to voice complaints. With the increasing fluidity of gender roles, the particular unfairness at issue is not as predictably associated with one gender or the other as it used to be. Thus, though it is still *usually* women who feel that too much of the responsibility of child care and household organization falls to them even though they are working full time, some men have a similar complaint.

The couple's differing ideas about fairness may fuel the resentments. They agree on the basic assumption, for example, that if one person has a more demanding job and works longer hours, then it is fair for that person to have fewer responsibilities at home. However, they may differ on the interpretation of that principle. It becomes complicated when one spouse feels the other, for instance, spends far more time at work than is actually necessary.

Gnawing resentments and not fully articulated feelings need to be addressed about what it means that one person in the relationship has or earns more money than the other. Sometimes the issue is raised directly but often it emerges in the context of an argument about something else. Thus, with one couple I worked with, the woman was angry that her husband wanted to have input on how the house they had just bought would be decorated. On the surface, it seemed odd that she would expect him to live with furnishings that did not appeal to him. Further discussion revealed that she felt a need to assert herself in this one realm because she thought he had made so many other important decisions autonomously, for example, deciding what kind of car to get or where to go on vacation; he earned far more than she and had come into the marriage with large personal assets. The husband disagreed that these had been autonomous decisions, but to his wife, the word *input* implied that he had power that she did not.

Some imbalances in relationships are partially self-imposed. Frequently, when one person resents being home with the children while the other goes out with friends or takes time for him- or herself on weekends, the partner's response is that s/he ought to do the same. But the partner who is at home doesn't actually *want* to be away from the children. This type of imbalance may be more about hurt that one's partner doesn't feel the desire for family time than it is about unfairness. Similarly, many issues about unfairness have to do with one person feeling bad that the other is looking after his or her own needs and does not having sufficient empathy and concern for what is important to the spouse.

PROBLEMATIC PATTERNS BASED ON AREAS OF HEIGHTENED SENSITIVITY

I try in the first few sessions to get a sense of how each partner *reacts* to the other's sensitivities, with the aim of being able to map out patterns of interactions that lead to escalating hurt and frustration. I start with the assumption that everyone, no matter how much individual therapy they may have had, has certain "hot buttons" that if touched can set off surprisingly strong emotional reactions. How spouses respond to their partner's intense reaction when an emotional raw nerve has been touched may play a big role in many of the couple's difficulties. The sensitivities couples bring to relationships can act like landmines—couples often know they are there but step on them nonetheless. What for one person may be a highly charged area may seem innocuous to the other, making it hard for the latter either to be fully empathic or successfully careful. Often one person's sensitivities may reverberate badly with the *other* person's areas of heightened reactivity, resulting in escalating hurts and accusations.

Quite frequently couples believe that the problems they are having stem largely from their partner's personality, temperament and emotional makeup. They may see their spouse as being excessively anxious and insecure, or too quick to take offense, or needing too much reassurance. The spouse may be perceived as too dependent on friends and family, or too moody, too angry, or too compulsive. Although it is certainly possible that one person does have more "emotional baggage" than the other, as I discussed earlier I end the first session by asking them *each* to reflect on the personality traits they bring to the relationship that make them *"not the easiest person in the world to live with."* This question helps create balance in the second session so that one person is not exclusively "the problem." It also provides some beginning information about how each person's personality traits interact with the other's. For example, if one person says, "I know I tend to be a worrier, and I guess that annoys my husband," and the other describes himself as someone who "procrastinates," the therapist can readily see that one person's procrastination increases the other's worrying and the other's worrying may in turn, for a variety of reasons, increase the partner's tendency to procrastinate. Or perhaps one person brings to the relationship a heightened sensitivity to emotional withdrawal and responds to perceived withdrawal with what the partner regards as a "demand" for attention; this "demandingness" can result in further withdrawal if the partner is particularly reactive to being controlled through guilt.

DIFFERENCES IN COPING STYLES
AND CHARACTERISTIC DEFENSE MECHANISMS

In addition to heightened sensitivities or hot buttons, differences in coping styles and characteristic defense mechanisms are often a source of tension and escalating conflict in relationships. For instance, one person in a couple may cope with concerns they are worrying about by wanting to talk about them and possibly planning for the worst-case scenario, while the other copes by compartmentalizing and not thinking about possible negative events until they actually occur. Conflicting coping mechanisms can cause tensions, but when they are tendencies about which they are both *aware* they are usually less likely to lead to spiraling negative interactions.

A common defense mechanism one sees in doing couple therapy is the use of projection and projective identification. One person may project disowned aspects of the self onto his or her partner and then be angry and critical of that trait. For example, feeling that one's mate is too angry, dependent, judgmental, hard on the children, and whatever may stem from the denial of any aspect of these feelings in oneself. The husband in one couple I worked with disparaged what he considered his wife's excessive caution about one of their children's food allergies. The wife was not only hurt but was also anxious about relying on her husband to be careful when he was the sole parent present. Exploration of this dynamic led to a discussion of the husband's childhood experience, at the age of 6 of being present when his father had a near-fatal heart attack. He spoke of being terrified at the time but then putting it behind him. On reflection, he realized that he didn't want to become immobilized by fear as his mother had become, even though his father had survived, and now, 25 years later, was still healthy. He described himself as rarely feeling afraid. He liked the adrenalin rush of skiing as fast as possible down a double-diamond ski slope, or of driving his car as fast as it was capable of going. For this man, his wife's cautiousness was too close a reminder of the fear he had repressed and defended against. Once this link was made, this man was able to get more in touch with *his own* concern about his child's allergies and no longer was so dissociated from his anxious feelings.

It is important to note that even when couples are initially *attracted* to characteristics in the other that they do not see or accept in themselves, those characteristics can over time or with changed circumstances become distressing because they stimulate emotions that have been defended against. This threat of disavowed feelings becoming conscious can lead to highly charged interactions. For example, Robert, who had been born when his mother was in her late 40s, adapted to being "an afterthought" by becoming quite self-sufficient. His wife, who was a self-described "caretaker" had, for many years, managed to be nurturing to him despite his being a "porcupine" who pushed her and other people away. Robert could "secretly" enjoy the nurturing while he consciously organized his life around not needing caring attention. But when life events changed—his wife needed to care for her elderly mother and a new baby simultaneously—she no longer made the efforts she had made to push through his prickliness. Instead, she took at face value what he himself believed, that he was self-sufficient and was fine without her attention. She no longer urged him to tell her what was worrying him when he clearly was stressed by something happening at work. She felt too exhausted to watch TV with him at night—a time when she would often rub the bottom of his feet. She no longer reminded him to make long overdue doctor's appointments. Robert was not consciously aware of missing her nurturing attention. Rather, he was annoyed with her for phoning him at work too often and for ignoring "the one thing" he asked of her, that she keep their home fairly neat. They seemed to bicker over everything, and Sara, his wife, felt that he had become critical and distant. She felt hurt and outraged by his constant carping. She was worn out by taking care of people and wanted him to take care of *her* "for a change," but was worried that it was not something he was capable of doing. Sara was touched and felt closer to Robert, when as a result of the couple therapy, he was able to *own* his wish for the tender attention he saw her bestow on their son. Sara, though still quite busy, found that she once again wanted to nurture Robert, saying, "It's a lot easier to do when he's not pushing me away and criticizing me all the time."

As I've been discussing, many of the conflicts that couples present can be more readily resolved when they are not taken simply at face value, but rather are also understood as a manifestation of more general, underlying concerns. For instance, a couple came to therapy because they were having fertility problems and were in conflict about the next step to take. The wife wanted to go the adoption route but her husband felt that using an egg donor made more sense. In talking about the disagreement, it became clear that he felt his wife was being selfish in vetoing what he wanted and didn't love him enough to give him a child who was genetically his. She, on the other hand, felt that this would be one more instance of an unfairness that she believed permeated the relationship in which "he always gets his way."

Another couple felt that a big source of conflict between them was that the wife was very unhappy living in the city but her husband "absolutely refused" to discuss moving to the suburbs. Though the particulars of the issue were of course important, they couldn't resolve their differences because they had different coping mechanisms. The wife's main reason for wanting to move was that she was afraid of crime. As their children were approaching adolescence and would need to be given more freedom, she didn't want to be worried every time they were out alone. Her husband felt she was overreacting since they lived in a very low crime area, and pointed out "that many of their neighbors even let their kids take the subway by themselves." The more intensely she expressed her anxiety by bringing up instances where their children had been exposed to some danger, the more he minimized her concerns and tried to convince her by marshaling statistics on the reduction of crime in their city. They were stuck in a pattern wherein each person's coping style exacerbated the other's and led to an escalation of a power struggle. The husband's way of handling anxiety was to tamp it down so that the more his wife talked about the dangers, the greater was his need to push his *own* anxiety away. But she coped by avoiding situations that made her anxious, in this case giving the children more freedom, and she felt a need to highlight and perhaps exaggerate the facts in order to justify her way of coping.

When couples get too bogged down in the details of one particular argument or disappointment, it can be hard for them or the therapist to see how the basic pattern or the basic sensitivities are the same as those discussed in a previous session or even 10 minutes ago. Instead of leading to productive work on resolving an underlying issue, the discussion is stuck in a fruitless "he said, she said" debate. It is one of the primary responsibilities of the therapist to help the couple extricate themselves from this immediately compelling but ultimately dead end of hashing over specific details. This may require the therapist to interrupt the playing out of the immediate interaction to help them gain a broader perspective. It's the dynamics that *underlie* the details of the particular interaction that need to be changed.

PREVENTING THE COUPLE'S DEMORALIZATION

In the first few sessions our goal is to get a sense of the difficulties and some of the underlying issues that may be a part of the presenting problems. The therapeutic challenge is how to get at long-standing, often unarticulated issues without leaving the couple feeling overwhelmed and discouraged by the "bigness" of what they are dealing with. Maintaining focus is one part of helping the couple feel confidence in the process even when much of the session may bring closer to the surface some of the most painful features of the relationship. Highlighting underlying recurring concerns and patterns can then take the session from a focus on one particular disagreement to issues that are more at the heart of the matter. As serious as the problems may seem, the couple needs to see that talking about these issues with the therapist can be quite different than trying to address them on their own. The therapist is working to ensure that when one of them has raised something that he had strong feelings about, the discussion does not devolve into mutual accusations or character attacks that leave one or both feeling more misunderstood, hurt, and resentful. Instead, by carefully considering what to respond to at the numerous moment-to-moment choice points, the therapist helps the couple to feel they are really getting somewhere in discussing the issues rather than being in the all-too-familiar experience of going around in circles.

The second thing that helps prevent the couple from becoming demoralized is that the therapist continues to also address their strengths even while the main focus of the session is on what is going wrong. As described in Chapter 3, these positive comments are often offered as almost incidental asides, not as a contradiction or minimization of the negative feelings being discussed. But even as minor notes, these brief positive comments help the couple experience the session as not merely dwelling on what's wrong. So, for example, when the wife in one couple I worked with talked about feeling that her husband was self-involved and gave little thought to her needs, I said, *"I know you're very upset about this, but before we get into it. I just want to say that I'm impressed by the way you're speaking about it. You're not being condemning—actually, you're speaking in a way that tells me you feel he's capable of being empathic and sensitive and hoping you'll get through to him. But tell me what goes on that makes you feel he's only thinking of what's good for him?"*

Or, in a session where the husband stated that he was jealous of his wife's relationships with male friends—some of whom were ex-boyfriends— and didn't think she found him exciting enough, I commented on his *also* saying, "I've always been insecure . . . maybe because I was a late bloomer and didn't have my first real girlfriend until I was 22 years old." *"I know what you're saying about your wife not finding you interesting enough is heartfelt, but I'm also struck by your ability to recognize that your feeling might be intensified because of your dating history. But tell me more about what makes you feel that you're not exciting enough for your wife."* Notice that in both cases I immediately return to the current feeling so that the person does not feel their upset is invalid or cannot be heard.

Lastly, even before the issues are fully understood, the therapist needs to look for things that the couple can *do* to start addressing the problems. Though it may be necessary for the couple to delve deeply into painful topics and to understand the complexity of each person's feelings, finding solutions cannot be put on hold until they are fully explored. Some beginning interventions, albeit very simple ones, must be incorporated into the work right from the start. By helping them *do something* different, the therapist stokes the embers of hopefulness that enable couples to tolerate what could otherwise feel simply painful and discouraging.

Let me be clear: doing something different does not necessarily mean enacting a big intervention. It can be doing something as organic to the work as getting the couple to listen with a mental set of trying to understand, join, and empathize rather than waiting one's turn to deflect and rebut what has been said. If the couple is able to do this, they have made an important first step toward addressing their difficulties, and by making note of this, the therapist reinforces the point that the therapy will aim for new ways of acting with one another, not just the voicing of upsets.

Other suggestions for what the couple can do at home also reinforce the idea that the emotional pain of the session can immediately lead to some small step in the direction of change. It's important, however, to make sure that the suggestions are small and doable. For instance, the homework after a second session in which the couple discussed feeling very alienated from one another might simply be for each of them to think about what they know they could do to touch each other emotionally if they *wanted* to try to warm up the relationship. They would not be asked to actually *do* anything, but merely *to think* about and write down a couple of things that are almost guaranteed to bring the other closer if they chose to do so. I might suggest that they try to recall some of the things that they used to naturally do for one another during the romantic stage of their relationship. This, it should be noted, is not meant to be a paradoxical intervention in which telling someone *not* to do something is intended to motivate them to actually do it. Rather, it is to get the couple thinking about what might be possible and how much each *individually* has some control over the situation.

Relatedly, with a couple who are very critical with one another, one could ask them to do a mental exercise in which they each try to notice every little positive that they can possibly find, including things they are so used to that they usually barely notice them. To facilitate this change in mind-set, I give them examples of the types of the things I'm talking about. Perhaps, in the morning, one partner always makes a pot of coffee using the beans that the other prefers rather than the ones that are his or her favorite. Or perhaps the spouse is very warm and friendly to the other's family. Or perhaps one's partner buys gifts that show a real knowledge of the other's taste, or is good at handling the landlord, or at helping the children overcome fears, or is the "go-to" person for friends in a crisis situation.

This chapter has focused on many of the common difficulties that result in couples seeking therapy. In the next chapter we look in more depth at how to begin to address these issues and how to make the transition from the first session, which gave us the "lay of the land," so to speak, to actually begin working on the problems that have brought the couple to therapy. Through clinical vignettes the reader will see how to apply the principles and methods described in Chapter 3 and Chapter 5 to the types of issues described in this chapter.

7

∽

From the First to the Second Session
Clinical Illustrations

When one writes about couple therapy, it can seem much more clear and straightforward in theory than it actually is in practice. In this chapter I present clinical material in a way that replicates as closely as possible actual sessions with couples. Though the couples are composites, I hope to present what I actually do and say. I am not always successful in getting couples to engage productively in the process. I make mistakes. At choice points I may choose a focus that in retrospect was not the best path to take. I may say something in a way that triggers defensiveness. I do not always "get it." My aim in presenting the following clinical vignettes is to show you how to put together the methods and ideas discussed so far in this book. But it is also an attempt to show you what I do when what I've said doesn't get the result I'd expected and how I try to change course and make the session more productive. To provide context for my discussion of my second session with these couples, I will also provide a fair amount of detail about the first session with each.

VIGNETTE 1: ROB AND RENEE

I have learned over the years not to fully trust my impression or assumptions about how the couple experienced the first meeting. Even though much of the first meeting focuses, if at all possible, on highlighting strengths and positives in the relationship, one or both partners may leave the session feeling less hopeful, rather than more so. And that is what happened with Rob and Renee.

The First Session with Rob and Renee

In the first session with Rob and Renee, they explained that they were seeking therapy because what had in the past been just annoying bickering had, in recent months, escalated to intense arguments. They had been talking about seeking counseling but finally decided to go ahead with it when, against all they believed in, they had had "a screaming match" in front of their 5-year-old son. He had been frightened both by the intensity of their anger and by hearing Renee sobbing in the bathroom. They were expecting another child in 4 months and were depressed and discouraged about their relationship. Renee had read recently that fetuses can be affected by stress hormones, and she worried that these arguments were not only harming their son but also their yet-to-be-born daughter. "I do a lot of yoga, and I meditate every day and try to let what Renee says roll off my back," said Rob. "I know she's pregnant and hormonal . . . but she's negative about everything I do . . . I just can't take it."

Renee agreed that she was often annoyed and critical but disagreed that it was due to hormonal issues. Rather, she attributed it to Rob's "total lack of responsibility for child care and the stuff that needs to be done around the house. I work full time too, but he acts like my job isn't nearly as important because I don't make as much money as he does."

When Rob started to protest and defend himself, I stopped him and reminded them of what I had said earlier: *"I just want to get a sense of what some of the issues are in a first meeting and then shift the focus to any strengths you may have as a couple, so that I have a clear understanding of the good things in the relationship before we delve into what's going wrong."* Even though couples are almost always relieved to hear that the therapy will not just be about what is wrong, it can nonetheless be difficult for some couples to go along with this structure.

Rob stated, "I know, but . . . it's just wrong what she's saying, and I think that's the problem . . . that she sees things that way."

"I know it can be frustrating not to respond right away to something that feels wrong to you, but I promise you we'll begin to sort all this out next time. And I also want to reassure you both, that I <u>know</u> people can see things very differently and I always get both people's perspective. But, if you can bear with me, for <u>today</u>, I want to spend just 10 minutes or so on getting some idea of the issues that bring you here. Of course, next time we'll go into them in some depth and put our heads together to figure out what's going on and to come up with some ideas for strategies to prevent

bad arguments from happening. So, as I understand it, you both agree that one of the big issues that propelled you here was that, whatever the cause—and I know you disagree on that—bickering has escalated to big emotional upheavals and you both feel bad about losing control in front of your son."

Before shifting focus to strengths and positives I asked Rob and Renee to tell me about other issues that concerned them. Rob stated that he thought Renee was angry at him for pushing her to agree to move from New Jersey to the city so they would have less of a commute. In response, Renee said, "I *don't* blame Rob. He's a forceful person—and I know he's right—that it's good that we'll both be home earlier and can even pick Timmy up from school sometimes. Rob was so sure it was the right thing to do—everything he said made sense and he was so enthusiastic—I think I *thought* I was persuaded—I could have said no, I guess. But now we live in a relatively small space without a backyard and worst of all, I have to work full time because now we really need the money—the mortgage payments are so high. Most people I know did the opposite—they moved from the city to the suburbs when they had kids—not the other way around!" Rob responded, "She says she doesn't blame me, but she's so depressed about it and keeps complaining about work and how she wishes she could work part time."

As I listened to this exchange I noted to myself—but didn't yet pursue—several of the core issues discussed earlier in this book. In addition to the more obvious concerns about dominance and submission, and maintaining one's identity and autonomy, I wondered if they had each split off parts of themselves so that they each expressed the other's ambivalence.

Switching to Strengths

Rob and Renee recounted a relationship that started out as a friendship. They had met when Renee was working as a temp to pay her rent while she was going to school for a degree in media studies. "I knew after I met Renee that I had to break up with my girlfriend. I laughed so much with Renee—we would go back and forth between bantering and the type of serious, almost philosophical conversations I had never had before. She was—still is—sexy and so interesting. I was never bored with her. All those things are still true—but now—I also see she's a fantastic mother. I hate that we fight so much. I was crazy about her then and even though she makes me so mad sometimes, I'm still in love with her—it's hard to explain, there's something really special about Renee—I've never met anyone like her. She's modest and at first people don't 'get it'—they don't see how talented she is. But when they get to know her they're blown away by her."

Renee stated, "I just didn't think it would work as a romantic relationship with Rob. But he was very persistent and persuaded me to give it a chance. He eventually broke down my resolve—he was learning to play the guitar and he wrote a song for me that was incredibly sweet. He was determined, and eventually we started dating. And he was right. Sex was really good. We had a lot of fun during that period, but when I had an interesting job offer in New York—maybe 6 months later—it felt like it was a good time to end it. He's a wonderful person. Very solid. Kind. And I could always count on him. But I just didn't feel I was ready to commit to him. I wanted my freedom. I'd been in a relationship for 4 years before him and I felt I'd gone from one relationship right into another. I knew I had to be alone for a while. I've always been with someone, and in therapy I realized that I tend to lose *myself* when I'm with somebody. But I did really like him a lot and thought that if I were ever ready to settle down, and he was still free, he'd be great to be with. He's ambitious, energetic, loves kids, and has a big, warm family."

They both went on to explain that about 2 years later Rob also moved to New York and again he pursued Renee. "He caught me at a time when I was feeling pretty discouraged about my career." She added laughingly, "And to be honest I'd been dating but had just been dumped by the one guy I actually liked—so it was good timing when Rob came back into my life. I had a lot of fun with him. He had all sorts of ideas about things to do in the city and even though I'd lived here for 2 years—actually in New Jersey—and he had just come, he introduced me to a lot of places and things that I hadn't known about. I would end up staying at his apartment a lot rather than going back to my apartment and kind of moved in 'temporarily.' Well, long story short—I got pregnant and though I was still uncertain about us as a *couple*, I knew I eventually wanted to have a baby and getting pregnant felt like a sign. I usually agonize over decisions—but not this time. I thought he'd be a great father and that was it—we got married."

Feedback at the End of the First Session

The first session ended by my restating what they had told me and acknowledging that indeed *"things have gone seriously awry in your relationship. It sounds like you used to have real fun together. Rob, I was struck by your description of how you and Renee would laugh a lot and have wonderful conversations, and Renee, by the smile on your face when you described how Rob introduced you to so many new things in New York even though he had just arrived. But now you are so frustrated with one another that when you <u>try</u> to talk about what you're feeling it becomes so intense that you temporarily forget about what is so important to you both—providing a peaceful and calm home for your son."*

By mentioning the fun they used to have in the context of how bad things had gotten between them, I was injecting a reminder of the strengths in the relationship without directly focusing on it. To make the reminder more powerful I reiterated some of the details that they'd described. Thus, instead of saying, *"You used to have fun together,"* I instead said, *"You would laugh and have good conversations, he introduced you to new things in the city."*

The reader might also have noticed that I used the word "frustrated" with one another rather than "angry" at one another. "Frustrated" implies that the feeling is variable and changeable rather than static, constant, and unmovable. I also highlighted that they were *trying* to communicate, and I further helped them *join* by referring to the value they shared in regarding a peaceful home as extremely important. Cumulatively, these slight differences in language contributed to maintaining hopefulness.

After stating that I understood the seriousness of their upset, I went on to briefly summarize their perspectives on the difficulties. Rob felt that Renee blamed him both for their recent purchase of an apartment in the city and for the stress she was feeling trying to juggle career and parenting. Renee said that she could understand why Rob might think that she blamed him, but actually she *didn't* blame him for what in retrospect felt to her like a bad decision. "His arguments made sense to me—we would have more time with Timmy because we wouldn't have to commute and we could pop out sometimes in the middle of the work day to go to things at his school. Somehow I thought it would be okay. But I'm pretty unhappy. I'm someone who likes trees and flowers—I had a little garden on my terrace in the apartment in New Jersey." But she did feel that she was often angry at him because in her mind she had the lion's share of the household and parenting chores. This signified to her a lack of respect for her work and an inequality in the relationship. Rob felt very misunderstood and felt unfairly blamed for what he regarded as Renee's bad moods. He interjected, "I don't know how to get her to see that *of course* I respect her—she's convinced herself that I think *I'm* more important and nothing I say changes her view."

Feedback about Their Strengths as a Couple

Once I was sure that Rob and Renee knew that I took their difficulties seriously, I then gave them some feedback about things I observed that I believed were relevant to the potential helpfulness of couple therapy. I noted that though they'd been very hurt and angry with one another, I noticed *"how you were able to access the positives about the other—Rob saying, for instance, that Renee still is sexy and interesting. Or Renee saying that he can talk about feelings and is very loving. You both said these things in the present tense. Some couples are so angry, and their love has eroded so much, that they actually don't remember or can't see the positives that drew them to the person in the first place. So far, the intense arguing and disagreements haven't changed your ability to experience the good things about the other that attracted you and ultimately led you to trust that you could have a good future together."*

I also noted that the things that drew them to one another were substantial, solid traits—for example, being emotionally steady, intelligent, and energetic, and that they had known each other as friends for a long time before getting together.

Lastly, I gave them some positive feedback about how they had acted in the session. *"It was interesting how you each went out of your way to mention that you knew the other sees it differently. So, even though you each feel that you are <u>right</u>, there's an acknowledgment that the other <u>sincerely</u> has a different perspective. That openness to hearing the other's point of view is a very helpful attitude when trying to resolve differences. You also were both willing to follow my plan for the session—and I know that isn't easy to do. Rob really wanted to answer your complaints but accepted my guidance on this—that it would be better to hold off until the next session when we would really start working on your difficulties together. That takes self-control and trust and I was impressed by both of you having the ability to do that. Again, that bodes well for couple therapy being helpful to you.*

"And even though you are here because the feelings you each are having are getting out of control, I'm not hearing you attacking each other in ways that go to the core of the person's character. Research has shown that expressions of contempt for the other in the heat of an argument are one of the characteristics that are predictive of things not working out for the couple. So far I'm not hearing that—as you've described it, even when you are furious with one another, you are not ripping the other to shreds and trying to humiliate the other. You probably take that for granted, but, in fact, many couples who come to therapy argue in a way that deeply wounds the partner."

Again, I was intentionally reminding them of the good feelings they had for one another by repeating the *specific* positives they had mentioned earlier—for example, intelligence, stability, and so on. I was also enhancing their self-esteem as a couple (described in Chapter 3) by highlighting some of the admirable traits that they may have taken for granted that not all couples exhibit. Additionally, by highlighting these traits—acknowledging that the other had a different perspective, not saying really hurtful things to one another even when angry—I was reinforcing productive ways of interacting with one another with the goal of encouraging them to continue to interact in this way. I've extended their each saying that the other sees it differently to include the idea that they see the other as *sincere*. Though they haven't said this explicitly, it is *implicit* in their acknowledgment of the other's different perspective. By using the word "sincere," I am helping them each to become conscious of a positive feeling that was there but unarticulated.

The first session ended with my telling them that in the next session I wanted to get a really clear sense of how things go wrong between them. I'd like them to give me some recent examples of an argument they had with as much detail as they can remember. I'd also like them to give me an example of when they have had that *"here we go again feeling"* even if it didn't actually end in an argument. And lastly, I concluded with telling them that I wanted them each to think about *"what you know about yourself that makes you not the easiest person in the world to be married to."*

The Second Session with Rob and Renee

I was pleased with the first session. By the end of the meeting, Rob and Renee seemed in much better spirits than when they had arrived. I felt that I had put their difficulties in perspective and that they had left the session feeling encouraged and hopeful. The fact that they both wanted to set up another appointment right then and there, rather than wait to talk about it, confirmed my feeling that the session had gone well. My feedback to them was genuine—I thought they demonstrated many of the characteristics that were associated with a successful outcome to couple therapy. I liked them both and, most importantly, I felt they really liked *one another*.

When I started the second session with *"I want to start by finding out how the last meeting felt to each of you,"* I was quite surprised, and frankly a little troubled, by Rob's response, since it was contrary to what I had hoped to achieve in the first meeting. Rob stated, "I felt terrible afterward, and all week I have been feeling really bad. I realized after the meeting how I was always the initiator—*I* made the relationship happen—I'm always the one persuading Renee, and suddenly it hit me—what if she's never really bought into it—not just living in the city, but me, the relationship? What if she's just given in and doesn't really love me? I knew Renee was still single, and to be honest, that was a factor in my taking a job that brought me to New York. Then I persuaded her to move in with me "temporarily," and I was so excited when she got pregnant. The pregnancy was an accident, but I was thrilled and kept talking about what great parents we'd be together." Rob repeated again that he had been really depressed all week and reiterated, "I just don't know if she's really bought into it."

I asked him to say more about what that meant: *"I'm not exactly sure what you mean—that maybe Renee hasn't really <u>bought into it</u>."* "I don't know if she really loves me or wants to be with me—maybe I just persuaded her and she doesn't actually love me. Maybe she wasn't ready to have a child yet either—she seems so stressed and unhappy about it. I know I didn't force her, but I can lobby so hard for something I want that maybe she just succumbed." *"Rob, before we get into that, I'd like to check in with Renee about <u>her</u> reactions to last week's session."* Renee said, "When we left, I felt good about it. I felt hopeful. But Rob was so upset about it that I really felt discouraged. I'm worried now that maybe couple therapy will only make things worse."

At this point, I needed to make a choice—to stick with my agenda, which would be to go back to what I had said we would do at the end of the first session (to ask for their answers to what each knows s/he contributes to their difficulties and to get more examples of how they get into arguments), or to address Rob's feelings and the issue he was raising, then and there. Since Rob was clearly upset I decided to stick with what he had said and to temporarily jettison my typical structure. After all, this is not a one-size-fits-all therapy and it would feel strange and insensitive to move on after such a heartfelt statement. But I also noted to myself that Rob's intense feelings had shaped the therapy and silently wondered if this is similar to what happens with Renee.

I began by asking Renee, *"What's going on for you as you hear Rob speak about this?"* She stated that she was surprised that Rob regarded this as a sudden realization, since he had said similar things many times. I pushed her a little more to talk about what she *felt.* *"How did you feel hearing it today?"*

"I feel bad about it. I understand how he could feel that way, because he does pursue what he wants pretty forcefully, but I *do* love him and I *wanted* to have a child with him. Maybe the timing wasn't perfect, but I did feel ready to have a child. But I thought we'd do it together—not that we'd end up having the traditional kind of relationship that it's turned out to be—where he 'helps out' when I ask, but taking care of Timothy and making child care arrangements is assumed to be my responsibility."

In response to Renee's comment, I said, *"I know this issue of how much real responsibility Rob takes for Timothy is a very important one, and it plays a big role in the tensions between the two of you. I'd like to put it on hold for now while we delve into what Rob said a bit more."* And to further reassure Renee that we were not ignoring her topic, I put a sticky memo note with the topic written in large letters on the folder of notes about the couple that I keep in front of me during the session.

The other side of the coin from choosing a focus is deciding what *not* to pick up on. In order to keep a session on topic, the therapist must ignore or explicitly put on hold obvious bids to move it in a different direction. Here, I chose to ignore Renee's slightly dismissive, exasperated statement that Rob has voiced his concern that she hadn't really "bought in" many times. On the principle that I'm trying to heal emotional wounds and not uncover every grievance, I decided it was best to ignore that statement. Had Rob himself responded to Renee's tone, I would probably have said something like, *"Let's put the issue of whether you voice that concern frequently, or too frequently, aside for a moment—we can come back to that later. Let's just stay for now with how you felt hearing what Renee had to say last session."*

Not picking up on Renee's complaint about the lack of equality in parenting and household responsibilities is another example of maintaining focus. Clearly, her feelings about these issues were intense but had I shifted to that topic at that point, we would not have had a chance to more fully explore the issue Rob had raised. As I described in Chapter 3, one topic *inevi-*

tably leads to another, and the session can feel unproductive if the therapist lets the session spontaneously drift from one thing to another as each partner responds to what the other has just said in his or her own particular way.

We spent the next 5 or 10 minutes on Renee's statement that she really does love Rob. I asked him if he can take that in, and he replies that he does believe her *today*, but often it doesn't seem like she does. I asked him to describe some of the times that he *does* feel loved by Renee. I then turned to Renee and asked her the same question. "I know he loves me deep down— but he doesn't act that way a lot of the time." I responded by saying, "*So, a lot of the time you don't feel he's acting in a loving manner—but deep down you feel he loves you. What makes you know that? Can you give me examples of the occasional times you feel he's acting in a way that comports with what you know—that he really loves you?*"

Before moving on, I commented that "*even though Renee states that she loves you and did want to have a baby, there seems to be a pattern in which you campaign for something and you [to Renee] go along with it in a way which leaves you <u>both</u> unclear about whether or not Renee is really on board. And Rob, being the one who needs to lobby for something may make it hard for you to get in touch with the complexity of <u>your own</u> feelings. It's confusing for <u>both</u> of you. We will need to look at this pattern in more detail.*" I then made another note in big letters to remind us all to get back to this pattern at a later time.

Here I am highlighting not only that there is a pattern that they get into, but that in a sense, they are both victims of this pattern. I also put on hold further discussion of the issue. I did this for two reasons. The first was that I thought that *some* progress had been made, and I wanted to stop while ahead. Additionally, I wanted to get back to the assignment I had given them at the end of the last session—for each of them to think about what makes him or her "*not the easiest person in the world to be married to.*"

Because we had used a good deal of the session to focus on Rob's concern and the question of if and how they each feel loved, there wasn't time (nor did it seem to "fit" with the session) to ask them about specific incidents where things go wrong between them. I explicitly put that issue on hold and focused instead on the question of what personality traits or issues they each bring to the marriage.

"*Last week I said that in this session I wanted to take a look at some specific examples of the kinds of exchanges that lead to big arguments. I'd like to put that on hold for now and get to the other thing I asked you to reflect on. What do you know about yourself that makes you not the easiest person in the world to be married to?*"

Renee stated that she can be moody and "though I hate to admit it, I think some months, but not always, I have bad PMS and get pretty irritable. But I try not to . . . and it doesn't happen all the time, and Rob has this way of dismissing things I'm upset about by saying I'm PMS-ing." Rob started to respond but then said, "Nevermind." I *didn't* suggest that he finish what he started to say. Often, as with Rob, I *don't* urge people to complete what they were about to say because I want to encourage self-control. But conversely, there are also couples and individuals where just the reverse is needed—where much of the problem may arise out of a *hesitancy* to say things that *need* to be said if one's needs are to be met. With this couple, Renee tended to acquiesce and often didn't know what she thought. Had she been the one to interrupt to insert her point of view, I might have encouraged her to speak.

"Okay, so you sometimes have PMS. When you said you were moody, did you mean aside from PMS as well?" Renee went on to say that she had suffered from pretty bad bouts of depression and during those times she went on medication. But even when she was not depressed, she could be moody. *"Is there anything else about yourself that you think might make you not the easiest person to be married to?"*

"I tend to keep things to myself. Rob is always asking me what I feel about things. He talks easily about feelings. I don't. Not just with him. Everybody close to me complains about that. My sister says she never knows what's going on with me. And my parents used to call me 'the clam' until I got mad and told them I didn't think it was funny." *"How do you understand that tendency in yourself? Do you have some ideas as to why you keep your feelings to yourself—what that's about?"* By asking Renee how she understood this tendency in herself, I was communicating that we can also address some of each person's individual issues. One goal of couple therapy is to enable the spouses to be sensitive to each other and to help one another resolve some individual difficulties. Renee responded to my question by stating that until a few years ago when her mother finally stopped drinking, she never knew what could set off her mother's temper. Renee also reported that when she was young, she was close to both her parents and she thought that she was quite open about what she was feeling. "But I became mistrustful. In a fit of anger, things I had confided to my mother would be thrown back at me. And if I shared anything private with my sister, my mother was sure to hear about it and then she would repeat it to my father. My father could be mean—and could take an innocent comment—like I had a crush on a boy—and twist it in a way that mocked and made fun of me."

Turning to Rob, I asked him what he had come up with in answer to the question about *"not being the easiest person in the world to be married to."* He repeated what he had said earlier in the session, that he realized he could be too persistent about something he wanted. *"And is there anything else?"* I asked.

"I seem to need more sleep than a lot of people, and when I don't get it I'm miserable. Same with exercise, if I don't get in a run every day I just don't feel well. That's hard for Renee, because sleep and running, and yoga, take time away from the family, but I just don't function well without those things." Renee interjects, "I know he really does need it, but it is part of what I resent. Maybe I'm being unfair. I think he drinks too much and that's part of why he needs these other things so much." Rob replies, "I don't think one thing has to do with the other. But Renee is right about the drinking. I'm working on it." Turning toward Renee, Rob asks, "Isn't it better the last few weeks. I've had one or two beers at night at most, right?" Renee nods yes and it's not clear if she's actually agreeing or just going along with what he says to avoid conflict.

Ending the Session

As the end of the session approached, I acknowledged their efforts to make the meeting productive. *"It felt to me that you both tried not to be defensive and both of you were quite open about your own issues. And I appreciate your letting me cut you off from time to time and put certain topics on hold. That's not so easy to do. So, I think we're off to a good start."* Then, even though we'd only just begun to identify and unpack one of the problematic patterns in their relationship, I gave them each some homework related to what we had been discussing. *"Renee, I'd like you try to notice when you are being persuaded about something. Even with small things. Try to notice when you've gone along with something, not <u>unwillingly</u>, but because Rob made a good case. For example, if you're choosing a movie to watch, or a restaurant to go to, or whether or not to visit your family—those kinds of things—try to notice if he's moved you along in a certain direction. And Rob, on your end, try to notice when you've swayed Renee about something—when you took the lead. If you notice it, how would you feel about saying something like, 'Renee, why don't you think about it before you agree?' Encourage her to take a little time to ask herself if she <u>really</u> wants to do something, or, upon reflection, might have a different idea."*

By asking Rob to help Renee think about what she really felt about something, I redirected his action orientation to something that could change the pattern between them. I wasn't suggesting that he hold back and not be as persuasive and forceful but rather that he *actively* work at making sure she has, to use his language, "bought in" to what she agreed to. Furthermore, I communicated to them both that Renee's difficulty with knowing what she wants and expressing it, though an individual issue, is not something she has to master completely on her own.

I then made one more suggestion: *"I think you both know what draws the other in and makes the other feel closer to you. Think about whether you might want to do some of those things even though there's a lot that's unresolved between the two of you and you get frustrated and angry with one another. Knowing that you are working on those issues in here, you*

<u>might</u> be able to set them aside and do some of the things that make you each feel loved. Think about it. Maybe you can do it." This suggestion was carefully worded as tentative because these types of gestures need to feel spontaneous, and not be experienced by the partner as the fulfillment of a homework assignment.

Rob and Renee left the session feeling hopeful and motivated to try some of what I had suggested. This was achieved both by focusing on the times they each *did* feel loved by the other (rather than when they did no) and by discussing concrete ways to break the problematic pattern that had been identified. This couple was rather cooperative and it was fairly easy to keep the session going in a productive direction. But as anyone who does couple therapy knows, couples are not always so responsive or considerate of one another, nor is it always so easy to keep the session focused and moving in a useful way. The next clinical vignette is intended to demonstrate some to the difficulties therapists encounter with more challenging couples.

VIGNETTE 2: DANNY AND LISA

The First Session with Danny and Lisa

Danny and Lisa were engaged in an obviously heated exchange when I went out to the waiting room to greet them for their first appointment. As they followed me down the hallway, Lisa said, "I guess it's pretty obvious why we're here." I suggested that they sit on the couch, but Danny ignored my suggestion and sat on the chair opposite it instead. Immediately, I was faced with a choice to make. Should I ask what's going on or should I proceed as usual? I felt it was important to provide structure and to take charge of the session so I said, "*Obviously, you're in the middle of something, but I'm hoping you can shift gears for the moment and help me get the lay of the land.*" I explained that in a first meeting "*I like to get just a brief overview of your difficulties and then hear about what brought you together—what the positives were—or what good stuff you might still have with one another despite the problems that have brought you to couple therapy.*" In response to this remark, Danny said sarcastically, "Positives? Good luck!" At this point I was very tempted to go with what was happening in the room. It was almost certainly no accident that they had had this disagreement right before entering my office. It was quite possible that the argument they came in with would demonstrate some of their key issues and the way they interacted with one another around them. Yet if I got into this right now we'd be off and running in a way that might too closely parallel what happened at home. I was still hopeful that they might be able to shift gears and that some strengths on which to build might emerge. In short, I was not yet willing to jettison the structure that I find generally gets the work going in a productive direction. I decided to make one more attempt at getting them to step back from their immediate feelings and instead to describe in a more general way what issues cause them difficulties. I asked if they could each briefly give me some idea of what was going wrong in their relationship. I turned to Danny and said, *"How about if you start?"* I thought he'd be happy to launch into his take on their relationship; after all, he was making it abundantly clear that he was feeling very negatively about their marriage. But instead, he said, "It wasn't *my* idea to come here. Let *her* start. She's the one who's *so* unhappy." This was the second time he had bristled at my suggestion—earlier, he didn't sit on the couch as I had asked. Again, I tried to move things along and I made a decision not to address this issue, or his belittling tone, just yet. *"Okay, Lisa, fill me in. From your point of view, what are the difficulties that bring you here today?"*

"To be honest, I guess it's a last-ditch attempt to work things out. I kind of understand why Danny thinks this is a waste of time, and I'm amazed and actually really appreciate that he agreed to come. We've been together 12 years and have been to couple therapy two other times, once when we lived in L.A. before we got married, and then after we moved to New York. I guess it helped a little, for a while, but basically nothing changed. I think we're both pretty unhappy. Maybe we're really here to break up—but we have two kids and I'd hate them to have to go through what I went through because my parents couldn't find a way to get along and just called it quits. I'm not a quitter—I think it might still be possible to work things out." I made a mental note to myself that she wasn't as put off by his sarcasm as I was and gave him credit for going along with her wish to see a couple therapist.

I asked Lisa to give me some sense of the nature of the difficulties between them. "I feel lonely. We hardly spend any time together, and he's not affectionate at all. At best, we're not arguing, but I don't feel we have any real relationship at all. He'd much rather go out with some of his guy friends than go out with me. Sometimes I think he just doesn't like women. I don't mean that he's gay—but he finds what I want to talk about boring. When I try to talk to him about something, he seems really uninterested. It seems like all he wants to talk about is sports or politics. And a lot of the time he rolls his eyes when I tell him something and acts like I'm stupid. And when I tell him he's hurt my feelings, he says I'm crazy—oversensitive." Danny was seething. He interrupted to say, *"Everything* hurts her feelings. She's way oversensitive. She's constantly wanting me to apologize."

At this point I explained that I know that he has another take on this topic, "but for now I'd just like to get a sense of how Lisa sees things. Of course, then I'll want to hear what you think is going on between the two of you." He replies, "But what's the point? She can say what she wants, but she's wrong." *"I know you see things differently, and we'll definitely get to that. But I wonder if you could try something."* I then explained to them both about listening for what they could agree with, what's basically right or even *a little bit* right, rather than waiting his or her turn to rebut. *"Is there anything right in what Lisa's saying?"*

"I guess she's right that I do prefer being with my friends. But that's because she's such a pain to be around. She's changed so much." *"Is there anything else that you "get" in what Lisa is saying?"* "I do roll my eyes sometimes, but that's because what she's saying is so ridiculous—she's gone back to school and thinks she's a psychologist." Mimicking Lisa, Danny says in a high-pitched voice, "You're passive–aggressive, blah, blah, blah."

Lisa then interrupts. "When I try to talk to Danny about how he doesn't act as if he likes me, much less love me, he gets furious and says, 'I make a good living, I take care of you and the kids, I wouldn't be here if I didn't want to be. What do you want from me?' I really think he doesn't get it—this just isn't enough."

Turning to Danny, I then asked him to tell me what *he* thinks are problems in their marriage. *"I'm not asking you to respond to Lisa right now—but rather, what do you think are the problems that if couple therapy could help with, you'd feel better about the relationship?"* "The way I see it, we have a pretty good life. We're financially okay, the kids are good kids—healthy, normal kinds of problems. So far our folks are healthy. I just don't think we have much to complain about. I think if Lisa were happier, we'd get along fine. But you know, as I said, she's always saying I hurt her feelings, or she's lonely—and then I get mad. Basically she's unhappy with me—I think ever since she started studying psychology, she wants me to be something I'm not. I tell her—see your friends, go out, maybe instead of working part time she should work full time—I don't know, but all I know is that she seems to think that it's all my fault! And I'm sick of it. She's always mad at me, and we haven't had sex in a couple of years! I've been shot down so much I've given up trying." Danny went on to say in a sarcastic tone that Lisa complained there's "no *romance*" and that's why she doesn't want to have sex. "Give me a break. How many couples who've been married 15 years and have kids have *romance*?" Lisa interjects, "That's *ridiculous*. That's *not* what I said—I just don't want to have sex with someone who doesn't act like he loves me or cares about me—it feels like it's just to meet your needs and has nothing to do with me. I could be anybody—basically just a body to you!"

I told Lisa and Danny that for now, I had enough of a sense of the tensions between them and as I had described earlier, I wanted to switch gears and find out more about what their relationship was like in the beginning, what drew them to one another, and what the good stuff was at that time.

Lisa spontaneously started and described that they met when they were both on a very challenging wilderness leadership trip in Canada. "We were in different groups, but every few days the groups would meet up at a campsite and though we'd all be wasted in the morning and not in good shape for climbing, we'd get blasted. The two of us would stay up talking for hours after the rest of the group hit the sack. A couple of weeks after the trip, he called me and, as they say, the rest is history." When I questioned Lisa about what made the relationship work and what about Danny made her feel that she wanted to marry him and have children, she responded that it was the right time in her life to settle down. After gently prodding her a bit more, she said, "It was easy being with him, he's very social and I'm kind of shy—and I liked his friends." Again, I tried to get something with more depth and I asked, "*So after dating for a while, you moved in together and then got married a year later. As you got to know him well, what made you feel you could have a happy life with him? You're an attractive woman and you were only in your late 20s when you met him—I know you were feeling ready to settle down, but why him?*" Finally, Lisa said, "Danny was—and actually still is—a really good guy. He never loses a friend—just keeps adding them, and literally has friends he's known since nursery school! He's fun. He made me laugh a lot. We broke up a few times. I *never* felt like I was much of priority. Everything was okay as long as I fit into his life. We hardly ever spent time alone. When we would break up, after a while I would reach out to him and we'd get together again. I don't know what would have happened if I hadn't reached out to him. He probably would have moved on. It was the same then as it is now—I'm just not that important to him."

Turning to Danny, I asked, "*What was it about Lisa that drew you to her?*" He too reported that they had fun. He also stated that "I thought she was adventuresome—we had met on this really difficult trek. Before we had kids we did some pretty cool stuff—we went to Costa Rica and sky-dived. A couple of times we tried hang gliding, but neither of us were that into it. And she got along with my friends—though she was jealous of ex-girlfriends who had become good friends. I know Lisa thinks of herself as shy, but I don't see it. We had people over all the time and she seemed happy about it—and everyone loved her. Now, she never wants to invite people over. She says they're all boring." Lisa interjected, saying, "We were young. We didn't have any real responsibilities. We partied all the time. Used a lot of drugs and drank. It never went too far though. I stopped it all when I got pregnant and Danny cut way back. But I think we both miss it. It's a lot easier to have fun when you're high!"

With both Danny and Lisa their discussion of good memories morphed into negative feelings. This is a common occurrence, and the therapist has to decide whether to pick up on these hurts and complaints at this point in the session. I decided to let their comments pass. They had said *some* nice things about one another and I didn't want to undo that positive by moving too quickly to their frustrations and hurts. I hoped too that perhaps I could get them to expand a bit on their descriptions of what was appealing about the other.

Turning to Danny, I asked him the same questions I asked Lisa. *"As you got to know her, what made you feel you could have a good life with Lisa—have kids, share the future?"*

In answer to this, Danny stated, "I felt she really loved me and would always be there for me. Before we had kids, she was interested in hearing about my work, or what was going on with my family—real supportive. I guess she paid a lot of attention to me and like I said, I felt like she loved me so much and needed me. But that's a thing of the past!"

I concluded this portion of the first meeting by asking whether they ever saw in their current life any of the things that they had with each other early on. Lisa volunteered, "We don't have much fun together. As I said in the beginning of our meeting, Danny spends a lot of time out with his friends, without me. He's still very social—but it doesn't include me anymore. Once in a while—usually if we've each had a couple of beers—we get into laughing jags like we used to years ago."

Danny concurred. Again, sarcastically, he blamed Lisa and said, "She's not a lot of laughs. I feel like she's not the same person I married. She's anxious about everything. Doesn't even want to leave the kids with a babysitter. Maybe I was unrealistic—but I thought even after kids we'd do some cool stuff. But she has no interest. It's all 'dangerous,' 'not appropriate for people with kids,' blah, blah, blah. She's always on her high horse—saying I'm 'childish' or her 'third kid.'"

I made a mental note that attachment themes were emerging for *both* of them. With Lisa, these issues were there right from the beginning. She never felt loved by Danny in a way that made her feel secure about his feelings for her. Danny had felt loved by Lisa and from his point of view this was a large part of the glue between them. At this point, however, he no longer feels her love and I speculated to myself that a significant portion of his sarcasm and verbal aggression came from his being hurt and threatened by her return to school and the new interests she's developed as a result of that change. His speech about how *Lisa* should be happy with the fact that they are financially secure and have happy, healthy kids may be more a speech to *himself* than to her. Maybe he's telling himself that *he* shouldn't complain about the loss of attention and the lack of a sexual relationship. Though in the session he is vocal about these issues and has no trouble airing his "gripes," nonetheless he doesn't normally focus too much on what he is missing.

Though their description of what was good in the past was tinged with more than a little bitterness about what had changed and what for Lisa had *never* been there, they had said some very positive things about one another. Interspersed with Danny's sarcasm were comments like "everybody loved her" or "she was always there for me." And Lisa not only admired him for his ability to have enduring friendships but said, "He made me laugh a lot." Lisa also was proud that they each behaved responsibly in regard to substance abuse once she became pregnant. I thought that when it came to giving feedback at the end of the session, I'd be able to acknowledge their ability to access some of the things they were attracted to in each other when they first met. But thus far, I was not seeing anything positive about how they interacted with one another currently. They didn't smile, nor did I see flashes of affection or humor. Danny's sarcasm was a danger signal (Gottman, 1999), though Lisa didn't seem to react to it as much as I would have thought. Again, I saw his snide comments as defensive. He experienced Lisa as putting him down with her psychological analysis of him, and by routinely saying he's "her third child."

Though I usually wait until the end of the session to ask couples to reflect on their individual contribution to the problems (the *"What do you know about yourself that makes you not the easiest person in the world to live with?"* question), I decided to ask the question earlier. I was hoping that perhaps I would get something to build upon and, frankly, I was not at all sure they would want to come back for a next session, since hard as I tried, no good feelings were generated in the first meeting.

In response to my question, Lisa said she'd been in therapy on and off for years because of anxiety. "It's weird, I'm not anxious about things like sky-diving—but I can get very anxious when people come over or if we're going out with people. I have a lot of social anxiety. Sometimes I think I should go back on Zoloft, but I don't want that to make me feel like everything's okay between us. The last few months I've been feeling pretty depressed, but it's for a reason. Our marriage isn't good and I don't want medication to mask that. Danny keeps telling me it's my problem and I should go back on meds." I asked, *"Is there anything else about your personality that's relevant here?"*

"I guess I have trouble letting go—maybe I'm a bit of a control freak. I like things done the way I want them, and Danny thinks I'm always criticizing him. I'm the one who does the cooking, and it annoys me if he puts pots away where I can't find them or just shoves things in the cabinet without caring if that's where I keep them." Turning to Danny, Lisa asked, "Is it such a big deal to put things away the way I like?" In response Danny turned to me and said, "What she's leaving out is that she's constantly rearranging the kitchen—I *try* to do it the way she likes, but that's impossible. I think maybe she deals with anxiety by constantly cleaning up and rearranging things."

"And what about you? What do you know about your personality that makes you not the easiest person to be married to?" Danny said, "My parents were divorced when I was 10. They hated each other, and each would try to get me on their side. I actually had to testify in court because they couldn't agree on custody. Who would put their kids through something like that? They're really selfish, and I don't have much to do with either of them. Each of them tries to guilt-trip me about their not getting to see the grandkids enough, and my mother is always complaining that I see Dad more than I see her—which isn't true, by the way! I'm someone who gets

very pissed off with guilt trips and people trying to control me. When we were in couple therapy before, that came out."

I asked, *"Is there anything else about your personality that's relevant?"* "I get bored easily. Sometimes I think family life isn't for me. One of our kids has ADD, and I think maybe I have it too. I need stimulation, I need excitement. I'm antsy if I'm hanging around the house too long, and it drives me crazy that even if we say we're going to take the kids somewhere—it's midafternoon by the time we get out of the house. I guess another flaw I have is that I don't have much patience."

Internally, I breathed a sigh of relief. Now I felt I had something to work with and also some positive feedback to give them. Also, I'm relieved that I'm liking Danny better. He's dropped the sarcasm, and I have a better sense of him as someone who is struggling with his own issues. Also, his explanation for why he doesn't put things in the right place puts Lisa's criticism in a different perspective. It's a very simple illustration of the homey adage that couple therapist know so well: "There are two sides to every story."

Feedback at the End of the First Session

As we approached the end of the first session, I stated that I'd like to give them a sense of how I saw things and whether or not couple therapy could be useful. *"The positive is that you both seem to be on the same page—that you would prefer to find a way to stay together. The fact that you are trying again, after having been in couple therapy twice before, tells me that you both want the relationship to work, but for you, Lisa, staying together with the way the relationship is now, seems untenable and you regard this as a last-ditch effort. Danny, it seems at times that you feel the relationship is good enough given all the other good things in your life as a family—kids, financial security, and the like. Nonetheless, you certainly don't seem <u>happy</u> with the way things are.*

"I also saw that you both tried hard to follow the structure I laid out in regard to how I like to conduct a first meeting. That wasn't easy for either of you. You both came in today in an adversarial mode—more interested in correcting and countering the criticism of the other than really listening. But to both your credits, you were able to make the switch and shifted focus to the issues that you know you each bring to the marriage. You were open and not defensive when talking about your own personalities and didn't blame the other for what you know are your own psychological sensitivities.

"If we continue, that will be a continuing challenge—to drop the angry, sarcastic response to what feels like an attack, and to really listen and problem-solve. It wasn't easy for you to do that today, but because you were able to be open about your own issues and contribution to difficulties,

I think with practice, you'll learn to listen nondefensively. I think you are both capable of doing that.

"Couple work would involve breaking out of patterns that you've developed that lead you each to feel hurt, misunderstood, and uncertain of the other's love. Though Lisa says she doesn't feel loved, it seems to me, Danny, that you're not so sure anymore how Lisa feels about you either.

"You also each have certain personality tendencies that right now are intersecting in problematic ways. So, for instance, Lisa, when you express insecurity, it touches on Danny's guilt button and he pushes you away. And Danny, even when you're not reacting to what feels like guilt-tripping, what you describe as your ADD or restlessness can feel to Lisa like rejection of her and your family life. And Lisa, your anxieties slow things down and add to Danny's feelings of restlessness. In couple work we would look at these patterns and come up with new ways so you can get out of these repetitive cycles.

"But a lot of the work would not be about stopping problematic patterns but about finding *new* ways of relating that are gratifying and lead to a feeling of closeness. You both know that the ways you used to feel close—through drinking and partying—are not something you can do now, and you stopped that as soon as Lisa was pregnant. Having adventures and excitement was important to both of you and is what initially drew you to each other. We need to see if there's a way to incorporate some of that adventure into your current life. By the way, it was noteworthy to me that when you first met you spent hours *talking*, so it wasn't as if the only way you connected was through drinking.

"The bottom line, though, is that right now neither of you feels there's much positive in the relationship. But you both don't want to put your kids through what you went through. We'll need to see what you can develop that feels good and makes you want to stay together not only because of the kids but because you are enjoying one another. And, of course, that includes seeing if you can get back to having a physically intimate relationship."

I've called attention to Danny's sarcasm by lumping it in with a general adversarial mode that characterized their interaction. By mentioning it in the context that they were able to *overcome* that stance, I made this feedback a bit easier to swallow and positively reinforced their efforts to allow me to guide them to a more productive way of interacting. I also gave them credit for their each being able to look at their own contribution to difficulties.

Although I reflected back to them that there wasn't much that they feel good about in their relationship at this point, I did so in a way that joined them in an attributional statement—they both know that the old ways of connecting don't fit with their current stage of life. By saying that we'd need to see if they could find new ways of being together that would be gratifying and incorporate some adventure, I gave them the message that it is *possible* to build something new. By pointing out that they did in fact spend hours talking without drinking, I highlighted that what was possible in the past is possible to attain again.

I ended the session by asking them each *"to think about what you might really like to have from one another in your relationship. If the couple therapy could help you have the kind of relationship you want, what would that look like? Even if right now that seems far-fetched, I'd like you to think about what you've seen in other relationships over the years that looks appealing—that makes you think, I wish we were like that."*

The Second Session with Danny and Lisa

It was 3 weeks since our first meeting when I next saw Danny and Lisa. They'd been away on a vacation with their kids and another family, and Danny started the session by mentioning that they'd had a great time. Lisa laughingly interjected, "Yeah, as long as we don't have to spend any time alone with one another, and there's no homework, and lunches, and getting the kids out in the morning, we're okay." I had a choice at this point as to whether to focus on one of the negatives in Lisa's statement—for example, it's much harder when they're alone together—or to ignore the negatives and focus instead on how they do get along in certain circumstances.

Danny replied, "Yeah, it's not just when we're on vacation or with another family—once we get out of the house and are doing something, we usually are okay." Lisa agreed. "He's right, the kids are great. They're like Danny, always up for doing something. We never have to drag them."

"So, how do you understand how this works? What makes it go so well? How is it that you're not getting into the kind of hurts and bad feelings that brought you here? What are you doing differently?"

Lisa said in response, "I think we both enjoy the kids so much. I don't feel lonely. And I don't really care if he's not talking to me." Danny interjected, "Lisa is great with the kids. She's a lot more relaxed when we're out of the house. It's not 'Danny, you didn't take out the garbage, Danny, why do you leave your shoes over there, Danny, you don't respect me' because I didn't put the dishes in the dishwasher the way she likes. When we're home, her mind is filled with trivia. That's all she thinks about."

Lisa responded, "He's so insulting and arrogant. Danny doesn't respect me at all. I'd love to talk to him about books I'm reading for school, or politics, but he looks down on me—like anything I say is naive or stupid. Danny is much better educated than I am—and always was a star student. He thinks my going back to school is a joke and that the classes I'm taking are all silly, women's stuff—poetry, psychology, art history." Danny responded, "I'm a math and science guy. She talks about feelings, and in a discussion of something she'll say something like 'Well, that's the way I feel about it,' when it's not a question of how she *feels* about something but what the *facts* are. She'll say, 'I feel like people will live on Mars one day.' And when I try to tell her the reasons why that's not possible, she'll just ignore me and say 'Well, I feel like we will be able to' without any facts to back it up."

"I'd like you both to notice what just happened. You both started out by saying something nice about the other in explaining why you have a good time when you're out as a family. Lisa said that the kids are like you, very up for doing things. And Danny said that you're great with the kids. But Danny, then you threw in a mocking comment about Lisa nagging you at home and Lisa counterattacked with saying you're arrogant, and then you countered that with saying she's illogical. And within 10 seconds you turned that nice moment into an exchange where you both were aggressive and hurtful—and not feeling good any more. And Lisa, though at this moment we could say that Danny started it, but earlier, in talking about the vacation, you said something similar—diminished the positive by talking about how it happened only because you weren't faced with daily stresses and didn't expect to spend time alone. You actually both have similar styles—you give each other little barbs—even when you are basically saying something quite positive." I asked them if they saw what I meant, and they both seemed to get it. Both agreed that what just occurred was fairly typical of a lot of their interactions. *"So, my job is to help you build on the good stuff—on the positive feelings. The old adage that your grandmothers could have told you is actually true, you catch more bees with honey than with vinegar. And another simple truth is that we want to spend time with and be close to people who make us feel good about ourselves, not people who see what is wrong about us. If you want to have good conversations, you are going to need to find ways to make the other feel good during the time you are talking, not feel inadequate, disregarded, or attacked. This is something you can learn to do and as part of our work I'll show you how to do that."*

At this point in the session I went back to the question I left them with at the end of the first session. *"What do you wish your relationship was like. What have you noticed about some other relationships that if you could have with one another would feel really good."* Lisa started by saying, "I thought a lot about that question. And you know, when I look at my friends' marriages, I wouldn't really want to trade what Danny and I have with theirs. It made me think that maybe it's just some romantic fantasy I have that nobody actually has." Danny jokingly responded, "Well, so I'm not so bad after all." They both laughed as he said jokingly, "You don't want to be married to Rodrigo or Frank?" [the husbands of Lisa's two closest friends].

I interjected, *"The way the two of you looked at each other and laughed gave me a glimpse of the chemistry the two of you had when you just met—*

for those couple of seconds you <u>clicked</u> and were getting a kick out of the repartee." This comment on my part is an example of how I'm noticing and underlining even the tiniest step in the right direction.

"*In my little thought experiment, you don't need to like everything about some other relationship. You can take bits and pieces from different relationships. For instance, maybe you find one of those men too bossy but you could still like, for instance, that perhaps he's physically affectionate toward his wife.*"

Danny said, "That's how I took it. I also couldn't think of someone as a whole that I'd rather be with. But sometimes I'm in a restaurant and I see a couple a lot older than us who seem really <u>into</u> each other—like they're happy to be out to dinner with one another and maybe filling each other in on the day." Lisa laughingly said, "I'd like that too. But I bet the guy isn't texting his friend about a football game during dinner!" And in turn, replying in a friendly tone, Danny said, "But I'm at least out—not glued to the set at home—you've gotta give me some credit for that!"

"*I've noticed how the two of you can sometimes kid around with each other and have the ability to say something important in a way that takes the sting out of it. The bottom line is that both of you have an image of a kind of engagement and attention from one another that you'd really like but seldom have with each other these days.*"

I asked Danny for other images he had of good relationships, and he said that it's what he and Lisa had before they had kids. "Lots of adventures and getting a little crazy together—but we're leaving out drugs and drinking, right? Well, I guess doing a lot of physical activities together—maybe rock climbing, biking, stuff like that. And yeah, let's not leave out sex. But I don't mean just going along with it because she knows she should, but being with a woman who acts like she's really *in to* me."

Lisa interjected, "Everything Danny says he wants is exactly the same for me."

I asked, "*Are there some things in addition to what's on Danny's list that would appeal to you.*" "I don't know, I have to think about it more. I guess more romance, a feeling that he thinks about me when we're not together, a sense that we're really a couple. That I'm his other half—something like that. And as far as sex goes—I want to feel it's about *me*. I guess some romance first."

I responded to these statements by underlining that they both noted that no relationship has everything and that neither of them felt there was some other ideal person out there. And it's striking how much overlap there was in what they each would want in a relationship. "*If you were going to try to make one of the things you each described actually happen—something small—like the kind of experience you each wish you could have when you're out together for dinner—what would you need to do?*"

Lisa said, "I don't know. Danny seems bored with what I talk about.

He always seems distracted and waiting to get a chance to check his phone." I asked Lisa to turn to Danny and tell him how she felt when he seems distracted. *"Talk from your heart. Tell him what's going on for you when that happens."* I chose this moment to ask them to talk directly to one another because I felt that the hostility between them had diminished considerably and that they each would be more likely to respond with empathy than they would have if I had asked them to talk directly earlier in the session.

Turning toward Danny, Lisa said, "I feel bad, like I'm just not that interesting or clever and that you wish you were with someone more like your friends from college. It's so disappointing. Every time we go out, I think it's going to be romantic—I don't know why I keep thinking that—and then after a few minutes I feel flat and empty and I don't even know what to talk about. I kind of go blank and end up talking about things that I know are stupid." Tearing up, she said softly, "I just wish I were smarter."

Danny reached over and tapped Lisa's knee. "You're fine, I just get bored easily. You *are* smart. But for some reason, you've decided you can't understand politics or some of the things I'm interested in. I used to send you links to some political things I found interesting, and you never mentioned them—I assume you never read them. You know I get bored easily. You shouldn't take it personally. Really, you're fine—smart. Your family made you insecure about yourself. But you're smart. I would never be with someone who I didn't think was smart." I commented, *"Danny, I saw how much empathy you had for Lisa ... you hated to see her feeling bad about herself."*

Getting back to the desire they have to be interesting to one another, I asked Danny, *"If perhaps you've done something similar to what Lisa does— told yourself that you're not interested in psychology or fiction or art—the kinds of things Lisa is studying now. I wonder if you've each become too set in your ways, too polarized. In your image of a dinner in which you're really engaged with one another, you would each <u>let</u> yourself become interested in what's important to the other."* I suggested to them that they might each try experimenting with expanding their interests a little bit. Perhaps before they went out to dinner, Lisa could give Danny a short story to read and she could read some short article on a topic that he found interesting. They might both find that they don't "get it," but then they could ask the other to explain. Or, if they didn't want to have to do preparation, perhaps they could at dinner each ask the other to tell them about something they're interested in. Danny might summarize some political issue for Lisa and she could ask questions about it. And Lisa could talk about something she's studying in school. By talking with them about *how* they might make dinner together a different experience, I communicated that these images of a good relationship are directly connected to things they each can *do*. Even if they didn't follow through on this suggestion directly, it is a hopeful message and orients them both to actions they can take as well as ways they can expand and enlarge their self-definitions.

Ending the Session

I ended the session by telling Lisa and Danny that they used the session really well. Instead of exchanging mutual accusations and barbs, they were able to refocus on what they would like out of their relationship, and they gave each other a couple of compliments along the way! I was also impressed by their willingness to hear what I had to say about the way they can each throw jabs at one another and then suddenly they're off and running with a hostile interaction. They were both open and nondefensive about that observation, and I felt that they worked hard not to repeat that pattern for the remainder of the session. In fact, I was impressed by how they were able to talk about some things that bothered them with a "light touch" and how supportive Danny was when Lisa opened up to him about her insecurities.

I then give them a "homework" assignment. *"I'd like you each to give some thought to what you know about the other after all these years that if you did it would draw the other closer to you. What warms the other's heart? Maybe it's things you used to do spontaneously years ago. Maybe it's things that once in a while you do even now. Don't talk about it. Just think about what you actually know generates warm feelings in the other."*

In this case example, we have looked at how to begin to move from hostile interactions in the session to a more productive way of engaging with each other. At first it seemed that there was little positive on which to build. But by focusing on some small positives, and by pointing out how each person's attack on the other leads to escalating tensions and a loss of any good feeling, the couple was able to have an experience in the session that brought them closer. They were able to talk about what they really wanted without being attacking, and Danny could experience himself as being able to be supportive of Lisa, who was openly expressing feelings of vulnerability.

But I do not want to paint too rosy a picture. Though this was a good start, keeping the couple on this path will not be easy. For years they have related in a hostile, attacking, and distancing manner, and undoubtedly, they will revert to that pattern again. Future sessions will in part deal with unpacking arguments and frustrations. But having had a session in which they articulated what they are wishing for will enable me to more easily shift them from the dissecting of arguments to "brainstorming" together, both about ways to avoid these interactions and about how to have more of what they both want from a relationship.

Gradually, my hope is that they will shift more and more to what they want, how to get it, and what gets in the way of their having the kind of marriage they would feel good about. A basic assumption I make is that the more the couple has some positive experiences with each other, the less they will focus on the things that annoy and frustrate them. It's not that these hurts, irritations, and disappointments will not be there at all—though they are likely to diminish in frequency—but that the overall *goodwill* that has been established will make them less important and will lead to a quicker recovery when they have hurt one another.

In addition to working on having more positive experiences with each other, future sessions will need to deal with both of their "hot button" issues—for Lisa, her insecurity about her intelligence, for Danny, his reactivity to anything that feels like "guilt-tripping." These issues would be addressed through further exploration of family history as well as by looking at the ways they are kept alive through current interactions and the unconscious enlistment of "accomplices" (P. L. Wachtel, 2014a).

Future sessions would also need to look at how what Danny called his "ADD personality" affects the family and the way that Lisa's anxiety interacts with his restlessness and need for stimulation. As described in Chapter 5, spelling out what actions can be taken to break these patterns is an essential component of the work.

The goal of the first few sessions is to learn more about the issues and patterns that need to be addressed while at the same time giving the couple an *experience* in the session that is positive and productive. These two vignettes are representative of the way the therapist can help the couple transition from mutual accusations to a focus on wishes and longings. The first few sessions implicitly educate the couple about the nature of couple therapy. Many couples assume that the couple therapist will act like a mediator, or even a judge, and that sessions will consist of rehashing arguments. Though they may have expected, or even wanted, couple therapy to be a forum for venting their grievances, most couples are quite relieved to discover that the session did not consist of a "he said–she said" review of arguments. Much of the therapist's skill consists of using particular incidents the couple describes as an entree into a discussion of more general concerns. But all couple therapists will encounter—with considerable frequency—cases where making the transition to general concerns and longings is difficult to do. In the following "Troubleshooting" section I discuss some common challenges that we encounter.

TROUBLESHOOTING

1. What if I Point Out the Attacking Pattern but Sparks Keep Flying?

When that happens, I try to get at least one person in the couple to reflect on and *talk about* their arguments. Even if only one person is able to do this, the escalating cycle of blame and retort is likely to diminish. I am attempting to mobilize each person's *thinking* self. This often works to shift the session to an examination of the exact nature of the couple's arguments, and the typical course they take. Instead of me telling them the pattern I see, I try to engage *them* in describing and analyzing what generally happens.

Often I will literally raise my hands and ask if they could stop for a minute and let me interject. Here are some of the questions I might ask: *"Is this similar to what happens between the two of you at home? Could you describe to me the course it usually takes?"* or *"If I were a fly on the wall in your home, what would I see? Would you be screaming at each other, throwing things, shoving, blocking each other, hitting—how intense does it get?"* or *"How do you each understand what makes your arguments escalate?"* or *"How long do you stay angry with each other?"* or *"Do you try to calm down? If so, how?"* or *"What happens once the argument ends? Do you try to talk about it later? Do you just go on with your life and put it behind you?"* or *"I would imagine that there are times when one of you is upset or annoyed about something and it <u>doesn't</u> turn into an argument. Is that right? How do you understand that? How does that happen? What might you be doing that prevents it from happening?"* or *"What have you tried to do to change the pattern?"* The question about what I would see if I watched them in their home is a particularly important one. If a couple doesn't control their anger in the session, it is likely that they are still much more volatile, and perhaps even physically violent, when at home. Including in the initial inquiry questions about how physical the arguments get is important, because couples often do not raise that issues spontaneously. They feel shame about it or are protective of their spouse.

It's very important to include in this inquiry the question about the exception to the rule. Reflecting on what enables them *sometimes* to prevent arguments from escalating can give them hope that they might be able to do this more often and gives both them and the therapist further useful clues about possible ways to foster an alternative way of addressing their differences. When people are upset, they tend to overgeneralize and see only the negative instances, and it's important for therapists to help both couples and individuals see the times when they were successful in changing course. Thus the questions need to help them not only to think about and better understand the pattern when things go wrong, but also to notice those times, infrequent as they may be, when they didn't argue but addressed their differences more effectively. Asking them to analyze *how* that happened makes it clear that they each *did something* that prevented a bad exchange from escalating.

The question *"How have you tried to calm yourself down?"* includes an implicit suggestion. Very often it hasn't even occurred to people to try to calm themselves down or to try to be less mad or agitated. These questions not only try to mobilize the couple to get some distance from the pattern and to see the pattern as something separate from them as individuals, but they are stated in a way that invites and assumes a problem-solving attitude.

2. What if I Can't Get the Couple to Switch from Arguing to Analyzing and They Keep Fighting in My Office?

There are times when it's almost impossible to interrupt a couple's argument, and when even if they do respond to the questions just described, they do so in a way that just continues the fight. They might, for example, be furious with each other about the answers each gives as to the nature of the pattern of their arguments and have the very same kind of argument right there in the office. "You hold a grudge"—"You're so cold"—"You want to talk endlessly about it"—"You never admit you're wrong"—"You never apologize." When this happens, I first try once again to give my little talk about listening for what you can agree with, what's basically right, what's even a little bit right and responding to that instead of what you disagree with. Sometimes this works, but with very angry, adversarial couples it may work for just a few minutes and then they are right back to having a heated argument.

Sometime when I'm not getting anywhere, I might sit quietly for a few minutes and then interrupt the couple with the simple question, *"Would you like my help?"* Unfortunately, with the situation I have just described, that question usually elicits a good deal of pessimism about couple therapy, perhaps with one person making it clear (again) that s/he agreed to come to therapy but really thinks it's hopeless.

I might respond to that attitude by saying, *"I can understand why you feel that way—the two of you really go at it, and I can see why you think it's just an impossible situation. But actually, you've been helping me see the things that each of you do and say that leave you each frustrated and feeling you're not being understood. If you could try to stop the back-and-forth and let me help, you might find that it's not as hopeless as it feels right now. I think you're both so angry because you're hurt and <u>want something</u> from the other that you don't know how to get. Couple therapy can often help people express what they are wishing for in a way that the other can better hear. But it does mean being able to stop the fighting long enough to let me help."*

Sometimes this approach works. But when it doesn't, I again sit quietly for a minute or two and then say to them that couple therapy may not be right for them at this point. I would invite them each to have a session alone with me before we decide whether couple therapy makes sense for them. My goal in these sessions is to determine how much each person actually wants to work on the relationship. Often one of them has a strong wish to separate but finds that s/he just can't get him- or herself to do it. The intense arguing that has occurred in the sessions is used to confirm and bolster that person's feeling that ending the relationship is necessary and inevitable. Sometimes identifying this issue has the paradoxical effect of enabling that person to engage productively in the couple sessions, and we are able to continue the work. Bur more often than not, individual therapy is necessary to help sort out why s/he is "stuck" and can neither separate nor work to improve the relationship.

Sometimes meeting alone with each of them enables me to share what I see about his or her role in how things escalate between them. Without the spouse in the room, it is more likely that the person can take in my feedback nondefensively. On rare occasions I might start the couple therapy by meeting a *few* times with each of them alone and then bring them together. I do this only when I feel each person will be better able to acknowledge his or her own part in the couple's difficulties when they are alone with me. I make clear that the individual meetings are temporary and are a part of couple therapy, not a switch to individual therapy. In order to be effective as a couple therapist, I find it is important that I don't know anything that the partner doesn't know. Thus, though I don't necessarily report back everything said in a private session, I need to feel free to share anything that I do think it is important for the spouse to know. I remind people at the beginning of the individual session to *"not tell me anything that I couldn't share if I thought it was important to do so."*

3. What if the Response to What the Other Longs for Is "That's Not Me"?

Sometimes that response comes when what the other person is asking for seems too big. I join with the person and say, *"Of course, we each have our own personalities, temperament, and styles, and it would be unrealistic to ask each other to be entirely different. But I don't think that's what your wife/husband had in mind."* This will lead to clarifications and perhaps a discussion of how one person feels that the other is fundamentally unhappy with the kind of person s/he is. At some point, I interject and ask, *"What changes "do" seem realistic to each of you? Do you believe those changes would make a difference in how you feel?"* The person who is being asked to act in ways that feel like "not me" may be skeptical that small changes would really matter. The only answer to that is to encourage the person to give it a try. It's also useful to explain that people are usually more capable of being different than they imagine and that part of the couple work is for each person to expand his or her sense of what's "me" or "not me."

Many people feel that people just "are who they are" and aren't capable of being different. Or they may explicitly feel it's *wrong* to ask their spouse to be different. I respond to this attitude by talking about the importance of change to keep marriages vital and note that in my experience people can and often welcome changing old definitions of themselves.

4. What if They Can't Come Up with Anything about Themselves That Contributes to the Problem?

This is an unusual occurrence but can happen when one person is convinced that the difficulties they are having as a couple are due to the behavior, or the unfair expectations, of his or her spouse. Not infrequently one person believes that the source of the couple's difficulties is fundamentally their spouse's "midlife" crisis, anxiety, or depression. A person who believes this sort of thing may be reluctant to open up about his own issues out of a belief that to do so would minimize the case he wants to make that the couple's problems are caused by the partner and not himself. Or the person may genuinely believe that she is easy to get along with, and it is only the spouse who sees her as deficient in some way.

The challenge for the therapist is how, at this early stage of therapy, to prevent one person's lack of forthcomingness from derailing therapy when it has barely begun. Thus, when I ask the couple what they each came up with about themselves *"that makes them not the easiest person in the world to live with,"* and one person says "I can't really think of anything" or responds in a way that's really about the other—for example, saying, "I don't handle her tirades well"—I try to move on without highlighting the person's refusal to really give thought to his or her role. I might say, *"I think it's likely that as we continue talking about the problems that have brought you here, you may come up with things about your own personality that contribute in some way to the difficulties."* I am basically trying to finesse the situation that has presented itself.

Another way I handle it when one person is not able or willing to reflect on his or her personality in a general way is to change the question to make it more specific to their relationship. I might say, *"Let me phrase the question a little differently and you can give some thought to it during the week. What do you know about your personality that is hard for your partner to deal with or accept?"* In order to avoid the couple getting into an argument, I prevent the person from answering it now, and say instead, *"It would be better if you give some thought to it and we can get back to it next week."* My hope is that if I can make the session productive, the discussion the following week will be more meaningful and not just another way to blame the spouse.

These impasses often arise when there is a history of one person feeling he is being blamed for all the marital tension, and as a consequence he is likely to respond with some intensity when his partner comes up with nothing in answer to my invitation to be self-reflective. Often the "accused" spouse will challenge the partner's view of his personality. For instance, John, who came to therapy with Douglas, said, "I'm an easy-going person, even-keeled—things don't bother me. I get along with people—I have lots of friends. I've never lost my temper the way I have in this relationship. This isn't who I am. Doug's not happy until he's provoked me to start screaming." And, not surprisingly, Doug responded, "He's easy-going because when something upsetting is happening—not necessarily to do with me—it could be a problem at work, or even something medical—he *detaches* from things. He loves Facebook—but when he's upset about something he'll spend *all day* on it and other stuff like it—Instagram, chat rooms. I mean it—a whole day! Basically, he goes into another world." When a retort like this occurs, I ask the other person to just give some *thought* to what his or her partner is saying. So, for instance, I would ask John, *"Can you see that? Does what Doug is saying make any sense at all?"* And again, in order to prevent couples from getting *stuck* on this debate, I generally will suggest that the person not answer my questions *now*, but rather spend some time thinking about it.

There are occasions when one *cannot* temporarily sidestep the issue, or the one who is being blamed will be so frustrated that she won't want to come back. At times, the therapist must be direct and confrontational about one person's refusal to see *any* role he plays in what happens in the relationship. For instance, recently the woman in a couple I was seeing responded with tremendous frustration and hopelessness when all her husband could come up with in answer to my question was that he left his socks on the floor sometimes. "This is so typical! He's always the sane, rational one—poor him—he has a crazy wife. It infuriates me. I thought if we came here it would be different, but he's doing exactly the same thing—this is useless."

I explained to the husband that being able to look at one's role in difficulties was absolutely essential and that it was maddening to his wife when he won't or can't reflect on his personality and what he may be contributing to their problems. Citing Gottman's (1994) research I explained about the dangers to couples when people are defensive or stonewall. In order to help the person identify some things s/he might be doing that contribute to the problems, I sometimes ask him or her to read sections of *We Love Each Other, But . . .* (E. F. Wachtel, 2000) with the mind-set of looking for him- or herself, not the spouse, in the dozens of case examples. I also ask them to look at the *list* of "hot buttons" in the book to identify what issues s/he might be particularly sensitive to.

5. Should I Encourage the Couple to Continue Talking about the Issues after the Session?

I generally don't initiate a discussion of this topic. One person may raise the question because s/he takes it as a bad sign that the couple didn't continue talking together on their own about the issues raised in a session. S/he may feel that the other "swept it under the rug." Or they may have tried to continue the conversation and it did not go well. Or, on the other hand, they may have talked about some of the issues in a way that they both felt good about. Whatever happened spontaneously is something that usually provides a good deal of information about patterns of interactions and coping styles. As psychoanalysts say, it's all "grist for the mill."

There are exceptions to my general laissez-faire approach. With couples who are unusually adversarial and emotional, I ask them *not* to attempt to discuss further what was raised in the session, as well as *not* to bring up for further discussion what was said in any argument they may have had. This, of course, is easier said than done for the very reason I'm asking them not to further talk about the argument—they are emotionally volatile. But by discouraging discussion at home for this stage in the therapy I am at least giving them guidelines. Hopefully, one of them will be able to end the unproductive discussion by citing what I have said in the session.

If a less volatile couple asks whether or not they should keep talking about the issues raised, I explore with them what they each would prefer to do and help them reach some agreement. As part of our discussion, we come up with a plan together for how to cut short the conversation if it is going badly. I make clear to couples that it is perfectly all right for them to defer discussion of difficult issues until they are in our session together. I assure them that one of the goals of therapy is indeed for them to be able to talk with one another in a productive way, but right now they are in couple therapy because they have *difficulty* doing that, so it makes sense that they defer discussion of difficulties until their session with me. Of course, if they'd like to try it, that's fine too, but they should have realistic expectations and not feel discouraged if it didn't go as well as they had hoped. I remind them that they have had years of communicating in a way that hasn't worked so well and that doing it differently will take some practice.

6. Should I Always Give the Couple Some "Homework"?

I've put the word *homework* in quotes because for me it has a slightly patronizing or authoritarian connotation. I think it's important to make suggestions to couples and sometimes it is useful even to use the word "homework," but only in a way that's respectful and doesn't trigger resistance. I might say, for instance, *"I have some homework for you which I think if you can try to do would be helpful."* There is no implication that this is compulsory or that I'll be upset with them if they don't do the "assignment."

Early in the work, the "homework" is not usually specific to the patterns that have emerged. That will come later and is discussed in Chapters 8 and 9. Here's a list of some of the suggestions I might make early in the work—some of which have already been touched upon. In addition to *"What do you know about yourself that makes you not the easiest person in the world to be married to?,"* I might in the first few sessions say:

> *"What are some things that you know if you did, would draw your spouse closer to you?"*
> *"What are some things that you used to do spontaneously that warmed up the relationship?"*
> *"See if you can do a mental exercise and notice positives about your partner. Keep a list—it's not necessary to share them."*
> *"Think about words or issues that are 'hot buttons' for you?"* (To help them think about this, I give them a list from *We Love Each Other, But . . .* [E. F. Wachtel, 2000].)
> *"Think about what are hot buttons for your partner?"*
> *"What do you see in some other relationships that if you could have you would like?"*

These early suggestions are for the purpose of heightening their awareness of themself and the other. They purposely do not ask people to try to act differently. At this stage of the therapy, I don't want to risk inciting more conflict by suggesting changed behavior, which if not done could add to despair and frustration.

This chapter has focused on how to make the transition from the first session to actually working on the problems that have brought the couple to therapy. The challenge is to make room for the negative feelings in a way that does not lead to an escalation of fighting or feelings of hopelessness. As I stated in Chapter 1, I'm hoping to leave the couple feeling better at the end of the session than when they walked into my office. This does not always happen, but it is my goal. It's particularly important to aim for this result early in the work so that the couple's frustration and despair does not lead them to drop out of therapy. As I said earlier, feeling better can simply mean that they have addressed their anger, frustrations, and disappointments in a way that feels different and more productive from what they do on their own. The first few meetings with a couple is when they learn how couple therapy works and when the therapist has an opportunity to reinforce a way of interacting in the session that will enable them to use the therapy time constructively. Tentative hypotheses about the patterns and issues of concern to each of them are offered. As the core issues are identified, the therapist and the couple gradually begin to work on them. Anyone who works with couples knows that there are a myriad of pitfalls with which therapists are confronted. Seldom does couple therapy go as smoothly as it may appear on paper. In Chapter 10, when I discuss the nitty-gritty of ongoing work, we will look, for example, at how to handle it when one person feels that you are siding with the other, or when one person doesn't follow through on what she seemed so earnestly committed to, or when the couple is fighting less but still doesn't experience much joy in the relationship.

A crucial part of my couple work involves helping each individual in the couple expand his or her sense of *self*. In the next chapter I discuss a way of doing a genogram that in addition to highlighting family patterns, provides a window into each person's values and worldview.

8

☙

The Genogram
A Window into the Psyche

*T*his chapter begins with a description of how to obtain information that helps us understand each individual in the context of his or her family background and social location (religion, culture, race, gender, sexual orientation), and how to do so in a manner that will elucidate aspects of the individual's personality and worldview that often have never before been explicitly articulated. With a complex and nuanced understanding of how an individual's assumptions, longings, and coping mechanisms have been shaped by his or her experiences growing up in the family as well as in the larger social–political–economic world of which the family was a part, we are better able to help the couple both to extricate themselves from the grip of unwittingly repeated negative patterns and to find ways to better meet each other's most deeply felt needs.

WHEN TO DO A GENOGRAM

Virtually every couple knows that each person's family background and culture plays a role in their marital difficulties. Though sometimes a spouse refers to differences between their families admiringly, or even longingly— for example, "I always wanted a big close family like hers" or "I'm closer to his mother than I am to my own—she's completely accepting and non-judgmental"—more typically, the contrast between the families comes up in the context of arguments. Couples implicitly understand "transference" reactions and will say things like "I keep telling her—I'm not your father— he's the one you should be confronting, not me" or "Every time I ask him to do something, he acts like I'm his nagging mother." Though there may be some truth to these comments, they are at best unproductive, and, at worst, add fuel to the fire of already volatile interactions.

In the first few sessions with a couple I do not focus very much on each person's family of origin. I prefer to delay getting a detailed family history— what family therapists call a "genogram"—until we have already begun to make a bit of progress. There are several reasons for delaying that inquiry until we have had a few meetings and made some inroads into the work that needs to be done. For one, the way I do a family history is time-consuming, and couples need to quickly start directly addressing their difficulties before they will have the patience to engage in this kind of effort. Moreover, as just mentioned, in the early stages of therapy, differences in the couple's families are often alluded to not in a way that promotes healing and mutual understanding, but in an aggressive and demeaning manner. One partner, for example, might say, "He grew up in a family where everyone thought it was okay to say nasty things to one another," or "Her family talks endlessly about every little physical symptom. They're a bunch of hypochondriacs and, let's face it, the apple doesn't fall far from the tree." Frequently, one person in a couple concludes that his or her spouse is acting very much in accordance in what he observed in his parents relationship—for example, "He doesn't think he needs to make any efforts to buy presents, since his mother seemed okay with getting almost no attention from his father and everyone including the kids treated her like a doormat" or "She's becoming more and more like her mother, who is constantly nagging—or should I say harassing—her father about what chores he needs to do."

In order to have some contextual information even before getting a detailed family history via doing a genogram, I will ask the couple to briefly *"fill me in if there is some part of your family history that's important for me to know right off the bat."* This simple request often provides a lot of information. For one, it tells the therapist what the individual *feels* is a crucial part of his or her story. "I'm a twin," or "My mother is manic–depressive," or "My father was one of only a handful of black kids in his high school," or "My father died when I was 2 and my mother never remarried," or "My mother is the only one in her family who married a non-Indian." By initially asking the question that way, instead of the more linear, conventional questions—for example, *"Where did you grow up? Are your parents alive? Do you have siblings?"*—I am learning not only about family background but, perhaps even more importantly, I am learning what that person *believes* to be the most consequential and salient part of his or her family background.

Often, because the context is couple therapy, the person will then volunteer thoughts about the relevance of these facts to the couple's relationship. As discussed earlier, an important element of my work is the encouragement of self-reflection about each individual's contribution to the couple's difficulties. For this reason, I follow up on these comments with questions that encourage people to also talk about how salient aspects of their background have contributed to their personality and values.

Thus, looking at the examples just given, if someone says "I'm an identical twin," I would ask, *"What are your thoughts about how being a twin has contributed to who you are and what you are like?"* Or if someone says, "My parents are both recovering alcoholics," I would ask about their history of alcoholism and how s/he thinks that affected what s/he is like as a person? How has it shaped who s/he is? Most people have already given thought to these kinds of questions, and that is *why* they are flagging these facts as important for me to know. The follow-up questions are essential because the therapist's assumptions about what it means to be, for instance, a twin, or a child of alcoholics, may be at odds with the meaning *for this particular person*. For instance, being an identical twin might lead someone to have expectations of or longings for intense closeness, or conversely, to have a particularly strong wish for separateness and autonomy.

It is particularly important to follow up when what has been volunteered about the person's family has to do with their place in the larger social and political context. So, for instance, if someone mentioned that his father was one of just a few black children in his school, the therapist would use that as an opportunity to inquire not only about the father's experience of race but how being part of a black family with that particular history has contributed to the patient's personality and worldview. More detailed inquiry about this topic will be obtained when doing the genogram, but it's important to address racial, ethnic, and social class issues as soon as possible.

Family and couple therapists routinely diagram a three-generational family history in order to look at the transmission of multigenerational patterns as well as the role that the sociopolitical environment (race, religion, gender, socioeconomic status) interact with families and influence family life (McGoldrick, 1999; Hardy & Laszloffy, 1995). Each person in the couple has grown up with assumptions about how families *are* and *should* be. There are unarticulated family rules that influence expectations and behaviors, and the clash of these often unconscious assumptions can create serious tensions in current relationships. For instance, are in-laws incorporated into the family, or do they remain outsiders? Were "family loyalty" conflicts between families of origin and new families a prevalent theme? Was allegiance to one's ethnic and racial background a dominant value, or was there an expectation or even encouragement of assimilation?

Of particular significance are the family's unspoken rules with respect to the permissibility of talking about feelings, arguing, and how conflicts are resolved. Is there a history of people staying together through thick or thin despite the quality of their relationship, or, conversely, are there numerous divorces, and, if so, how are these regarded? Similarly, if there are significant tensions between parts of an extended family, do they remain in contact with one another, or are there one or more "cutoffs," in which for years, or possibly forever, family members no longer speak? When it comes to looking at the extended family, there is never just one family pattern, but there are myths and stories that are influential even though they selectively ignore aspects of the family that don't fit the pattern but are "exceptions to the rule."

It is similarly important to look at how the patient's nuclear family differs from or is similar to the extended family or even the larger social context in which they are situated. So, for instance, Jane's mother, who identified herself as a "feminist," had told Jane and her two sisters stories of women in her family who had been totally dependent on men who, though initially successful, "got greedy and eventually lost all their money." Jane's mother, Rebecca, had vowed to herself both to always earn her own money and to marry a man who was conservative and not "looking to make a killing." Although one could say there is a family pattern that might have some bearing on Jane's marriage, it is essential to take into account how Jane *processed* both the stories of dependency, greed, and failure in the account of her *extended* family and the quite different narrative that underlay her nuclear family.

Families have *ideas* about themselves, a way of thinking about their family in relation to other families, and these concepts are absorbed by children at an early age. So, for instance, the individual's nuclear family may have differentiated themselves from other families by seeing their family as "not as conventional," "more concerned about social justice," "more ambitious," "more cultured," or "more middle class" than their extended family or the ethnic or racial group with whom they are identified.

The point here is that the *factual* information obtained is often less important than the opportunity the genogram gives us to better understand the worldview of each member of the couple (E. F. Wachtel, 1982). Because talking about one's family is easier for many people than talking about their own psychological makeup, the genogram is a good vehicle for helping people open up. Through descriptions of family members we can learn about an individual's unarticulated, or even unconscious, assumptions, wishes, fears, and values. Discussing family relationships, comparing oneself to one's siblings or others in the family, describing personality and character traits of a variety of people, provides a structure that enables many people to discover things about themselves that they may not have consciously articulated previously.

Diagraming one's family tree and conducting a genealogical investigation in order to find out more about one's roots has become a popular pursuit. Sometimes when I tell a couple that I'd like to learn about each person's family background by constructing a genogram, they propose that they do it themselves at home, or that they come in separately to give me the family history that their spouse already knows. I explain that I like to do it in the session both because I'll be asking them some things about their families that they may not have thought of before and because I'd like them each to participate in the discussion of the way each partner's personality and values developed in the context of his or her family background. I describe what we'll be doing as not just diagraming a family tree but rather creating a *psychological* genogram, an account of how family members through generations behaved in and experienced the world.

I frame the inquiry in terms of what I might learn about them as *individuals*, and I am careful not to say something like "how it impacts your marriage" or "how it contributes to the issues between the two of you." Because it is so common for couples to pejoratively refer to the negative impact on the marriage of the other's family background, I do not want to raise the specter of this being what the history taking might lead to. Though of course I *will* be making links to issues in the couple's relationship, I don't preview that effort, since when I do make those links it will be in a complex, nuanced, and nonaccusatory manner.

HOW TO DO A GENOGRAM

Doing a genogram in the way I am about to describe can be quite time-consuming. It will take a minimum of two sessions to do properly. I try to complete both sides of one person's family in one session, but that is not always possible. And doing the other person's family the next session, though ideal, is also not always possible. Sometimes urgent issues have arisen, and completing the genogram, or starting to do the other person's, has to be temporarily put on hold. Later in the chapter I describe how to do an abbreviated version of a genogram that, although not as wide-ranging, will still provide insight into the individual's psychology.

The first decision that has to be made is with whom to start. Often I have a preference. If possible, I like to start with the person whom I don't "get" as well. Perhaps one person in the couple has been more guarded than the other. Or one person's feelings and behaviors seem extreme and not proportional to the current situation the couple has been describing. Or perhaps I am having trouble empathizing with one person or, despite my efforts to be systemic and nonjudgmental, find myself silently thinking that one person is more "at fault" than the other. Getting a family history almost always helps me understand and like the person better, not only because I see him or her in context, but because many people open up and are much less defensive when talking about themselves in the context of providing family history.

When I have a preference, I casually say, something like, for instance, *"Briana, how about if we start with you?"* I don't give any particular explanation, and if the person objects to going first, I don't push or explain my suggestion, but rather turn to the other person. Though I might have liked one or another of the couple to go first, it is not worth making that person uncomfortable or more defensive and I certainly don't want to engage in any power struggle.

Before starting the genogram I explain that I'm going to ask the spouse for input from time to time about family members of her partner that she may have met. Interestingly, sometimes, a spouse is quite close to some members of her partner's family and actually can add information or stories that the partner has never heard.

Initially I diagram a very basic three-generational family tree with the most simple key information. Basic information about the family is obtained first—ethnicity, divorces, deaths, remarriages, religion, social class, and so on. Since I am hoping to use all this *factual* information to understand more about the individual's psychology, I always ask (and include on the chart) how old the person was at the time of various events. I want this information because I am looking for events that may have influenced the patient in some way consciously or unconsciously, and thus knowing the patient's age at the time of various life markers is crucial basic information.

Family Stories and Personality Descriptions

After this initial charting, I begin asking for personality descriptions and family stories that will help me get to know more about the unique and idiosyncratic worldview of the person doing the genogram. I ask the person to give me some adjectives that tell me what the family member is or was like. So, for example, I would say, *"Tell me about your mother [grandmother, stepfather, etc.] . . . give me some adjectives that describe her."* Frequently people will mention that the person has changed considerably with age. To this, I'll reply, *"Tell me what she was like when you were growing up and how she is different now."* In order to really get a sense of what these adjectives mean, I pick a few and ask for a story that illustrates what is meant. So, for instance, I might say, in response to some description like "controlling," "passive," "energetic," "nonassertive," "charming," "very smart," or "anxious," *"Give me an example, a story that will give me a good sense of what she's like."*

If someone never knew a grandparent—or even a parent—I ask what s/he imagines the person to have been like. *"From stories you have heard, or even bits and pieces of information here or there, what do you think [her grandmother] was like?"* Not infrequently, someone will say they know absolutely nothing about a grandparent or an absent or deceased parent. When that is the case, I'm interested in the person's thoughts about the absence of information, and would ask, for example, *"Why do you think your mother never talked about your grandmother?"*

Often discussion about one set of grandparents spontaneously leads to descriptions of the other. When that happens, instead of working on just one side of the family, I switch to the other grandparents and ask for adjectives and stories that flesh them out too. Regardless of whether we discuss one set of grandparents or both, I generally switch to the person's siblings before getting descriptions of aunts and uncles. The purpose of these questions is to get a better sense of the individual, and thus there really are no hard-and-fast rules about the order in which the inquiry occurs. Because I don't do a genogram until I've worked with a couple for at least a few sessions, I already have some issues in mind that I want to explore, and when I hear something that seems relevant to that issue, I am likely to deviate from my plan and follow my clinical instincts.

Questions about Relationships

Genograms provide therapists with an opportunity to expand their understanding about how an individual thinks about various couples' relationships—what his or her image is of a good or bad relationship, what relationships can offer, and how people adjust to and cope with one another. Thus, I not only ask about the personalities of family members but what their relationships were like. For example, when someone is describing grandparents, I would ask such questions as *"How did your grandparents get along?"*; *"What do you think they got from one another?"*; or *"How did your grandmother handle your grandfather's irritability?"* Often the person doing the genogram does not know very much about his or her grandparents' relationship. Here again, I encourage speculation and fantasies, and this is perhaps even more relevant to the couple's issues than so called reality.

Because of the structured nature of the questioning, factual information about the extended family often emerges that would not be likely to have come up spontaneously. For example, when Liz described her aunts and uncles she mentioned that one uncle died in his mid-40s from complications of routine hernia surgery. Or when Donald described his cousins he mentioned that "one was a perfectly normal kid who became schizophrenic when he went to college and now lives on the street." Whenever a fact is volunteered, I ask the person how old s/he was at the time. Often this takes some figuring out because when the event that occurred did not happen to an *immediate* family member, the person has usually not thought about that occurrence as an event in his or her own life. So, for instance, Liz, after thinking about where she lived when she heard of her uncle's sudden untimely death, was able to calculate that she must have just started second grade in a new school. Later, further discussion of this event led to an understanding that her mother's grief at the loss of the sibling she was closest to meant that Liz was more on her own in a new situation than she had ever been before, and that "abandonment" issues she had when her husband was "tense and preoccupied" were probably related to this period in her life. And, similarly, Donald realized that his cousin's breakdown when Donald was 16 had played a role in his being "so uptight around people smoking weed and acting crazy," and that this may contribute to how disgusted he gets when his wife very occasionally "has one drink too many and gets a little tipsy."

Participation of the Spouse

Involving the listening partner whenever one can is important for several reasons. First of all, it is difficult for many people to passively listen for an entire session. Even though the material gathered is likely to be quite relevant to the couple's issues, that isn't necessarily apparent until I give feedback at the end of the meeting. Even when the stories and descriptions of family members are unfamiliar, the spouse may feel that this isn't about them as a *couple,* and thus that his or her presence seems unnecessary. Thus, I tell the couple in advance that I'm going to ask the spouse for input about family members that s/he knows or has met. Knowing that at some point s/he will be asked to give input facilitates active listening. Often the person doing the genogram will spontaneously turn to the partner for corroboration and elaboration of the descriptions. Of course, this is likely to happen only in instances where the partners are in general agreement about a family member. When this does not spontaneously occur, I might turn to the partner and ask, *"Can you add anything to the description?"* or *"What have* you *observed about how your wife's parent's interact with one another?"*

Sometimes this contribution by the other partner, and the sense of both that the partner sees what might not be obvious to an outsider, heightens the sense of the couple being a "we," with shared experiences and perceptions. At other times differences or conflicts emerge, and when that occurs, I make a note to get back to the issue in another session and continue with the genogram.

When a spouse describes a family member or relationship differently than his or her partner does, the therapist has an opportunity to learn something about the dimensions of personality and relationships that are particularly meaningful to the person's partner. For example, Cheryl described her mother as insecure, and part of what she got from her father was his calmness and ability to take charge of situations. Her husband, Rick, saw Cheryl's parents' relationship somewhat differently. He felt that Cheryl's mother resented her husband for being such a "take-charge" person and was acting more helpless than she actually was as a way of punishing him. The "truth" here is not knowable, or even particularly relevant. Each person's interpretation of what they see in the relationship tells us a great deal about his or her sensitivities and concerns. So, I would ask myself, does Cheryl wish that Rick would be steadier when she is anxious? Is Rick inclined to see some behavior as a "passive–aggressive" expression of resentment? These are very preliminary thoughts that I would jot down for further exploration, knowing full well that they could easily be incorrect; not every difference in perception is a personally meaningful projection.

At times, a spouse is aware of a glaring omission in his or her partner's narrative. The things that have been omitted can range anywhere from instances of sexual or physical abuse in the family, to a family member being engaged in some criminal activity outside the family and having been incarcerated, to a parent having had affairs or even a second "secret family." I assume that shame plays a big role in the person having omitted the information, so I try as best I can to prevent the spouse from blurting out something, and instead ask the one doing the genogram if it's okay for his or her partner to talk about what has been left out. Responses can range from "I'd rather not talk about that—I don't think it's relevant" to "Sure, you can mention it, be my guest." Most often, however, once the spouse broaches the subject, the person is likely to be okay talking about it then and there, but if not I'll ask if meeting alone for a session would make it more comfortable to discuss what is being referred to.

Though it is essential for the spouse to participate, the therapist needs to be prepared for heightened defensiveness and an increase in conflict if what is said is experienced by the person doing the genogram as overly critical. It's a common phenomenon for people who feel okay about expressing anger, frustration, and sometimes even disdain for a member of their family to resent their spouse saying the same thing. The spouse may feel she is simply joining with her partner and being supportive and doesn't understand the angry and defensive reaction that has occurred. When this happens I defuse it by normalizing the reaction, saying something like *"Yes, this happens all the time. One person feels, 'It's okay for me to say it, but when my wife jumps on the bandwagon it feels like piling on.'"* Additionally, I explain that often reminding one's partner of some *good* things about his family is very much appreciated. But, of course, it is a delicate judgment call, since that can be seen as a lack of empathy for the spouse's negative feelings.

Additionally, in the context of adding his perspective on the other's family, a spouse may heatedly point to a complaint and a dynamic in the couple's own relationship that is a source of considerable hurt, anger, and conflict. For instance, Peter described his wife's parents as "snobs who think they know better than anyone about everything—and Susie [Peter's wife] is completely dependent on their opinions about things. It really infuriates me—she'll ask them for advice about something before she asks me, and what *they* say counts a lot more than anything I have to offer." Or Bianca said of Leona's parents, "They're very phony—particularly her mother—I know she gossips about me, and though she acts warmly when I'm there she's really homophobic and hates that I'm 'butch.' And Leona is so concerned about pleasing both her parents that she insists I wear a skirt when we visit and gets really mad at me if I touch her at all—even taking her hand—in front of them." When obviously important topics like this arise, I note them down and assure the couple that we will get to this issue later but for now I'd like to continue with the genogram.

Siblings

Ideally, I would ask the same type of questions about siblings as I did about the parents and grandparents—for example, adjectives that describe them, stories that bring to life the adjectives, what their relationships are like, and so on. But realistically, there is seldom time for this much detail. Instead I start by getting basic information—for example, ages, marital or relationship status, children, where they live, and the like. Then I simply ask *"What do you think is important for me to know about each of your siblings—what stands out about them?"*

I ask too what the relationship with each sibling was like when they were growing up and what's it like now. Since my goal is to learn as much as possible about the individual concerns and perceptions of the person whose genogram I'm doing, I also ask questions that encourage self-reflection. So, for instance, I might ask, *"Which of your siblings do you think is most like you?"; "Most different from you?"; "What characteristics do you share?"; "How did your family background affect you similarly or differently?"* Comparative questions such as these often help the person talk about how they see their strengths and weaknesses. Oscar, for example, the principal of a charter school that had recently been cited as one of the most successful ones nationwide, described his sister as "much smarter than me"—a comment that surprised his long-time partner, Carmen. This was a deeply held belief by Oscar, despite the fact that he had an EdD as well as an MA in public health and had clearly more than made up for his mediocre performance in grade school. Similarly, when Jaime said in a self-disparaging tone that his brother was braver and more of a risk-taker, his wife concurred, but saw this character trait as an asset of Jaime's not a deficit.

In general, with siblings too, I regularly ask for input from the listening spouse. *"What's your take on this? How do you see their relationship?"* Often the spouse basically agrees with how the siblings have been described, but nonetheless, s/he may add a detail that enhances the portrait presented. For instance, John said of Sarah's brother, "He's good-hearted but more out of it than Sienna realizes. I think because she's used to him she just doesn't notice how strange he is—like when he visited us during our vacation at the beach and sat under the umbrella wearing a jacket and tie!" Or Marie said of Anthony and his brother: "Yes, I agree that his brother can be a bully and they butt heads—but a lot of the time they're like kids having a fight—they roll around on the floor and wrestle with each other—and when one of them gets hurt accidentally, they scream at each other just like my kids. And Anthony left out that when they're together they drink a lot, and that's how the fights start."

THE GENOGRAM AS A PROJECTIVE TECHNIQUE

Perhaps the most interesting use of the genogram in the context of couple therapy is the way it can function as something akin to a method of obtaining projective material. Descriptions of family members, as well as the "family stories" remembered and transformed in the telling, act as a map to schemas, assumptions, and intrapsychic conflicts about which the individual is often not fully aware. The yield of the genogram involves a mixture of reality information and the individual's unique "take" on the facts. The large amount of data generated by the genogram provides both explicit and subtle clues to the unspoken and perhaps unconscious fears, wishes, and values of the individual.

The choices people make as to what to focus on when selecting from the myriad of possibilities available when trying to describe many people tell us a good deal about their concerns and the perhaps unconscious schemas that influence their experiences and ways of being in relationships. For example, the first thing Ariana said about her mother was that she had lost her father when she was only 7 and it had been a great hardship to her mother to have lost a parent at such a young age. That Ariana chose this story of loss as one of the most significant facts about her mother tells us something about her mother, but also possibly suggests that Ariana herself is deeply concerned about issues of loss and abandonment. We might also speculate that Ariana was the mother's "caretaker," so to speak, and that seeing her mother as hurt by loss made it difficult for Ariana to "abandon" her by fully committing herself to her husband and their marriage. One might also wonder if it made it difficult for Ariana to have her own needs for nurturance attended to. In a different vein, Rhiana's description of her grandmother as "a smart lady, who, even though she was a single parent working a night shift and didn't get home until midnight, was so determined that her kids would go to college that she'd wake them up at 5:00 in the morning to study with them" tells us as much about how Rhianna values ambition and determination as it does about her grandmother.

Inferences are drawn, of course not just from *what* is said, but from the tone of voice and the accompanying affect—Is the story told with pride? With contempt? With dismay? When Duane, for example, described his older cousin as "the family nerd," his smile made it clear that he *admired* him for not succumbing to the family's—and the neighborhood cool kids'— antipathy toward "geeks." Or when Emilia described her aunt as someone known in the family for "never letting herself get pushed around by men," her shrug made it clear that despite her positive feelings about this attitude, she also had concerns about her aunt having a bit of a "chip on her shoulder." And when Genevieve described her grandmother as someone who was so self-confident that "she'd walk into traffic because she assumed cars would stop for her," her affect made it clear that she felt very negatively about this kind of arrogance. All of these hypotheses and speculations must, of course, be evaluated in light of the observations that accrue in the course of the work. But often we only notice what we are prepared to notice, and the provisional hypotheses afforded by the genogram can help us to see what we might otherwise have overlooked.

In addition to seeing the particular *selection* of family stories as conveying what is meaningful to the individual doing the genogram, it is also helpful to notice the characteristic *dimensions* on which people are described. Family members are often compared and distinguished from one another around specific features—an indication that these character and personality traits are ones to which the individual is especially attuned. But like any projective method the genogram only gives us hints or *inklings* about concerns and internal conflicts. These then need to be further explored to assess their actual relevance to the person's individual and relationship issues. Craig, for instance, described the women in his family (on both sides) in terms of how competent or incompetent they were. Some were described as hapless or dependent, some as dynamos, self-starters, or brilliant. But almost all were depicted along the dimension of competence or incompetence. Though Craig had always known that it was important for him to be with a strong, independent woman, he had not quite registered just how important an issue this was to him until doing the genogram. Upon further exploration it became clear that his encouragement (or "pushing," as his wife described it) for her to go back to work soon after their first child was born was much less about financial pressures than it was about his anxiety that his wife would become too dependent on him.

Melinda described many family members according to whether they had married for love or "for money." This was clearly a family theme and she had grown up with the story of her parents having eloped and although having had to struggle financially for much of their marriage, being proud of having married for the right reasons. She heard too, in contrast, how uncles on both sides of the family had explicitly rejected "romance" and had married for "convenience," or money. The fact that these marriages were now of 20 to 30 years duration, and seemed, at least on the surface, fairly good, in no way seemed to alter her mother's—and consequently her own—critical stance in regard to the uncles' marriage choices. The characterization of marriages along the dimension of "love" versus "convenience" proved to be an extremely relevant issue in the tensions between Melinda and her husband and one that had never explicitly been talked about.

Often, as in the case of Melinda, family stories seem to have been swallowed whole during youth and remain undigested by the adult. Such stories can have a powerful effect because they have never been examined by mature critical intelligence. Not infrequently, it is not until relating the stories as part of doing the genogram that the individual actually *thinks* about the validity of what s/he has implicitly accepted as true for his or her whole life.

For instance, one man said that his father had almost died from a heart attack because he "worked too hard to support his ailing mother, wife, and three children." This was the family story he first heard when he was age 9 and never questioned. Now at age 39, Henry believed this narrative as thoroughly as he had during his childhood. A very intelligent man, whose work involved analyzing complex data, Henry somehow mentally separated this story from the rest of what he knew about his father—that he smoked, was overweight, and was very sedentary. Recognition of the lesson learned in childhood that "domestic responsibilities can kill you" provided an important insight into his apprehension about the prospect of having a child. The belief that the pressure of taking care of a family might literally kill him was unconscious until brought to the surface by the genogram.

GIVING FEEDBACK

At the conclusion of the genogram I share some of what I have noticed about the characteristics that are important to the person doing the genogram. Frequently, people are intrigued by this feedback, because they haven't been quite aware of the centrality to them of certain personality traits. So, for instance, I might say *"I noticed how you described many of the men in the family as 'kind,' or 'gentle' or sometimes quite the opposite, but what struck me is that 'kindness' in men—its presence or its absence—is an important dimension to you. It's something you value and take note of when it's absent."*

Or, to a man who included in his list of adjectives about numerous women in the family words like "clear-headed," "very together," and "calm," or conversely, "hysterical," "emotional," "bonkers," and the like, I might say, *"It strikes me that a woman being rational and even-tempered is something that really matters to you and you notice where women in the family fit along that dimension."* I may offer at that time some tentative thoughts about possible links to the couples' difficulties but won't do so if I think that it will stir defensiveness or may stimulate or reignite an argument that has been temporarily put on hold while we examine family history.

As the reader has seen throughout this book, I am always on the lookout for opportunities to address the person's most painful, or conflicted, or vulnerable experiences in a fashion that will feel constructive—and, importantly, will be *heard* rather than warded off. This is just as important in giving feedback about the information gathered in doing the genogram as it is in all the other aspects of the work. As I talked about in Chapter 1, it is all too easy for therapists to focus on pathology. Although, of course, in doing the genogram we see some of the ways that experiences in the family of origin have negatively affected the person's current relationship, we must also look at the material gathered with an eye toward identifying strengths that evolved out of the family experience and potential alternative foundations for new ways of relating to one's partner.

Interestingly, even when people feel quite negatively about how their parents treated them or the kind of background they came from, they generally welcome feedback that also is attuned to whatever features of their family or its values and characteristics they may be proud of, as long as that feedback does not deny, minimize, or contradict their primary experience. Kim, who came from a severely dysfunctional home—both her parents were alcoholics who put Kim, the oldest child, in charge of the younger ones "while they were out partying and getting drunk"—was startled but receptive when the therapist noted that *"in light of all that was wrong, I was struck and a little surprised about your description of the family going to church together on Sunday mornings and then out for a buffet lunch at the local hotel. It seems that when your parents were sober they had some wish, at least for a couple of hours, to be a family. And I'm even more surprised at how they wanted you each to give your opinion about the sermon. It seems that they really encouraged you all to think for yourselves. Of course, that doesn't really change the reality of your family life, but it may be part of why you are such an independent thinker."*

In a similar vein, the therapist might note the absence of something negative that the person has taken for granted. For instance, after Stefan described family get-togethers as fraught with tensions and family feuds, I commented that *"in your family there could be serious, and at times very nasty discord, but somehow everyone stayed connected and tried to work things out. From what you've told me it seems like nobody ever cuts off contact—nobody refuses to go to family events. That's not true in every family where there is conflict, so it's noteworthy."*

Josie, who described her parents as having a bitter divorce, was surprised when I said, *"It's striking that even though your parents got divorced when you were quite young and your father lived in a different city, both he and your mother made sure that you would see a lot of him. My impression is that they could put aside their own hostility to one another to do what was best for you and your siblings. Is that right?"*

It is also can be helpful and affirming to give feedback about the way a person has dealt with a difficult family situation. For instance, Shawnta, in talking about her mother, said she hadn't had "had much to do with her for years. She has a bad temper and when I was a kid she was physically abusive." She went on to say that a couple of years ago she started seeing her mother more frequently. "I really have forgiven her—it was how she was brought up. She actually thought whacking a kid was the way to make sure they didn't go bad. I reconnected with her but I have very firm boundaries and she's careful how she talks to me. I never leave her alone with my kids." Part of my feedback to Shawnta was that *"she seemed to be someone who wanted to* <u>understand</u> *and thus temper her anger as long as it didn't put herself or her family at risk."* Or, when Rita described learning to get along with her "certifiably borderline" sister by reading some self-help books on the topic, I said, *"I'm impressed not only with your wanting to do that, but that you were actually able to use the advice. Are you generally like that—a problem solver—taking ideas and running with them?"*

In giving feedback, a general rule of thumb is to be careful never to "pile on" or exaggerate the negatives that a person is expressing. Though it is important to acknowledge and affirm that a person was mistreated, it is easy to go too far and trigger defensiveness. An important therapeutic skill is to be able to join with a patient without overdoing it. Experienced therapists will recognize the phenomenon in which you think you have just restated in slightly stronger terms what the patient has said, but their reaction is to say something like, "It wasn't *that* bad." Most people do not want to see themselves as victims or as having been deeply scarred by the events of their childhood.

Particular care needs to be taken in this regard when doing couple therapy. The couple dynamic may be such that the individual who has been hurt by his or her family does not want to be seen by the spouse as the "damaged one." In individual therapy, the therapist might use the defensive, recoiling response as an opportunity to examine the patient's need to minimize the harm inflicted on him or her. In couple therapy, that approach can be tricky and can fuel a combative response by the spouse. Thus, one might not highlight this in the same way unless minimization of emotional harm is a theme in the couple's relationship.

I might on occasion also give some feedback to both the listener and the person whose genogram I've been doing in regard to how they interacted during the process. Early in the session Felicia, Julia's soon-to-be wife, interrupted her narrative and said, "Come on—be real—you know that your dad had affairs—tell the truth." Felicia didn't get angry, but firmly set boundaries, saying, "It's my family history—I'll tell it the way I want to." When I gave feedback, I mentioned that though there was clearly some tension between them at that moment, they both handled it well. Felicia said, "Back off," and Julia said, "Sorry," and in the rest of the session asked permission to add something if she saw things differently. Not infrequently a spouse may chime in with a *supportive* comment, like "She's being kind about her brother—he's much more difficult to deal with than she's describing—but somehow Caroline hangs in there." Later, I might point out that it was clear that he admired how his wife persists in trying to have a relationship with her brother and how he had made a point to voice his admiration. Or I might say to someone, *"I was struck by how interested you were in hearing about your husband's family even though a lot of this family history is probably pretty familiar to you."*

USING WHAT WE HAVE LEARNED

The genogram provides us with data that we might not otherwise have when people relate their family history in the way they have told it many times before. Not infrequently, the person whose genogram I am doing is startled by what can seem like almost an uncanny accuracy about what has come to light about his or her assumptions, concerns, and values. But the truth is that there is nothing mysterious about what the therapist can infer from the material that has been generated. The genogram per se does not magically give us useful information. It simply provides us with a type of information that gives us more to work with; the usefulness of what may be surmised depends on how skillfully we use it clinically. Thus, as I collect family stories, descriptions of family members, and the dynamics between them, I jot down on the side of the paper one- or two-word notes to myself about how some of what I am learning might be of use in my work with the couple.

Here are some of the ways the information obtained in the genogram informs my clinical work.

Deepening the Couple's Understanding of Problematic Patterns and Increasing Empathy for One Another

Having a rich historical narrative that provides some context or explanation for the clashes they are having helps them be less blaming of one another and enables them to more easily step back and *externalize* the conflict and say something like "Oh no—the pattern has taken hold of us again." Though insight into the pattern they are engaged in is helpful, *avoiding* these automatic actions and reactions is, of course, even better. In the next chapter we look at active interventions that can enable the couple to resist the pull of habitual ways of interacting.

In addition to elucidating the source of negative cyclical interactions, the genogram enables the therapist to make connections that explain an individual's psychological makeup in ways that both partners can readily "get." When the therapist underlines the stressors, events, and family dynamics that have understandably left their mark on each person's psyche, many couples are able to have more empathy for one another and feel less angry and frustrated by behaviors and needs that derive from these experiences.

Learning Each Person's Language

Another important benefit of doing the genogram in the way I've described is that it not only highlights attributes and values that are of concern to the person, but also enables us to use the specific language that is most likely to "speak to" and be accepted by him or her. An awareness of the emotional meaning of particular words can help the therapist and the spouse avoid talking about something in a way that will trigger resistance, and conversely, can help us say things in a way that is more likely to "reach" or make sense to the person. By noticing the words and phrases that have been used repeatedly, the therapist is better able to couch statements in a way more likely to bypass defensive reactions. For example, when describing men in his family, Roberto would frequently use the word "sweet." He talked about his uncle as "a tough businessman who was very *sweet* with his kids." His father, though demanding, was "basically a sweet guy." This was particularly noteworthy because Roberto was quite put off when his wife would complain that he wasn't "nurturant" or "sensitive" to her when she was feeling upset about something. Insulted, he rejected her claims and countered that "I'm your husband, not your mother." The genogram helped to explain his defensiveness. Roberto felt that he, like the men he admired, was basically "sweet," and when I raised this issue, his wife said, "Yes, of course, he's at heart a real softy—very sweet." In fact, it was in large part because she *knew* he was sweet that she wanted more nurturance from him. Once they could talk about what his wife was longing for in terms of incorporating into their relationship the "sweet" self that was already there, the couple was able to join together to find ways to enable his "sweetness" to be expressed more overtly.

As I discussed in Chapter 3, helping couples convert complaints into wishes is a central component of the work. Often the person doing the genogram will use words that are quite compatible with what their partner is longing for. For instance, Jayne felt her partner, Len, with whom she had lived for the last 6 years, was "becoming a couch potato." Jayne was concerned about how bored she was feeling in the relationship. She loved Len, but felt their life together was too insular and isolated. She wanted more excitement and stimulation. Len was very hurt by Jayne's "complaint" and worried that they were just too different. Yet, in doing his genogram, Len described numerous men and women along the dimension of whether or not they were "fun-loving." And Jayne had used this phrase to describe her initial attraction to Len. By saying to Len that something was getting in the way of his being his "fun-loving" self, I was able to address the issue with Len in a way that countered his feeling that there was nothing he could do to change how Jayne was feeling.

And of course just as we learn useful words to *use*, we learn too what words both the therapist and the spouse should *avoid*. Some words are inherently negative—for example, *controlling*, *self-centered*, *arrogant*—and we don't need the genogram to tell us (and the spouse) that talking in this way will only elicit a negative response. But sometimes in doing the genogram we can see that words that might be neutral for most people have a negative connotation for that particular person. For instance, Andrew described his father as having no time for his kids: "He was *ambitious*—making it big was the only thing that really mattered to him." Or Francine described many women in the family as "*charming*," but this was said in the context of seeing them as more concerned with appearances than "what was real."

Clues to Unexpressed Parts of the Self

Often a source of tension in couples is that one person feels negatively about a personality characteristic of the other. I am not talking here about traits that have a direct effect on the partner—for instance, one person might find the other too controlling, or too concerned with neatness, and so forth. Rather, I am referring to personality characteristics that by and large do not have a direct impact on the relationship per se, *except for the fact* that one person is disapproving of the other. So, for instance, Sophia was very embarrassed by what she regarded as her husband's lack of tact—for example, saying to someone at a party, "I can't believe you liked that 'chick-lit' book"—and often after an evening out they would argue about the appropriateness of how he had acted. Or, Carla, who worked at a very demanding job, would be extremely hurt and withdraw when Jack responded to her occasionally taking a "play hookie" day by sarcastically commenting that she was "spoiled."

Sometimes the negative feeling about something one's spouse does represents a true difference in values. For instance, Pema, who was Tibetan, came from a family and culture where "self-promotion" was frowned upon and she found it distasteful and "wrong" when her husband, Thomas, would talk about some of his accomplishments. But in many instances, the dislike of a trait in one's spouse derives from the denial of that inclination in oneself. So, for example, the person who derides any expression of anxiety in the other may be so adamant about it because he has not made room for that feeling in himself. Or the person who sees his spouse as too needy may be denying his own need for reassurance and care taking. In other words, sometimes the criticism is not a clash of values but rather a reflection of internal conflict about one's own longings.

If the therapist can help a person get in touch with and accept denied aspects of his or her self, s/he will be more comfortable when seeing its expression in the other and usually will not feel as much need to criticize or denounce the way the partner is acting. The genogram can be a "safe" way for people to explore aspects of the self that they have not been paying attention to. Descriptions of relatives in the genogram can provide useful clues about conflicted impulses that the person may then be able to recognize and acknowledge. Alex, for example, described a number of uncles in terms of how much or how little fun they had in life. By noticing his smile and animated expression when describing one uncle as "a little wild—like a kid," it was possible to point out to Alex that he seemed to long to be a bit more that way himself. This led to a discussion of how he had told himself he had to "grow up" when he became a father but did miss "getting a little crazy once in a while." That insight eventually led to a discussion of how his wife could help him get a little bit of that old self back, and it was the beginning of his being less judgmental about his wife's "irresponsible" occasional shopping sprees. Similarly, Ester, who clearly admired a cousin whom everyone else in the family regarded as a black sheep, was receptive to the therapist's comment about her perhaps wanting to conform less to her family's expectations.

Pointing the Way to New Ways of Interacting

If we listen with an ear to latent meanings, we often get a sense of some possible solutions to difficult interactions that had not heretofore been seen. Sam recognized that he was "obsessive–compulsive" and perfectionistic. But despite his awareness of these traits, he continued to comment about and critique his wife on numerous things that she didn't do "correctly." When describing various relatives, Sam spoke of an uncle of whom he was particularly fond as "a wonderful man, but he can be pretty rigid some times." As an aside he added, "My aunt knows how to deal with him when he gets that way—and they're really close. She'd tell him quietly that he's being 'stubborn as a mule,' walk away, and then a few hours later he'd change his mind. No fighting about it—she just basically told him 'cut it out.'" Though this situation was not directly parallel to his own, it led to a discussion of his thoughts about how his partner should "handle" him when his perfectionism results in his being controlling and critical. He believed that if his wife could disengage, it might really help him to gain perspective. If instead of angrily snapping back at him "when I'm being a pain," she simply said something like "You're being *too much*," he thought he would quickly "get it," stop, and even apologize. He recognized that this was asking a lot of his wife, and that he needed to work on controlling *his own* behavior, but nonetheless realized that "in the best marriage I've ever seen, that way of responding worked really well."

Conversely, the genogram can also illuminate how a way of handling difficulties that was learned from interactions with the family of origin does not work well in the current relationship and needs to be changed. For instance, Laura described her nuclear family as one in which her sister and her parents were "at war." In relating her family history, almost every family she described had at least one child who "was a terror" and others who were "sweethearts." Laura had learned that it was "of course better to be someone who goes along to get along." She was often told by her mother that she was the "bonus baby" in her family in that she was cheerful and easy-going in contrast to her siblings, who were difficult. Her easy-going attitude served her well in most of her life. She had many friends and was well liked in her workplace. But in her relationship with her husband, Kenneth, her "cooperativeness" felt more like disengagement than just being easy-going. He wished she had some stronger preferences and found it burdensome to be relied upon to plan all weekend activities, vacations, and other features of their life. Her "cooperative" stance also sometimes resulted in her going along with rather big decisions that she would later resent. This is clearly a dynamic that would have been obvious even without the genogram. But, for Laura, seeing how her world growing up was divided into "terrors" or "sweethearts" highlighted for her how powerful the inclination was to be "agreeable" but at the price of fully knowing and expressing herself.

The genogram generates a good deal of material to work with. But we need to use the insights gained and the goodwill generated to help the couple actively address their relationship issues. The therapist must help couples translate their new understandings of themself and their partner into changed ways of interacting. Thus, the next chapter focuses on the numerous ways that our hypothesis about the influences of each person's family background can be both further explored and utilized to help them interact in ways that are more gratifying to them both.

9

❧

"The Things They Carry"
Working with Legacy Issues

*T*he concept I am trying to convey by the term "legacy issues" is perfectly captured by the evocative title of Tim O'Brien's novel *The Things They Carried* (1990). Whether via a genogram or from a host of other ways in the course of conducting sessions, the therapist gradually develops a keener understanding of what each person "carries" into the relationship—the particular mix of values, cultural expectations, fond and painful memories, aversions, longings, vulnerabilities, strengths, anxieties, and assumptions about love, trust, and marriage. These, in toto, make each person unique. It is not, however, the mere knowledge or understanding of each person's individual psychology that leads to new ways of feeling and acting. For deep and lasting changes to occur, new, emotionally resonant *experiences* must be generated. In couple therapy, these new experiences include the couple interacting in a new manner with one another. But these changes are not merely behavioral; the couple, and each partner individually, come to *feel* differently about themselves and their partners.

This chapter describes a range of interventions that can generate the kind of change that makes a couple's life together genuinely different and enhanced. The interventions are designed to move the work from *insight* to *action*. But the relationship between the two poles is reciprocal, not sequential. That is, the interventions not only build upon the insights gained in the work, but the new ways the couple interact enable each partner to know and actualize parts of the self that may have been tamped down, denied, or disassociated.

In the way of working described here, each intervention with a couple is in a sense custom-designed by the therapist and the couple collaboratively. As I said earlier, this is not a "one-size-fits-all" approach. There is not a singular set of interventions that work, say, for couples dealing with abandonment issues or another package of interventions to be employed when there is fear of dependency, or a third "prescription" to be used with couples in which one person dissociates when angry. Instead, the therapist helps the couple explore the sensitivities, expectations, schemas, and coping mechanisms that are causing difficulties in the relationship, and together they come up with individualized ways to prevent the vicious circles that can result from the ways that each partner's vulnerabilities intersect with the other's.

Even when one person's emotional problems contribute more to the couple's difficulties than the other's, that person does not have to be "fixed" or "cured" in order for the impact on the relationship to be significantly lessened. For example, one partner may suffer from severe anxiety or depression, is too quick to get angry, or has a strong tendency to feel rejected. That does not mean the individual suffering from these issues does not need to work on them or that a referral for individual therapy or a medication consult might not be called for. I often say to couples, *"All of us are stuck with emotional baggage from our childhood, and even after individual therapy these issues still have a hold on us. In our work together, we will try to find ways to not let these issues affect the relationship quite as much as they are right now, but also we'll see if there are ways you can help one another with these issues. In other words, in a good relationship, your problems are not yours alone, and you do not have to solve them entirely by yourself."*

In what follows you will find a "sampling" of some of the active strategies that have worked with couples to change dysfunctional patterns that derive from individual sensitivities, self-definitions, problematic narratives, and unconscious schemas. Often a good deal of experimentation is required before a solution "takes." When a couple doesn't follow through on a plan that they have come up with, or when what they tried didn't work very well, or wasn't done in the way we had talked about, I take that to mean that the "solution" that made sense in the office wasn't really right for their real-life situation. I take it as my responsibility to make sure that the couple does not feel that *they* failed and that they do not blame one another. I model for them a problem-solving, trial-and-error approach, and I say something like *"If you couldn't get yourself to do what we had planned, then it just wasn't the right approach, and we need to keep working on it. Let's put our heads together to see why it wasn't realistic, and see what else we can come up with."* Alternatively, I might say, *"Obviously, this plan needs fine-tuning. Let's look at what you each could do that would make it more effective."*

Throughout the process I am the voice of realism. So if someone says, "I just have to try harder," I might say, *"Maybe, but I think the problem is probably not that you didn't try hard enough, but that what we came up with wasn't quite right. Let's see if we can come up with some things that feel easier for you to do and more compatible with who you are."* The bottom line here is that I do not automatically assume that the plan didn't work because of "resistance" or a wish on one or both of their parts to keep the status quo. It is not that resistance is never a factor in why the couple is stuck. There are times, for example, when progress isn't being made because one or both partners are quite ambivalent about whether or not they want to stay together. One or both of them may hold back from trying to interact in a different way because s/he feels concerned that it will make it seem like s/he is more committed to the relationship than s/he actually feels or may be (consciously or unconsciously) worried that the marriage will improve just enough to make it hard to leave but still be only "tolerable," and not genuinely gratifying.

PROBLEMS WITH ANGER

Vignette 1: Suzanne and Matt

Suzanne and Matt came to couple therapy at a point when Suzanne was seriously thinking that it might be time to end the relationship. She still loved Matt and believed that he loved her too, but felt that she couldn't respect herself if she continued to live with the verbal abuse that spewed out from him when he erupted in rage. It's not that this happened very often—maybe twice a year—but when it happened, he said "such cruel and vile things that I feel crazy for staying with him. What kind of woman stays in a marriage after someone who supposedly loves them says such vicious things? He seems to want to put a knife in my heart. I *think* he really loves me, but then I think I'm kidding myself—I'm just convenient for him—and what he *really* feels comes out in those explosions. I deserve more, and unless I know that this will never happen again—and feel that he really loves me—I'm going to have to move on in my life. We have two great kids and I really love Matt, but these horrible outbursts hurt me so much. I just can't get over them."

Matt felt great shame about what happened when he "lost it." He never hit Suzanne, but "after cursing at her and saying things that I know will really destroy her, I sometimes am in such a rage that I go in another room and start breaking things—my stuff actually—things that matter to me. I never break anything of hers. She's rightly furious, but she tortures me by not talking to me for days. I tried anger management therapy for a while, but clearly it didn't help—maybe because most of the time I'm not an angry person. I don't feel anger coming on, but suddenly I'm in a rage. I've gone to a neurologist to see if there's something wrong with me, and he had me get a CT scan to see if there might be something pressing on my brain. I was fine. And anyway, this isn't a recent thing. It's happened for years and used to happen in my first marriage too."

In the first few sessions, we had looked at some of the strengths in the relationship as well as some of the concerns either might have in addition to Matt's explosions. They both agreed that they had enormous respect for the other's values and intelligence. "He's a really good man. Really honorable. I respect how he handled his divorce—how civilized it was. And he's a great father to our two boys, and to his teenage daughter—not an easy kid to parent. But he hangs in there, and he's consistent about seeing her even though she pushes him away and is still angry about the divorce." Matt similarly said that there could be no better mother than Suzanne. "She's great. Everything runs smoothly at home because of *her*."

They both described a problematic dynamic that was there almost from the start of their relationship. "I'm not a very expressive person," said Matt, "and I know she's disappointed a lot. When I've hurt her feelings—unfortunately, that's frequently—she wants to talk about it and I'm not good at that." Suzanne added, "I don't know how to get through to him about how hurt I am by the things he says sometimes—not just the couple of times a year when he explodes and says *vile* things—but the more ordinary routine way he says things that hurt my feelings."

As discussed earlier, in addition to focusing on their problems, I try to get the couple to describe some of what they might like or wish for other than just the elimination of the negatives. The line between what one wishes for and what is a problem to be eliminated is not always so clear; sometimes they are two sides of a coin. But Suzanne had no trouble answering this question. She wished that Matt was more attentive and showed his love for her more explicitly. She felt that she wasn't on his mind at all. For example, he often didn't remember to ask her about important things in her life. Even when he had helped her prepare for a job interview, he "forgot" that she had it and didn't ask how it went. And though she remembered all *his* doctor's appointments—he had a number of chronic medical conditions that he needed to stay on top of—he never asked about her appointments, even when she had made it clear that it was something she had some anxiety about. Matt admitted that he had a hard time keeping these things in mind. He felt that Suzanne was right to expect that kind of attention, and, again, was upset with himself that his resolve to try harder never amounted to much.

Matt's response to my question about what he might wish for was "that Suzanne was happier with me." I explained to him that what I was looking for was some thoughts he might have about what he might like to *have* from Suzanne—not just the elimination of the negative—that Suzanne wouldn't be disappointed in him. Though Matt's initial response was "I have nothing to complain about," he was, with some encouragement, helped to understand that what I was looking for was not a "complaint" but rather a "wish." With that reassurance, Matt was able to say that it felt good when he actually did something that made Suzanne happy and he loved when they laughed together.

The information obtained from doing the couple's genograms hinted at some things that they each might wish for in addition to what they had described and were consciously aware of. Additionally, it provided information that was useful in devising interventions to address Matt's rage reactions and his inability to stay consistently connected to Suzanne.

Matt's father was a career military man, and the family had lived on bases all over the United States as well as in the Middle East. Matt had grown up as an only child "after my baby brother died of crib death when he was 8 months old." Matt was 4 at the time. "I don't *remember* having a brother, but the family story is that I was crazy about him, and there are pictures of me holding him."

Matt described his family as "*Waspy* . . . through and through." His father was of German descent and his mother's side was Scottish. According to Matt, both sides of his family were sort of "boring." Everyone got along but they didn't see each other much, and everyone was "very private." When encouraged to offer adjectives and some family stories, it was clear that there was much more to be said about his family. His initial assessment that they were "ordinary" was more a reflection of how difficult it was for Matt to talk about personalities and feelings than it was about the nature of who they were. But with the structured questioning of the genogram, Matt was able to provide a good deal of richly evocative material. For example, when asked for adjectives that described his mother, Matt said "stoical," "strong," a "just-get-on-with-it" kind of person. A story that illustrated her "stoicism" was that when, a few years ago, she found out that she had breast cancer, she never told anyone even her closest friends, until she had already had a mastectomy. "I don't know for sure how she handled losing the baby, but I guess it was in the same way. I've never seen her cry about it, and though, as I said, I've seen pictures of him, my mother and father never talk about him or how it was for them afterward."

Matt described his father as a strong "military" type. When asked to elaborate, he said, "It's not that he was strict or authoritarian, the way so many military people are, but just that he's very traditional. He left all 'home' issues to my mother." He went on: "My parents gave me a lot of freedom. From as far back as I can remember, they trusted me and I did my thing and they did theirs. They didn't comment much on my achievements—that's the WASP way. Not overly effusive . . . not big on compliments. Occasionally they'd tell me they were disappointed in my school performance—but basically they didn't comment much about me one way or the other."

Matt expressed a lot of admiration for an uncle who retired in his 40s. He'd made a lot of money in business and though he had never complained about the pressure, decided he'd had enough and didn't want that kind of stress in his life anymore. He became a "stay-at-home dad, so to speak—though his kids were already in high school—and wrote short stories, which he's had some success in getting published."

Because nothing had come up spontaneously about anger, I asked Matt how people in his family dealt with anger. He had already discussed his mother being stoical. *"Was she able to maintain that or did she explode sometimes?"* I asked. According to Matt, he never saw his mother explode, but he wondered if at times her "migraines" were due to stress. His father also never exploded, but he could be very firm and a bit scary when Matt engaged in typical teenage stuff "like drinking and smoking weed."

At this point Suzanne interjected, "They are the most controlled, unexpressive people you can possibly imagine. I love them. They've been wonderful to me. And I know they love me too. But don't ever try to talk to them about a feeling. I know why Matt is so closed off emotionally. But still—when I met him he was so different from them. And he still is, with the kids, but not with me. I've tried to think about when it started to change. It was gradual, but I think after we had kids all that emotional stuff got expressed to them, rather than to me."

Suzanne's family couldn't have been more different. She came from a close-knit Italian family and grew up in Brooklyn on the same block where her grandparents and aunts and uncles on both sides of her family lived. Like Matt, she was an only child, but she had 13 cousins, and they were in and out of each other's houses all the time. "I wasn't lonely, but I definitely think being an only child affected me. I got a lot of attention. My parents focused everything on me. They lived for me. I had no privacy. They watched every expression I made, and asked me what was wrong if there was the slightest sign I was upset."

In describing aunts and female cousins, Suzanne frequently mentioned whether or not they *let people walk all over them* and related this to the person's self-esteem. For instance, Suzanne was very close to her mother's sister, but "it upsets me and my mother—actually my father too—how she allows people to use her and take advantage of her good nature." A cousin was described as "having low self-esteem—it took her years to get out of an abusive relationship," and another aunt was characterized as having given up a good career "to be treated like a doormat by her husband." Conversely, she included in her descriptions of *good* relationships "They had a lot of respect for one another" or "They were really supportive of each other and proud of what the other accomplished."

Another dimension that repeatedly entered into Suzanne's descriptions of her extended family was whether or not they were able to have fun. One uncle "knew how to have a good time." Or an aunt "always had a smile on her face." A much older uncle "always was a kid at heart." In contrast, her grandmother frequently seemed "anxious" or "worried." And the brother to whom her mother was closest always "looked like he had the weight of the world on his shoulders." Suzanne's parents were "fun-loving." They "looked for any opportunity to celebrate something and it seemed like almost every weekend they were inviting people over to celebrate *something*. I'm exaggerating a little, but [turning to Matt] isn't that basically the truth?" Matt agreed that Suzanne's family was extremely social and liked to laugh. It was always fun being with them.

Suzanne went on to say that the one place where they weren't easygoing or fun was when it came to her. "They watched me like a hawk and wouldn't let me date while I was in high school. When I was younger it used to drive me crazy how controlling and overprotective they were—but the other side of the coin is that no child was ever more loved and praised than I was. As far as they were concerned I was the smartest, most beautiful child that ever walked the earth." Because they were so protective, she'd hidden from her parents "that Matt and I were practically living together before we got married. It was hard for them to accept that Matt had been married before and had a daughter. But they love him, and they'd be completely devastated if Matt and I were to break up. They'd be shocked and horrified if they knew the kinds of things he says to me and how out-of-control he can be."

My Feedback

I shared with the couple some preliminary thoughts I had about the way their family backgrounds had affected them and were played out in the relationship. To Matt I said, *"You really learned in your family not to need much—not to want approval or attention, and to take care of yourself. It's a devastating experience to lose a baby, not only for the parents but for the siblings. You had no permission to express that. And in addition to losing your brother, you also lost your parents—in the sense that even though they handled it—they were grieving and it's hard to be fully present when your heart is broken. Perhaps when Suzanne wants attention it touches on a desire that you've forbidden yourself to have and that's part of why you block it out.*

"The other thing I wondered about is whether you were too stoical about Suzanne's attention shifting to your kids when you became parents. Again, perhaps wanting her attention is something that feels wrong to you and that's why you started to be less "there" for Suzanne after the children were born.

"In your family, you learned that being angry was unacceptable and had to be dissociated. Understandably, your parents emphasized what a loving big brother you were. But children have mixed feelings about younger

siblings, and it's likely that you also were angry at your parents for the loss of attention that having a baby brother entailed. Maybe that's part of why you explode. You're not comfortable expressing—or even knowing—that you're angry and then it takes you by surprise."

The thoughts I had about Suzanne's psychological makeup were not as new to her as Matt's were to him. She'd been in therapy, and was in general a more "psychologically minded" person. Even though she "knew" a lot of what I reflected on, hearing these observations underlined and elaborated was helpful to her. I observed that she had grown up with an awareness of women who had passively accepted mistreatment and so that added to her upset about Matt's rage reactions. Was her concern that she was perhaps being like some of the women she had described? This was confusing to her because she believed herself to be someone who had high self-esteem yet this sense of herself didn't fit with her staying married to a man who could, at times, be verbally abusive.

I also reiterated that though she was very close to her parents, their focus on her also felt at times stultifying and controlling. In an earlier session, Suzanne had mentioned that when she first met Matt, she found it appealing that he was not "clingy" or "controlling" at all. He respected that she was a separate person and that was a nice change from other boyfriends who had tried to possess her. *"Hearing about your parents, I really get why feeling loved by Matt but not underline{owned} by him was so deeply appealing. But clearly, the separateness now has gone too far. Before it was in the context of his sending you love letters, but now it just feels emotionally disconnected."*

In giving feedback about the genogram, I focus on observations and hypothesis that I think the person may be able to accept, and carefully word my statements in a way that is least likely to trigger defensiveness. So, for instance, when speculating about Matt's way of handling the diminishment of Suzanne's attention to him when they had children, I said, *"Maybe that's why you were less underline{there} for Suzanne"* rather than saying something like *"Maybe you were really angry at her for not giving you the attention you used to get before you needed to share it with the children."*

From a psychodynamic perspective, one could readily see Matt's "forgetting" as a passive expression of unarticulated anger. But even if that was the source of his behavior, "uncovering" this motive would trigger defensiveness and would do little to move the work forward. Instead, as I discuss below, I focused on his being able to express the other side of the coin from anger—the banished wish for nurturance that his "mature" self disallows.

Active Interventions

Given the speculations just described about the psychodynamic issues underlying Matt's explosions, the first order of business was to help him to get more in touch with his longings. He had been educated in stoicism, self-discipline, and self-sufficiency. Matt's explosions were seen not so much in terms of the holding in of things that annoyed him until he finally exploded, but rather that he had needs and wishes that he was unaware of and didn't feel he had a right to express.

As we have seen, a major theme that came up in Matt's genogram was that one didn't show upset or stress but just "soldiered on." With this in mind, I asked Suzanne if Matt seemed stressed by his demanding job. She said that he never talked about work. "I know he must be stressed . . . he has a couple of beers as soon as he comes home—but when I ask him how was his day, he just shrugs and says 'the usual.'"

In a light but serious tone, I said to Matt, *"We have to help you <u>complain</u> more. When you were a kid, did you complain to your parents about teachers, or too much homework, or some annoying kid in your class?"* Of course, as I expected, he replied that just wasn't "done" in his home. He had changed schools often, and was expected to—and did—adapt easily. This led to a discussion about how Suzanne and Matt's kids do talk a lot at dinner about what's going on, and some of it is complaining exactly the way I had just described. I gave Matt some positive feedback about that, saying, *"I'm struck by how you overcame your own legacy to allow your kids to do what you didn't do as a kid—and don't do even now. I really think it would help you to not eventually explode if you could have a little time alone with Suzanne to be able to unload from the day."* Not surprisingly, Matt initially rejected this idea, saying that they were all so busy at night and that he didn't want to burden Suzanne. I asked Suzanne what she thought—"Was it realistic? Would it be too hard? Would it be a burden?" She said, to the contrary, she'd *love* to spend a little time alone with him. "The kids are eager to leave the table after dinner, and as soon as they get up, Matt starts clearing the table. I'd love it if we could sit for 10 or 15 minutes at the end of the meal. But if we did, I'd probably be the one talking about my day."

I asked them if they'd like to try changing that pattern, and together we came up with a plan. They agreed that if they slipped into the old routine, as soon as Suzanne caught herself she'd be the one to stop it and ask Matt to tell her something "annoying" about his day. Of course, it would be best if Matt could interrupt Suzanne and remind her that he was supposed to do the "complaining." But given how ingrained it was in him to keep negative feelings to himself, it might be difficult for him to "demand" attention. Hopefully, in time he would become more comfortable talking about the stresses and strains of his day and would not need Suzanne's encouragement to do so. Suzanne's helping him with this difficulty is an example of what I discussed earlier; even though something is an individual issue reflecting psychodynamic conflict and ambivalence, it does not have to be resolved entirely on one's own, but rather can be worked on together as a couple.

In the genogram, there was also a hint that Matt wished he had more time to relax. He spoke of an uncle who had retired early so he could have a less stressful life. I raised this issue by saying, *"I know you aren't in that position or in that stage of life, but is there any way that the two of you could figure out how Matt could make room in his life for relaxation, and perhaps even creativity; you mentioned earlier that he used to write poetry."* Suzanne eagerly picked up on this. "He never relaxes. Every weekend he feels he has to fix things around the house and does all these self-imposed chores which then take a lot longer than he thought they would, and then he gets incredibly frustrated and stressed. And besides that, he's available 24/7 to his clients—I know that other people in his office don't do that—I've spoken to their wives."

Matt then said, "I'm a little OCDish, I guess. I feel guilty if I'm not working at something. I do enjoy doing some of the chores—it feels good to clean out the garage. But I never feel okay if I'm just relaxing—I feel like I 'ought' to be accomplishing something, getting something off my checklist."

"Can you think of any way that Suzanne might be able to be of some help to you with this problem?" Not surprisingly, Matt, so accustomed to taking care of himself, answered, "Not really—it's my problem. I just need to figure out how to stop being so compulsive. I should go to yoga more regularly." *"Yes, yoga and meditation could be helpful. But you don't have to solve this totally on your own. Perhaps there's a way Suzanne could help a bit."*

Suzanne interjected, "He's pretty good when we're all out of the house. Maybe I could plan more family activities on the weekends, when the kids don't have so many activities. Usually Sunday is fairly free. I know he loves movies, and the kids are old enough now that there are adult films we could take them to. And Matt likes museums, which the kids actually don't mind going to once in a while. I don't plan those kinds of things because I know he's always got some project he's going to be working on. *"Matt, what about that idea? Would that help you? Is Suzanne right that you relax more when you're out of the house?"*

This led to a preliminary action plan that would undoubtedly need to be fine-tuned. Should Suzanne remind him not to start a project if they were going out later? Would that feel like being taken care of or like nagging? How could it be done in a way that would feel good to Matt? Can Suzanne help with his compulsion to check his phone and answer emails right away? Eventually they came up with a plan to help Matt be "less OCDish," but as always we discussed it as a first attempt that would need to be evaluated and modified after seeing how realistic it was and how it worked in practice.

At this point readers might be wondering about *Suzanne's needs*. So far, all we've been focusing on is Suzanne helping *Matt* to access disowned parts of himself—a dissociative process that we have hypothesized has led not only to explosions but also to his "forgetting" about the things that are important to Suzanne. So, after coming up with these ideas in regard to helping Matt, I asked Suzanne to talk more about what *she's* been upset about and what she's been feeling has been missing *for her* in the relationship. Suzanne started by saying that she had always been aware that, to use her words, she was a "high-maintenance" person. She laughingly said, "I'm used to being told how wonderful I am and being the focus of attention. As I said, my parents thought I was a princess. And I guess I have good self-esteem because I did very well in school and have always had boyfriends who thought I was great and wanted more of a commitment from me than I did from them. I know my expectations are probably too high—we have kids and a million things to take care of—but I feel hurt that I don't seem to be on Matt's mind at all. I try to let a lot of things go, but it just sits inside me until he does—or I should say *doesn't do*—one more thing, and then I can't hold it in anymore, and I tell him how much he's hurt me. He's always apologetic, says he understands, says he'll try harder, and for a day or two he seems to pay more attention to me."

My aim was to help the couple break this pattern in which Suzanne feels hurt and Matt chastises himself and temporarily tries harder. The information obtained in the genogram generated some ideas about alternative narratives and possible new ways to approach this issue. I had been struck by how much of Suzanne's time in growing up had been spent with her cousins and aunts and uncles. I said to Suzanne, "*I know you grew up with a lot of attention from your parents, and you think because of that you're high maintenance. But you also spent a lot of time being part of the 'gang of cousins.' I don't have the sense from what you described that the focus of the cousins was particularly on* you. *You were one of many. So, actually, under the right circumstances, you're fine with not getting much attention. So I'm curious what you meant when you said that sometimes you wonder if perhaps your expectations are too high?*"

We then explored what Suzanne thought was appropriate to expect and what was perhaps "too much." "I think it's weird that he doesn't remember important events in my life and doesn't ask me about them, and I don't think that's asking too much. But maybe when I'm hurt that he hasn't called during the day to ask how I'm doing [Suzanne was a freelance journalist and worked from home] that's asking too much. I know he has back-to-back appointments all day. I'm also hurt when he's so busy with his projects that he 'can't' take time away to have breakfast or lunch with us on the weekends. I know that it's his being a little OCDish, but I still don't think it's *right*—it's not the kind of family life I want." I then asked, "*Is there anything else that would go in the category of* maybe I'm asking too much?" Suzanne replied angrily, "I *don't* think it's asking too much of him to want him to be 'present' when he's with us and to stop checking his phone."

Suzanne had mentioned that Matt had been so different in the early years of their relationship. I asked Suzanne to talk directly to Matt and to tell him again what she was craving and what she remembered about how he acted with her at that time. By asking her at this point to talk to Matt about the good things she remembers rather than her hurt, I am hoping to minimize the defensiveness and shutting off of warm feelings that often accompanies criticism.

Turning to face Matt, she said, "You seemed so *into* me. Like you'd remember that I had a dentist appointment or something, and you'd surprise me and pick me up. Remember when you used to leave little notes for me in funny places where I would just discover them? Sometimes you even wrote poems. I know we're well beyond that stage in our marriage, but I really wish you'd at least remember to ask me about important things."

As Suzanne spoke, Matt gently touched her leg and said, "You're right. I'm sorry I'm not that way anymore." I asked Matt to think about what he could come up with to give her a little bit of that feeling again. *"Think about what you know warms Suzanne's heart. What does she find endearing? What do you know makes Suzanne feel loved?"* To preserve the feeling of spontaneity and romance I did not ask them to *plan* together some of the things he might do to recapture some of that lost feeling. For this same reason, I did not encourage him to say aloud his answer to my questions. In fact, as Matt started to answer, I said, *"Just give it some thought—no need to talk about it—that way you can surprise Suzanne."* Matt seemed quite on board with this—*"I know what to do—no problem—it will be easy."* Frequently, however, someone expressing good intentions of this sort does not actually follow through on the plans or commitments that s/he has made. In the next chapter I discuss some ways therapists can work with the anger, disappointment, and at times frustration with oneself that is generated when this pattern repeatedly occurs.

As the work with this couple progressed, the deeper understanding of each of their individual needs, in part derived from the genogram, led to discussions of other things they could do differently. For instance, I was able to explore with them the contrast between Suzanne's childhood, which was filled with people, and the way their life was structured now. For a number of years, she had worked from home, and thus had been deprived of companionship and good feedback from colleagues. Because of their kids' activities and Matt's weekend home improvement projects, they didn't socialize nearly as much as Suzanne would have liked. Together, they discussed various ways to remedy this situation.

A discussion of the differences in their backgrounds led to a focus on how rarely Matt was complimented. Though he disavowed any need for "a pat on the back," we discussed that in general the more that couples give each other positive feedback, the better their relationship. They agreed to each try to consciously notice and comment upon things about the other and the way s/he acted—with family, colleagues, friends, neighbors, or even strangers—that they admired or were impressed by. In short, they *both* needed more compliments—for Suzanne, because she had grown up with them and missed them, and for Matt, because he had never had them.

We have been looking at Matt and Suzanne's legacy issues and how to address them in couple therapy, but the reader should keep in mind that this is only one part of the work. Matt needed to learn to recognize signs in his body that are precursors to his rage reactions and to find some methods to calm himself down physiologically (Fishbane, 2013). I discussed this problem with the two of them and made some recommendations about "instant calm" (Wilson, 1995) methods and also suggested that Matt take a course on mindfulness meditation. Future sessions need to address too how they can deescalate conflicts if Matt has *not* succeeded in preventing an outburst of anger.

Vignette 2: Dani and Brewster

Dani, a woman in her early 50s, frightened by the anger she was feeling at her husband, worried that she "was going crazy." Until the past year or so, she considered herself happily married to a man whom she "revered" as a brilliant, highly successful businessman. Throughout their 24 years of marriage, she had wished that they'd have more leisure time together because when he was available, they both agreed, they enjoyed each other tremendously. But there always seemed to be a new crisis at work which, he claimed, when it was resolved, would enable him to work fewer hours.

Dani heard these claims with a grain of salt. She knew that despite Brewster's complaints about the long hours and the stress that he was under, he loved not only the recognition and financial success he enjoyed, but also the intense stimulation of his work. Though she had been frustrated that there was always something that made it impossible for him to get home early or to take more than a few days of vacation time, she was basically content to be there for him, and to "keep the hearth burning," so to speak. His ambition had resulted in their being "very well off." They lived in a large house in the suburbs and also owned a ski cabin and a beach house, but they barely used either vacation home because Brewster could never get away. To make it up to her, Brewster would, from time to time, come home with a gift of expensive jewelry.

A year ago their son, their only child, had gone to college on the other side of the country, and only came home on long school holidays. "I'm lonely. I don't like waiting until Brewster gets home at 9:00 to eat dinner, and I'm angry that my life revolves around him so much—but it's not his fault. He loves work—I think more than he loves me—and that's just the way it is. I have to accept it. He's just made that way. He is who he is. I can't ask him to be someone he's not. But I can't take everything being about him anymore. I've been exploding at him—and that's just not me. I feel like I'm losing my mind. I almost never get angry, but lately I feel so mad and say really nasty things to him. He's right when he gets mad back. I have nothing to complain about. He's a great provider and I'm being unfair. He's the same as he's *always* been. I guess I have to start traveling by myself or with my single women friends. But that's not what I want. That's not for me."

Brewster responded that he was completely devoted to Dani and that he was very upset that she was so unhappy. They'd always been very close—"kind of two against the world, I guess." Even though he was the one out there "taking on the giants," he thought of them as a team. From time to time he would look to her for advice about dealing with various situations, and he generally felt that "she's the only one who has my back—it's very cutthroat in my world." They didn't socialize much except for business events because they preferred just being with one another whenever they had a chance. Brewster sheepishly admitted that he was glad to have his wife to himself even though he is "crazy about" his son. "I don't know what's got into her. I can't take her yelling at me and saying nasty things. Maybe she's drinking too much. Maybe it's her hormones. But I'm not going to let anybody talk to me like that, even her!"

Here's what the genogram illuminated: Dani grew up in a milieu where people were quick to be angry and where conflict was "resolved" by cutting off all contact with the person who angered you. On Dani's mother's side of the family, numerous relatives had stopped speaking to one another. And although Dani's father's family didn't fight with one another, he was so emotionally removed from them that she saw her grandparents, aunts, and uncles on his side only once or twice a year at most.

Dissension permeated Dani's immediate family, both when she was growing up and in the present. Her parents, who divorced when she was a young child, had never attended a family event together—including Dani's wedding. And Dani's mother hadn't spoken to one of Dani's brothers for at least 8 years. Much to Dani's dismay, a year ago, her mother stopped speaking to her as well. Dani had always been the most easy-going of the children. What precipitated the rift with her mother was Dani's refusal to cancel some prior plans when her mother called and wanted her to drive her to a shopping mall. "I guess she was shocked—since I'd always change everything in my life around if she, or even my brothers and sisters, asked me to do something. I tried to talk to her about it, but she went into this rage about how unappreciative I am, how I don't treat her with respect—and then she just stopped answering the phone when I called. In a way I wasn't surprised—I think I always knew everything was all about her."

And a few years ago, her older sister, the sibling whom Dani was closest to, got angry at Brewster and refused to come to their house anymore. Though she would see Dani privately, she wouldn't even come to her nephew's high school graduation. Dani felt that she really didn't have a family. Ingrained in Dani was a belief that you can't count on love. Connections can be fractured quite easily if you're not completely selfless. With her mother there was "no money in the bank" so to speak. As soon as she asserted herself, all the years of being nice counted for nothing.

Brewster too was a caretaker. He was an "accident," born to older parents, and his siblings were almost grown when he was born. The first thing he said when I asked him about his family history was, "When I was 8 years old my father died suddenly of a stroke, my mother was not only very depressed but she also suffered from extreme high blood pressure and diabetes." Brewster had two much older siblings. His sister lived on the West Coast and was a "druggie," and his older brother went away to college when Brewster was 6 and never really came back. "So, when my father died, it was just me and my mom. I was pretty mature for my age and 'raised myself.' My mother was very sweet and loving, but 'out of it.' She trusted that I knew what I was doing when it came to homework and other things— she'd never dream of telling me, 'Do this,' or 'Don't do that.' She'd talk to me about her worries about my sister, and as I got older I was happy to look after her. By the time I was 25, I had made enough money to buy her a new house. She died a few years ago. I still miss her a lot."

From Brewster's genogram we could see that he placed a high value on being strong and independent, and described people in his family and extended family along that dimension—for example, "Aunt Martha really know how to take care of herself" and "Grandfather Arthur was a self-made man." But combined with this view was Brewster's self-image and pride in being a devoted person who looked after people. It had given him tremendous pleasure to provide for loved ones, and he said that even with all he had now accomplished, buying his mother a house was one of the greatest achievements and pleasures of his life.

Active Interventions

It was very obvious to Dani that she was exploding at Brewster because she was angry at him for all the years that he had done what he pleased. She knew that she had never pressed him to work shorter hours or to take time off for vacations. She felt that "she had been totally at his beck and call." Sobbing softly, she said, "I've realized lately that I've actually been *scared* all the years we've been married—scared that if I pushed him he'd get angry and that would be *it*. Even if he didn't actually leave—which I don't think he'd do because of our son—he just wouldn't love me anymore. I know in my head that this is *my* problem and that it's not true. But honestly, I'm not actually *sure* about that. I'm really afraid. Brewster is used to having his own way. He's been getting really angry at me lately."

Brewster was startled by Dani's crying—a rare occurrence—and reached out to hand her a tissue. The thought that she felt afraid that he wouldn't love her stunned him. She continued, "But it's true that you don't like anyone telling you what to do—and I never have. And you've been furious at me lately when I've gotten mad at you." Brewster's angry response was, "I've gotten mad because of the way you're talking to me—with a chip on your shoulder. Maybe I'd be more willing to accommodate to you a little more if you'd be nicer about it!"

After talking more about this challenge, Dani resolved to take a chance and said she would try asking for things *before* she got mad. And, in turn, Brewster said he didn't want her to be unhappy and would try to be more responsive to her needs. It can be tempting to assume that the couple, having "gotten it," will now be able to change this pattern. But habitual patterns, especially ones based on deeply held assumptions about relationships, are not, even with the best of intentions, so easy to shift. After all, Dani's hesitancy to assert herself was based on feeling real anxiety, and it will take many experiences—not just cognitive understanding—to disconfirm her deeply felt expectation that disagreements will lead to a loss of love. And conversely, it is unlikely that it will be as easy for Brewster to change course as he thought it would be. His demand that Dani ask "nicely" for him to even *consider* accommodating to her request only confirmed how much they both were still operating within the familiar parameters and expectations that not much accommodation should be expected of him.

So, with that in mind, I said to Dani, "*I think you really get it, and I'm hopeful that you'll try trusting in Brewster's love for you. But often, these old ways of acting with one another are more difficult to change than one expects. Let's put our heads together and think of some ways to help you remember, or get up the courage, to try putting out there what you want or don't want.*"

I also tried to increase the odds that Brewster would indeed be able to tolerate the lack of total autonomy that would be the consequence of Dani being more assertive. I linked his positively responding to his wife's requests to what I knew he took pride in: that he was generous and took care of those he loved. Thus I said, "*Brewster, if Dani does ask you to do things for her that you don't particularly want to do, and you say yes—that would really be more than just doing what she asked. It would be giving her something she never had. You'd be providing her with a corrective emotional experience so that she can learn that it's safe to be less accommodating and more assertive, and that the marriage you and she have made is very different from the relationships she experienced growing up, and that you won't become emotionally cutoff from her because she's asking something of you.*"

It was also important that when Brewster asked something of Dani, that she not *automatically* agree to his requests. She needed practice in actually taking stock of what she was feeling and what her actual preferences were. I asked them both if they thought it might be helpful for Brewster to *remind* Dani to take some time to think about what she wanted rather than be her

usual "go-along-self." I suggested this because it would give Brewster something *active* to do, so that it would be less likely that he'd feel controlled. With
this encouragement and reminder, Dani was more likely to push through her
anxiety. Of course, by his asking her to think about what she really wanted,
Brewster was also lessening the "risk" she was taking, since the very question
implied that he'd be okay with a "No" answer. But it was essential for her to
say "No," to be assertive about what she wanted, *even* if he'd be annoyed by
her decision. For this reason, I reminded them both that it would be important for him to ask her to reflect on what she actually wanted, even for things
that he *really* cared about. Over time she'd need to be able to do this without
being prompted, but for now, dealing jointly with what she had called *her*
problem would give her the support that would make success more likely. An
added benefit of this strategy was that instead of Dani's request being only
something that Brewster had to adjust to, this approach gave him something
to actively *do*, which fit not only with his "take-charge" style but also with
his wish to *give* to those he loved.

As we talked further about ways to put the insights she had into action,
Dani said, "I need to remind myself of how different Brewster is from anyone in my family and that there's no reason to expect that he would act the
way they do." That comment led to the suggestion that she make a list of the
ways he is different from them and put it someplace where she'd remember
to look at it regularly. Although cognitive challenges to entrenched schemas
are usually not sufficient to break ingrained patterns of interaction, they are
useful in helping someone "get over the hump," so to speak, so that they
can begin to accumulate new experiences that contradict old assumptions
in a *felt* and *lived* way.

It's also useful to plan for negative scenarios. For one thing it normal-
izes setbacks, so that if they do occur, the couple will not feel shame or discouragement. So, I said to them, *"Let's think together about what to do if
despite all this, things don't go according to plan."* I said to Brewster, *"What
if on a particular occasion Dani has not been as outspoken as she thought
she'd be, and when she finally speaks up there's been so much pent-up frustration that she blows up at you?"* Dani interjected, "If he'd cut me a break
and not yell back at me, I know I'd apologize later. But that's asking lot of
him—not to get angry even though I've been horrible."

I asked, *"What do you think, Brewster. Is that realistic?"* He was forthright in his response, saying, "I could try I guess—but I burn up if she starts
insulting me." Because it's important to be a realist and work with people in
a way that is accepting of how they actually *are*, I said in response, *"Okay,
so that doesn't sound so realistic. Maybe all you can do is try to shorten the
blowup by each going your own way for a while and trying to calm down
and gain perspective. Remind yourself that it takes time to change and temporary setbacks are part of the process."*

I also alerted the couple to the possibility that even when Dani is more assertive in a nonangry way, Brewster may feel annoyed at having to accommodate her. Or, conversely, Dani may make a request and Brewster may ignore it or say no. I told them that the *"main issue here is that Dani did speak up loudly and clearly, and nothing terrible happened."* Even if Brewster was annoyed or didn't agree to what she was requesting, this is a very different response from the emotional "cutoff" that Dani feared. That is not to say that it was all resolved. Clearly we needed to talk more about expectations, compromise, and flexibility, but nonetheless, some progress will have been made in challenging Dani's expectation of fracture and catastrophe.

The two case examples just discussed were intended to give the reader a detailed sense of how active interventions can be used to address legacy issues. They are but a small sample of the types of issues one is likely to encounter in work with couples. Although each intervention has to be custom-tailored to the specific couple, I thought it would be useful to offer some sense of the kinds of strategies that I have used with a variety of difficulties that derive from individuals' sensitivities, projections, transference reactions, ambivalences, and unconscious conflicts.

OVERREACTION TO ANGER

Some people who have been traumatized by growing up in a home with an angry or explosive person may react even to minimal irritability as if it were the equivalent of rage. It is not realistic to expect a spouse never to be annoyed, angry at something, or just simply irritable. Nor is it realistic to expect an irritated person to carefully choose his or her words. Solutions that require great care in how one speaks can make sense in one's office but are not realistic in the heat of the moment in a couple's relationship. But one can learn to respond to the spouse's *reaction* in a different way so that the legacy-based overreaction can more quickly be corrected. For instance, one couple came up with a phrase that the husband would use in response to his wife saying, "Why are you yelling at me?" Instead of forcefully responding "I'm *not* yelling at you"—the usual response, and one that only confirmed the wife's feeling that her husband *was* in fact extremely angry at her—the husband would say instead, "I'm annoyed, not angry," or "I'm very frustrated, but not angry," or "I *am* angry, but not the way your father was angry."

It is generally easier for a partner to change his or her way of responding to a "transference" reaction than for the person who has the primary reaction to control his or her behavior; that is, to *stop* the reaction. But again, there are no hard-and-fast rules, and sometimes it is important to be alert to the *exception*. One woman in a couple I worked with felt that she needed some tools *of her own* to not see every eruption as "catastrophic," like it was in her family of origin. She had once been in cognitive therapy, and thought it would be useful to go back to some of those methods. She felt that if her husband could resist the temptation to respond angrily to her when she said "Stop yelling at me," she would be able to calm herself down and remember that she was an adult and not a terrified and trapped child.

A person who knows that her family background has resulted in her being highly reactive to perceptions of anger can feel in a *particular* instance that she is *not* in any way overreacting. Couple therapists often encounter the following kind of stalemate: one person insists that the other was clearly angry, and the other person with equal adamancy claims not to have been so. This rather common scenario can leave the therapist feeling "stuck," particularly if she finds herself siding with one person's perception over the other's. Therapists need to remember that, generally speaking, their task is to help change *future* interactions, not to sort out and reach consensus about what has already occurred.

One woman, turning to her husband, said, "You spoke to me in such an icy cold way—really meanly—how can you say you weren't mad!" In this instance I asked the woman to imitate how her husband sounded and asked him if he recognized himself at all in her imitation. Although he didn't believe he actually had sounded quite the way she had imitated, he did acknowledge that there was a bit of an edge to his tone. He continued, however, to assert that "she's reading into it. I was a little impatient, not angry." My first approach to this dilemma was to see if the couple could accept that this is not a discussion or argument that will get them anywhere. I talked to them about "agreeing to disagree." I asked the husband if he'd be comfortable, if this type of disagreement arises in the future, saying something like "Sorry, I didn't mean to speak in a way that sounded angry," and could prevent the debate from continuing by not adding something like *"because I'm really not angry."* Of course, the wife too would have to be willing to move forward without the satisfaction of an admission of anger. This matter-of-fact way of handling the situation is unlikely to work, however, if in fact the spouse actually *is* angry and is either unwilling to admit it or is actually out of touch with what he is feeling. When the therapist senses that this may be the case, it is best to schedule an individual session with the person to explore further what might be going on. And similarly, if the wife is unable to move forward without the husband conceding that her perception was correct, an individual meeting with the therapist can help the person explore why confirmation of her feelings is as important as it seems to be.

ANGER, DETACHMENT, AND REPAIR

Many people, when angry, hurt, or intensely frustrated about getting through to their spouse, emotionally detach and go into psychic states in which they have lost touch with positive feelings toward their partner. The intolerably painful feelings they are having result in their temporarily not being able to access or simultaneously hold in mind feelings of love, empathy, or concern for the person whom at other times they feel they love. This mental state involves splitting off and not having access to loving feelings when the hurt or painful state of mind is dominant. For some people this emotional cutoff is short-lived, while for others it can go on for weeks at a time.

One woman who had this pattern could sometimes in sessions say things like "I have no feeling at all toward my husband. I feel nothing toward him—I'm in a black hole that I can't get out of." This extreme feeling of detachment was only evident toward "*him.*" With her children, friends, and coworkers she was emotionally present. She described being so frustrated with what she regarded as her husband's extreme defensiveness and unwillingness to hear about the hurt she felt he was causing her that she had "withdrawn into a cave." Another woman described feeling like she was looking at her husband through a "wall of ice."

Sometimes this type of withdrawal is obviously a way to severely punish the partner. At other times it is self-protective, because permitting strong positive feelings toward the partner would be extremely painful or infuriating. Often the withdrawn person feels that it "just happens" to them and is not something that they intentionally or willfully do. But whatever the cause, the experience of the person is one in which "no feelings exist." Often with the help of the couple therapist, the "no feeling" state can disappear in the session. But connecting and repairing in the session is not enough. The couple needs to develop new patterns of interaction so that such extreme hurt is less likely to occur.

Another related but different form of detachment occurs when a person, in anger, says things that are so hurtful that it is hard for the other partner to feel there is any love left for them at all. In their state of rage, these people want to crush and destroy the person that in other states of mind they love. This was the case with Matt described above. Often the attacked partner is left feeling that the brutal words represent the spouses' true feelings because "If he really loved me, how could he possibly want to hurt me so much? He wants to make me feel completely worthless. You don't do that to someone you love." And because the attacking words are coming from a dissociated part of the psyche, the raging person often does not understand how hurtful his or her words are, or why they cannot be easily forgotten or dismissed as just a lashing out, and not the *truth.*

I start with the assumption that although people do not *consciously decide* to split off their loving feelings, there are still some things they can do that at times can help them come out of that quasi-dissociated state more quickly. And they may be able to stop themselves from disconnecting in the first place. How much "will" (or self-indulgence) is involved in this kind of rage reaction is unclear. But it's been striking to me that many people who get into these kinds of split-off mental states with their spouse never do so with their children. That is not to say that there aren't plenty of instances where people feel emotionally burnt-out with children and get into a state where they feel they are numb and don't care anymore. And, of course, there are verbally abusive parents whose words leave the child feeling completely worthless and unloved. In cases where a person rages against a spouse but not his or her children, I'll point out this disparity by saying something like *with your children you're able to be extremely angry and yet remember the love that is there and don't want to make your child feel worthless.* Pointing out this reality challenges the person's feeling that his rage reactions are not within his control. It also offers some encouragement because he *already knows how* to be very angry without going too far.

Splitting off loving feelings, either through detachment or in the context of rage reactions, is a major contributor to many couples' difficulties. Therapists need to brainstorm with the couple to see if there is anything they can do to prevent the emotional "cutoff" and find ways to help the person who has disconnected more quickly reintegrate into consciousness the positive feelings that have been split off from awareness. Some people who have previously tried verbal cognitive techniques—for example, trying to *argue* with their "withdrawing self"—find that a nonverbal reminder, such as looking at a particularly endearing photograph, is more effective. One couple thought they might put together what they called a "rescue" photo album that the husband would put on his phone. But, of course, remembering to look at photos when hurt and angry is quite a challenge. One woman who felt ashamed at how "verbally abusive" she became when she "lost it" decided to put photos of her husband playing with their children on the side of the bathroom mirror because she often retreated to the bathroom after they'd had a screaming fight.

When someone is "in a cave" or feeling emotionally cutoff from his or her spouse, it can be helpful to speak to a friend who can remind the person of the warm and empathic feelings that have been temporarily walled off. It can be useful to think through in advance which friends are most capable of helping the person get in touch with the loving feelings that have been banished. Some people I've worked with decided to talk to the friend in advance to set up a "withdrawal hotline," so to speak; the person being called would then know beforehand that what was needed was to help the person remember loving feelings.

Some people have found it helpful to practice—when s/he is not hurt or angry—visualizing his or her spouse doing something that has very positive associations. One man would close his eyes and picture himself lying on the couch watching TV with his wife rubbing his feet. Regular practice bringing this image to mind helped him access it when he was feeling very angry and allowed him to express his anger in a way that kept the whole person of his wife in mind.

When terrible things have been said, the person who lashed out needs to repair the damage that has been done as soon as possible. Often it is not enough to apologize or even to express remorse. It can be very difficult for the hurt partner to believe that what was said does not actually represent the other's true feelings. One sometimes effective way to "undo" the hurt, or to at least mitigate it, is to elaborate more about why what was said didn't represent what one truly feels when one is not in a dissociated, rageful state. The person who has been verbally abusive needs to give detailed and specific examples of how what was said was not what she truly felt. Thus, for example, when Drew lost it, he would accuse his wife, Kari, of being a "parasite" who "was spoiled" and "only thought about herself." Kari was deeply hurt by these accusations. Though she knew that these were "legacy" issues for Drew, and that in fact he was expressing feelings he had about the women in his family of origin, she nonetheless worried that deep down Drew really thought of her that way. When Drew not only said he didn't mean it, but elaborated by saying that he was very aware and appreciative that she worked at a job she disliked in order to bring in some extra money for the family, and added that "you're more likely to buy *me* something than to buy something for yourself," Kari could finally accept that what Drew had said did not reflect his true feelings.

ANXIETY ABOUT DEPENDENCY NEEDS AND ABANDONMENT

There are a number of different ways that anxiety about dependency needs and attachment issues can manifest themselves. Some people will not let themselves "need" anything from their spouses, and this "not needing" can result in a buildup of resentment, loneliness, or detachment in either partner. It can also result in a great deal of anger when, on the rare occasion that a need *is* expressed, it is not heard or responded to in a satisfactory way. In order to best devise a method to help with this issue, the particular reasons for this anxiety need to be understood.

For example, Dwayne, who was African American, had as a small child been the object of much ridicule by his older brothers for being a "crybaby" who would complain to his mother about how he'd been hit, pushed, or insulted by his siblings. The family at that time lived in a tough inner-city neighborhood, and his father too worried that Dwayne wasn't thick-skinned enough to handle the normal teasing and rough-housing and fighting he was likely to encounter in the schoolyard as he got older. When Dwayne was 6 years old his mother was diagnosed with cancer, and though she did in fact survive, she had needed very aggressive chemotherapy and a bone marrow transplant. Perhaps in response to the stress the family was under, his older brothers became even more aggressive toward him, and his father, whom he described as "having his hands full with working two jobs, looking after us kids, and taking care of my mother," became furious at him if he so much as sniffled. One day, without any discussion, Dwayne was "shipped off to live with an old-lady aunt." After begging and promising that he wouldn't be a "cry-baby" anymore he was allowed to move back home. "After that, I learned to take care of myself and things just sort of calmed down at home. A big part of what initially attracted Dwayne to his wife, Felicia, whom he had met in college, was that she was the person everybody came to when they were upset and needed a shoulder to cry on. Now, 18 years later, she was still the person everyone came to with their problems even though she, according to Dwayne, using the same phrase he had used to describe his father's situation, "had her hands full" juggling her career—she had become a pediatrician—and raising kids. Because Dwayne was extremely hesitant about expressing needs, and conveyed that he could take care of himself, he had become "last on her list." It was unrealistic to think that the clarity with which he understood the issue would in itself result in him being able to let himself "need" Felicia. A better approach was for his wife to take the initiative and *ask* him if she could help him. This could be in small, practical ways as well as in the deeper ways that she was so good at with her friends. So, for instance, if he had broken a glass and was cleaning it up, she could volunteer to help, and if he said something like, "No, it's okay," she should persist and do it anyway. Small gestures like that often can be quite meaningful. When Dwayne seemed stressed or worried about something, his wife should not so quickly accept, his "No, I don't want to talk about it." On his end, he needed to notice how he set up "tests" for her that she would fail and thus confirm that he was right not to depend on her. For instance, after she had her coat on and was about to leave for her office, he would sometimes ask her for a favor, for example, taking some things in to the cleaners for him. Understandably, she would not immediately respond in the affirmative, since she was now in an "I'm leaving" mind-set and would feel interrupted. Each time she failed one of his tests (or better, "pop quizzes"), he would be more convinced that it was better not to ask for any help.

Sometimes fear of dependency is related to a history of traumatic losses. One woman sensed that she "held back" because her heart had been broken when she was a young girl when her father, who had a volatile relationship with her mother, walked out and "basically abandoned me and my brother." The couple came up with a humorous way to remind the wife that her husband's personality was very different from her father's. When he and his wife were texting one another about the logistics of taking kids to their practices and lessons, he would sign his messages with "notyourDad." And though he couldn't always do it, even when he was angry, he'd try to remember to say, "You're stuck with me. I'm not leaving you but I'm really mad."

There were times, however, when it was difficult for the husband to be supportive in this way. He felt hurt and sometimes even incensed that his wife, who feared he'd leave *her*, would during an argument *herself* say things like, "Maybe this just isn't working" or "I've had enough" or "I can't take this anymore." Sometimes he felt that *she'd* one day just announce that she wanted a divorce. In one session I raised with her the possibility that in those moments she was converting fear of abandonment into her doing the rejecting, so she would not be so vulnerable. I encouraged her to say instead "I'm afraid about what's happening between us right now," because that statement more accurately reflected the despair and hopelessness that the argument was evoking and could more readily be heard by her husband.

SENSITIVITY TO CRITICISM

Some people seem to react very defensively to even the slightest *hint* of criticism. It may be that they were criticized a great deal as a child and they learned to anticipate and immediately deflect and discount "attacks," sometimes with counterattacks. They may still not feel very good about themselves and some minor criticism can set off a cascade of self-doubts. As discussed earlier, criticism erodes love, and so the less of it in a relationship, the better. But, nonetheless, minor comments, like "I wish you'd take your stuff off the dining room table" or "Hey, you were supposed to get home early tonight," are an inevitable part of being in a relationship. When comments even as relatively benign as these are experienced as assaults by the other, the relationship will inevitably be under challenge. In response, the other partner needs to work hard to find ways to defuse the potentially hurtful experiencing of what would ordinarily be run-of-the-mill expressions of annoyance. Even simple requests like "Have you made the appointment for Timmy?" (if he hasn't) can be experienced as if the spouse had said, "You don't even care about your son."

In one couple the wife knew that her husband took any slight criticism as meaning he was a selfish, inconsiderate person—the criticisms that had been leveled at him by his physically and verbally abusive parents. If she prefaced her statements with something that addressed this issue, she made it more difficult for her husband to reflexively hear what she was saying as

"I'm worthless." She said, for example, "I know you try hard about a lot of things, but you're still leaving the table a mess" or "I know you help me out in a lot of ways, but it makes me mad that you forget to call me to tell me you'll be late getting home."

Often these minor criticisms are defended against by a countercriticism which then leads to an interaction that *is* hostile. By responding defensively, the sensitive spouse creates just what s/he has been trying to avoid. It is almost impossible for a partner who feels that she has a legitimate complaint to respond to a countercriticism without intensifying and amplifying the original complaint.

One woman who knew that she was extremely sensitive to criticism came up with a system in which her husband would rate his complaint from 1 to 10, *10* being extremely important and a *1* little more than a preference. In this couple, the husband was "a little compulsive" about neatness and cleanliness. Though this strategy seemed a bit strange to me, it did work well for the couple. Thus, the husband might say, with a fair amount of irritation, "I don't know why you can't load the dishwasher the way I showed you. . . . It's only a 3 but it really bothers me." The husband was concerned that the things he rated fairly low on the scale wouldn't be done because he had made it clear that it wasn't actually that important. But it turned out that seeing his complaints more realistically resulted in his wife being able to respond to them without so much emotional baggage, and she did in fact try noticeably harder to accommodate to his standards.

CONFORMITY, PASSIVITY, MERGER

One couple came to me when they were trying to see if they could get back together after having been separated for over a year. But the woman, Janine, was concerned that she became very passive when she was with a strong man like Benjamin, her boyfriend. In the year that they had been separated, she had been in her own individual therapy and now recognized that she had a tendency to lose herself in close relationships. This happened with women friends as well as with her boyfriend. Janine held a responsible position at work and easily took charge and made decisions. "But in personal relationships, especially romantic ones, I become childish and dependent. It's very peculiar. It's not a put-on. I really *feel* like I can't handle things, though I handle very complicated things at work." She also described herself as a "chameleon," blending in with the environment she was in.

Benjamin, who also had been in therapy, agreed that "I've been a bad influence. I would persuade her to spend money on trips she couldn't really afford, and to go out drinking on week nights—which left her hungover the next day." Benjamin asserted that he had grown up a lot in the year they had been apart and that he was a lot healthier than he had been a year ago. Janine was happy that he no longer drank as much and felt hopeful that perhaps they'd be on the same page if they did get back together. But she knew that *his* being better about pushing her wasn't really the issue.

Though we all agreed that Janine needed to continue working on her problems on her own, the three of us strategized about ways they could also work on this issue together, without it paradoxically becoming just another thing that Benjamin took charge of. I suggested that Benjamin should not make this too easy for Janine, and I did not mean this paradoxically. She needed to develop the ability to be her "outside, professional self" in relationships even when the other person was strong. So, basically, Benjamin should be himself. Janine should not ask him to be less forceful, nor to stop volunteering to take over difficult tasks. Her ability to be mature and differentiated from him should not depend on how *he* acted. Janine "got it." She had decided that when he asked her to do something, she was going to try not to answer right away. Instead, she planned to say, "I'll think about it for a little while and I'll let you know soon." The only change she did want to ask of him was that he not "lobby" her for a "Yes" and that he respect her need for time to think about how she really felt about something. "I know I ought to be able to hold my own even if he is trying to persuade me, but I think that would be just too hard for me."

In another case, a married gay couple had taken on very stereotypical heterosexual gender roles. Dimitri took care of repairs on the car, did their taxes, did most of the driving and generally took charge of things. Zachary worked freelance and ran their household—arranging play dates for Eddie's 5-year-old son, who lived with them, and organizing their social life. Zachary felt he had become too dependent and no longer had a life of his own—he seldom went out with his own friends, and basically fit seamlessly into the life Dimitri had created before he'd met Zachary. Zachary did not blame Dimitri for this. He'd done this before—merged with a partner and adopted his life and friends, leaving his own behind. "I don't want to break up, but I don't know what to do. When I try to assert myself, Dimitri feels hurt and doesn't understand it."

Zachary didn't understand why he tended to lose his "self" in relationships. After doing a genogram, it became clear that in Zachary's family differentiating and being together but separate wasn't acceptable. On family vacations, even with adult kids, his parents were hurt if they didn't do activities as a group or eat every meal together. On both his mother's and his father's side of the family, people who didn't conform were "black sheep" and were regarded as "ruining the family." Interestingly, Zachary's family had no trouble accepting Zachary as gay. What was important to them was that Dimitri and Zachary have a conventional life together and they were delighted when they were able to marry.

As we discussed these issues, Dimitri understood that he needed to actively counter Zachary's assumption that being in a family meant merger and conformity. He was honest about this attitude being hard for him. It was probably no accident that Zachary fell in love with Dimitri, who in many ways had the same assumptions about family life as did Zachary's family; he too liked "togetherness," perhaps because he had come from a large Greek family where three generations lived relatively peacefully in the same two-family house." Dimitri loved Zachary, and assured him that he could cope with Zachary becoming more independent. They decided that the roles they took in their life together needed to be more fluid, and as part of this Dimitri arranged to work from home 1 day a week so he could take over some of the child-care responsibilities. He said jokingly, "Even though I'm a better driver, I get it—Zachary needs to drive half the time." Zachary was also going to start seeing some of his old friends and would plan some ski weekends with them. If he "forgot" to do these things, Dimitri would remind him and ask him if he was feeling anxious or worried about his separateness from Dimitri.

CREATING AN EMOTIONAL ENCOUNTER IN THE SESSION

Frequently, couple sessions focus on deeply felt and painful emotions, so the therapist's aim is to help the couple repair a rupture in their relationship. One or both partners may feel deeply hurt by the other. Sometimes there's been a been a specific blow to the relationship, like an affair, but just as often there's been an accumulation of smaller hurts that have resulted in the couple having "grown apart" and questioning whether or not they still love each other or should be together. Some couples get along, but are troubled by an emptiness or flatness in their relationship. It's not uncommon to hear one person describe feeling "lonely" even when s/he is with his or her spouse. Couples often report feeling more like friends or coparents running a household than people who are romantically attached to one another. Many couples feel troubled that they barely, if ever, have any sexual intimacy, and one or both partners may not even want to try to get that started again until they feel a greater emotional connection to their spouse.

What I want to focus on in this section is that often a turning point for the couple is that, in the session, one partner hears the other say something that s/he has not heard before and is deeply touched by it. Expressing love, empathy, appreciation—as well as hurt—can powerfully affect their experience of one another, and can be the catalyst for new ways of interacting and being together. So often I hear people say, "You've never said that before," and so often the response is one of surprise and dismay: "Really, I thought you knew that." Sometimes *what* was said was not entirely new, but it has been said in a slightly differently way that had a different impact, or the therapist has helped the spouse more fully register it as meaningful.

Couples are able to be open and vulnerable with one another when they feel "safe." They need to trust that if they open up about their feelings, things won't spiral out of control. In individual therapy, trust is more easily obtained than it is in couple therapy. Individual therapists are trained to respond therapeutically and to provide those conditions of safety. But when one opens up to *one's spouse*, s/he may react in ways that are disappointing and hurtful. For this reason, I wait until the work with the couple has progressed enough that they are genuinely listening to one another with the intention of trying to *understand*, not debate and rebut, before encouraging people to open up about feelings that have not been spontaneously volunteered. Furthermore, by waiting a while before focusing on unspoken feelings, I allow the couple time to develop trust in me and in the therapeutic process. They will have had numerous experiences of seeing that I generally move sessions in a positive direction, and, as they gain confidence that I use whatever is revealed *constructively*, they become more comfortable opening up about what is going on for them emotionally.

There are a number of ways in which couple therapists can facilitate emotional connectedness in the sessions. One way is for the therapist to underline and help them each attend to and really hear emotions that are embedded in what the other is saying. Another is for the therapist to help the couple put into words feelings that they have not explicitly articulated. Finally, the therapist can specifically encourage a couple to turn to one another in the session and speak from the heart.

Noticing Embedded Feelings

Not infrequently someone says something emotionally powerful in a fashion that is so brief or offhand that it is easy to miss. For instance, Mary, in discussing her frustration at the long hours her husband, Hank, worked, stated, "I was really angry, that again, I had to go to a family event by myself—that's no fun!" As we have seen throughout this book, we have a choice to make about what to respond to. One could ask Mary to elaborate on how she feels about these family events, or about the anger she feels toward Hank. Or one could ask Hank about how he feels about these events, or what goes on that he can't (or won't, or doesn't want to) set limits on his work hours. But any of those responses would miss an opportunity to pick up on something not only more positive, but potentially more self-revealing. Instead, I said, *"It's more fun when Hank is with you?"* Mary then went on to say, "Yes, Hank is good with my family. Everyone loves him." I then invited her to elaborate on this by saying, *"They love him?*

What's he like with them?" After Mary, with a smile on her face described how Hank "can get a smile out of even my stodgiest relatives," I said, *"It sounds like you really get a kick out of watching Hank in action with your family and really miss him and wish he were there."* I then went on to underline this situation for Hank and make sure he really took it in. *"Hank, I just want to make sure you are registering this. Mary is upset that you're not with her, not for the sake of 'appearances' but because she really enjoys you in these situations and is proud you're her husband."* Turning to Mary, I said, *"Am I getting that right?"* And to Hank, *"What's it like for you to hear that?"*

In another case, Arturo was angry that his wife, Angie, sought advice from her sister about some work tensions, rather than turning to him. In a loud voice he proclaimed, "I *get* it that Angie's sister knows more about it because she's also a nurse, and that Angie doesn't want me to worry that she may be fired, but still, I'm angry, it's wrong. And embarrassing. What does her family think? That I'm not important! I'm her husband!" Again, the therapist must choose what part of the statement to respond to. In choosing what to focus on, I keep in mind that my goal is to encourage the expression of emotions that usually get short shrift or are not part of the conversation that the couple is accustomed to having. Thus I tend to skip over the more obvious emotional content—in this example, Arturo's anger or his embarrassment—in the hope that by focusing on something *less* evident and more embedded, the couple will have the experience of hearing something *new* and learning something about the other that will foster intimacy. Thus, I choose to respond to his feeling that his wife was being protective of him even though that statement was embedded in the main point and delivered almost as an aside. I asked, *"So, Angie doesn't want you to worry? What do you mean?"* In response to that, Arturo said, "She knows I'm worried about money and doesn't want to give me something else to worry about." Turning to Angie, he said, "Do you think I can't handle stuff—that I'm weak?" Angie was taken aback, and said "Weak, *you* weak? You're the strongest person I know!" With my help, the couple continued to talk about what they both had been feeling—what Arturo meant by *weak*, why he was concerned about his wife perceiving him that way, what she *was* feeling that led her not to share her anxieties with her husband, and so on.

Asking People to Talk about What They Are Feeling in the Moment

Another way to encourage the expression of feelings is to ask about how people are reacting to what is being said in the session. This approach asks people to focus on what they are feeling in the present, rather than reporting about feelings they have *had*. So, for example, when Neil said that he felt he and his wife, Marnie, "could never agree on anything—we're like oil and water," I asked Marnie what was going on inside her in reaction to what Neil just said. Typically, people will respond with their cognitive, intellectual self and say something like, "I agree . . . we're very different," or, in a less agreeable, more defensive mode, "I think he's exaggerating," or "That's because he'll automatically disagree with anything I say." But if the therapist points to a focus on feelings—"*What's going on inside you right now? What are you feeling? You have your arms wrapped around yourself, what's going on for you?*"—most people are able to make the shift.

In response to these questions, Marnie, teared up and said "I feel hopeless . . . I think Neil has made up his mind that it's over." Turning to Neil, I asked him to "*see if you can get in touch with what's going on inside you?*" He said, "Honestly, I know I should feel bad that Marnie's so upset, but I'm numb, or maybe angry. It feels like a manipulation. She knows I cave when she cries!" "*So, you don't want to cave this time? What else do you feel? Take a minute, go inside yourself—what comes up for you?*" After a long pause, Neil said, "I feel guilty. I care a lot about Marnie, I don't like hurting her, but I'm not happy in this relationship—I don't know, maybe she's right, maybe I've given up?" Though the exchange was very painful, they both were relieved that they had spoken honestly to one another instead of engaging in their customary accusations and counterclaims.

In another case, Rhima talked about her husband's lack of sexual interest in her. Disdainfully she said, "He prefers porn—he'd rather imagine sex with bimbos than with me." By asking her to explore what feeling come up for her about that, she was able to get beyond anger and expressed her insecurities about her body. "I've always felt bad that I'm flat-chested and not the type that men look at. But I thought that didn't matter to Ron. But now I see it does. I feel really terrible—the way I did when I was a teenager and I developed much later than my friends and even then could barely fill a bra!" Ron expressed amazement that she could imagine it had anything to do with her body. "You look great. I've got a problem. I've become addicted to porn." Rhima couldn't accept this explanation. "Oh come on—do you think I don't notice how you look at women with big boobs—did you think I haven't noticed?" Ron, in response, said, "Okay—so I look—every man does. But *that's* not the problem. Your body is fine. I just feel that you're really not interested in me—sexually and in other ways too. You say I'm not interested in *you*, but it's you who's not interested in *me*. When you come on to me I feel like you're just going through the motions—that you think we ought to have sex once in a while. But there's no spontaneity or real interest. It depresses me to think I'll never have genuinely passionate sex again." My asking Rhima to talk about what she was feeling led to Neil opening up about how *he* felt, and they both came away from the session having heard things from one another that had never been said in quite that way before.

If people have difficulty shifting to discussing their feelings, I sometimes use some methods borrowed from Focusing. I might ask a person to search inside his or her body and ask where s/he feels the tension and what word or image matches what s/he is *sensing*. *"Can you let your body talk to you? What is that feeling in your stomach saying to you? Let your body tell you what that feeling is."* Another useful approach borrowed from gestalt therapy is to notice something in the person's gestures and ask him or her to focus on what his or her gestures might be saying. For instance, I might say, *"I noticed that you're squeezing your hands together as your husband is speaking. What is your body saying? Could you put words to that feeling?"*

Having the Couple Talk about Their Feelings Directly to One Another

In the examples I've given thus far of how to enhance the experiential component in the couple therapy, the couple has been talking to *me* and describing emotions *in the presence of* his or her spouse, not *to* the spouse. In much of the work, the therapist acts as "translator," so to speak. I might say, for instance, *"Did you hear the sadness in Ignacio's voice?"*; or, *"I hear Malena saying she relies on you a lot and trusts that you'll be there for her."*; or, *"Did you hear that Kevin is saying that he feels scared when you're driving late at night on country roads?"*

Sometimes, in the course of answering *me*, the couple spontaneously start to speak directly to one another. That is an indication to me that they now feel safe with one another and don't need me to "run interference" so much. But often the direct exchange is brief and they revert back to speaking with me. And often, after stating something really meaningful and emotionally powerful, people *undo*, or go on a tangent that makes it easy for the most meaningful part of the statement to get lost. The role of the therapist in these instances is to get them back on track and highlight what is significant (or potentially points to change) in what was said.

But although in much of my work I am the sounding board to whom each speaks, and, as noted above, the "translator" or refiner/articulator, it is also important as the work proceeds to make sure that the couple speaks directly to one another in a sustained way. Frequently, I'll ask a couple to turn toward each other and speak to one another directly, not to me. If they have trouble doing that because they have become used to talking to me, I tell them that I'll look down and doodle on my pad, so they can forget about my presence for a few moments. Often my asking that the couple talk to one another is in the service of highlighting something important that has just been said. *"Could you tell MaryAnne <u>more</u> about what you said just now about needing her . . . talk from your heart . . . tell her so she can really take it in."*

Sometimes, when I have "translated" something one of them has said, the other person will turn to his or her spouse and say, "Do you really feel that way?" Generally when couples do this, I go with that structure, and interrupt only now and then to help keep them on focus and to make sure that they are really understanding one another. However, if the couple isn't talking productively, but rather is engaged in mutual blame and attack, I ask them to resume talking to me, not to one another. I explain to them that it takes a lot of effort and practice for people to break these entrenched patterns of communication. Together we look at how what started as a good conversation evolved into the "accusation–counterattack" mode. I then encourage the couple to start the conversation again with a "joining," "what-can-I-agree-with" frame of mind.

Lastly, although sharing emotions fosters intimacy, and thus is useful for its own sake, much of the continuing work of therapy involves doing what was described in the previous chapter—helping the couple *use* what they have learned about one another to better their relationship. Though sometimes just the voicing of feelings leads to change in the way a couple interacts, usually, unless they learn to put their new perceptions into action, they are likely to revert to old perceptions and behaviors. Thus, just as I have described how to devise active interventions to address legacy issues, so too do I work with the couple to use the self-disclosures each has made to change deeply ingrained habitual patterns of interaction to ones that they each will find more gratifying.

In this chapter, we have looked at how the couple can incorporate into their interactions an awareness of their own and their partner's "legacy" issues. When couples understand the unexpressed needs and heightened sensitivities that each brings to the relationship, they are better able to interrupt repetitive negative cycles that have been disruptive to their relationship. People often behave in ways that end up "confirming" their anxieties, transference reactions, and problematic schemas, inducing their spouse (as well as others) into behaving in ways that make them an "accomplice" in perpetuating their partner's fears (P. L. Wachtel, 2014a). Finding creative interventions to address each person's individual issues can help the couple better avoid stepping on each other's emotional landmines, and, at best, can provide the spouse with a corrective emotional experience that contributes to healing old hurts and deepens the love between the partners.

10

Deepening Connections

Sometimes couples benefit greatly from just a few sessions, but more typically progress takes working through multiple issues, many times, and with a variety of different approaches. In this chapter we look at the wide variety of matters that come up in couple therapy as the work progresses. Often the issues discussed in the previous chapter will come up again in another context or in a slightly different form, and this repetition will give us an opportunity to further deepen our understanding of how each person's sensitivities interact with the other's in problematic ways. But in addition to these legacy and hot button issues, sessions may focus on topics as diverse as a couple's frequent intense arguments; chronic bickering; inability to resolve differences in a way that doesn't leave the other feeling resentful; perceived power imbalances; feeling emotionally disconnected from one another; not feeling loved or attended to enough; the inability of the couple to enjoy spending time with one another; not having a physically intimate relationship; and, in general, a lack of vitality in the relationship. As extensive as this list is, it is by no means exhaustive—couples may also be facing profoundly difficult and complex issues around finances, fertility, serious illness, or aging, to name but a few.

In this chapter we look at how to address some of the more common difficulties that are encountered, but it is important to bear in mind that the fundamental *principles* discussed throughout apply to almost all of the difficulties couples bring into therapy. If, for example, the couple therapist looks for strengths on which to build, helps the couple hear and understand one another, and helps them learn to tackle problems collaboratively, even seemingly implacable differences are often resolved. Nonetheless, *applying* the basic principles in specific cases or with specific problems may require a good deal of resourcefulness and creativity. It is with these specific applications that this chapter is concerned.

TALKING WITH THE COUPLE
ABOUT THEIR SEX LIFE

As I discussed in Chapter 4, many couples are extremely hesitant to talk about sex with each other or with me. I have two goals when it comes to discussing sex with couples. One is to help them become more comfortable *talking* about it. And the other is to help them revitalize their sex life by focusing on how to increase desire and expand their sexual repertoire.

Even when couples are connecting somewhat better emotionally, having fewer arguments, and are generally feeling happier with one another, they often do not resume having a sexual relationship. One or both of them may not really be interested in having a physically intimate relationship. For some couples, their sex life with one another has never been very gratifying. For others, though they once had a strong sexual relationship, it has faded into a distant memory. Many couples would like sexual intimacy to be part of their life together, but it's been so long since they related that way that they are awkward about how to get started again. One person may have made overtures that the other has rejected. The other person may feel that the partner's approach was more dutiful than sexual and thus not at all inviting, much less arousing. Although couples who have made some progress are more likely to raise these issues than they were at the beginning of therapy, it's important for the therapist to check in with them periodically about this aspect of their relationship. One or both of them may not be mentioning their concerns about the lack of sexual intimacy because they feel that it may lead to hurtful things being said that may undo the progress that they have already made. Or they may feel that it *should* or will happen naturally and is not something that they should have to "work" on in therapy. When the therapist raises the sex issue, it's important to do so in a way that does not pressure the couple to address something that they would rather not confront. There's a fine line between being intrusive and being "inviting." Often the first order of business is to get some agreement between the couple on *if*, *how*, and *when* they would like to address this issue. So, when Adriana said, "I think it will happen when it happens. I don't want to force things. I think we're getting closer and it will just happen," I ask her husband, Brad, *"Is that okay with you?"* Sometimes it's a simple yes. But often, as was the case with Brad, the response will be something like "Even when we were getting along we barely had a sex life." It is tempting then to inquire more about how they understand that. But to do so would be to override one person's wish not to discuss their sex life at this time. It's important for the therapist to acknowledge this wish and ask the person who was reluctant to talk about the topic if s/he is *"okay with us talking about what has gotten in the way of sex happening naturally."* Almost always, the reluctant person agrees to this level of conversation. But I am careful to keep the initial foray into the issue quite brief.

Often, a couple begins the discussion by talking more about logistics than issues of sexual desire or the quality of their sexual interactions per se. So, for instance, the couple who are rarely awake and in bed together because one is a night person and the other is an early riser, might discuss some solutions to this problem. Or the couple who feels that they are always busy doing separate things when they are at home together can share some thoughts about what might make a natural transition to a sexual relationship more likely. Though I am aware that there may be a lot more to this problem than being out of sync with their scheduling, I do not push the issue at this point. During the discussion I also mention, as I had when I asked about their sex life in the first session, that if there are issues around feeling desire for one another, or keeping sex lively, or making the sexual experience better, we could also discuss *that* at some point: *"Many couples talk to me about not feeling much desire for one another after having been with each other for a long time. There are some things you can do about this problem, and I'm very comfortable talking to you about these things in a lot of detail, if at some point you would like to do that."* Again, I am normalizing something that they may be hesitant to talk about and letting them know that I have something to offer them in that sphere too. I am hoping that their curiosity will enable them to be more open to discussing the topic.

Working on Issues of Desire

The first stumbling block for many couples is that one or both of them no longer feels much spontaneous desire for the other. When I explore with the couple the quality of their sexual interaction when they *do* have sex, they often say that they enjoy it. And not infrequently both partners assert that they enjoy sex very much. That makes it all the more puzzling why so much time elapses between one sexual encounter and the next. It seems that they are all too ready to go back to relating to one another in a nonsexual way.

For most couples it is not that they don't feel sexual at all, but rather that they satisfy their sexual urges by masturbating. Many men frequently masturbate to pornography. And though many women like pornography, they more often masturbate to arousing books and sexual fantasies. Opening up a discussion of if, how, and when each of them feels sexually turned on is often a little embarrassing to one or both of them. But usually the awkwardness passes and even by just being open about this topic, they are already relating to each other in a new, less-inhibited manner.

Frequently women feel that they can't compete with the images that arouse their spouse when they watch porn and need reassurance from their partner that real sex doesn't have to be like pornography to be satisfying. Many other topics emerge from this first line of inquiry. Sometimes one person has thought his or her partner didn't have any interest in sex at all, and is surprised, and possibly hurt, to hear that s/he masturbates. Sometimes the issue of being addicted to porn comes up, either by the person who watches porn or by his or her partner.

At some point in this discussion, I ask the simple question *"Do you think you'd like to try turning to each other some of the time for sexual fulfillment rather than satisfying yourself?"* Often the answer is that though masturbating is okay, they would actually like to have a sexual relationship with their partner, but there is a lack of the preliminary warmth, affection, and physical contact that would make that seem more natural. This can be true even though the couple is getting along better and many of the issue that originally brought them to therapy have been largely resolved. It is helpful for the therapist to normalize this state of affairs by saying something like *"It seems like the tensions that existed, or just the day-in and day-out stresses of life, have resulted in you getting out of the habit of being physical and warm with one another."* And if the couple have children, I might add, *"Many couples relate to their children in a warm affectionate way but forget to be that way with each other."* I explore with them what each of them pictures if they were to start to be physically affectionate with one another. Often it's something as simple as snuggling a little while watching TV or hugging each other in bed before they go to sleep.

Though being warm and affectionate with one another may be a necessary preliminary to wanting to have a sexual relationship, it is not the same thing as stirring desire in oneself and in one's partner. If the couple is in agreement that they would like to have sex with one another on a more regular basis, they need to keep sexuality in the air, so to speak. Here's what I say: *"You've gotten out of the habit of relating to each other as sexual beings. Probably when you were first dating, you touched each other in an erotic way even when you couldn't have sex. What I am suggesting is that you go back to doing that. So, when you have a minute alone with one another, you can touch each other in way that's a little bit of a tease and a reminder that you are both sexual people. I'm not talking about touching as a way of getting sex started. But rather, touching each other when you couldn't possibly have sex. So, for instance, sometimes having a quick sexy kiss goodbye instead of the usual peck on the cheek. Or rubbing your partner's backside during a hug. Or coming up behind your partner while she's at the computer and gently kissing the back of her neck. Or, when nobody's looking, rubbing the inside of his thigh or touching his crotch. Or briefly licking or sucking her finger. Or caressing her breasts for a brief moment."*

This usually leads to a discussion of the kind of erotic touching they each like and don't like. To make this feel like a long, slow tease rather than something intrusive or annoying, each needs to know what's appealing and what is not. For instance, many men say they try to do just what I'm suggesting by coming up behind their wife while she's cooking and squeezing her breasts, only to get rebuffed. But perhaps if it was a gentler touch or a kiss on the neck, it would feel erotic, not intrusive. I emphasize that people need to do not what *they* find erotic, but rather what their *partner* finds arousing. I reiterate to couples that in order for it to be a *tease*, it has to be clear that this is not an overture to having sex right at the moment. It's just meant as a reminder that they each are sexual and that at some point they may have the time and the inclination to act on the desire that's being momentarily stirred.

Often, just my mentioning the various erotic things they could do to each other in the course of their daily life stirs desires that they have boxed away. Frequently there is laughter, or comments like "sounds good" or "maybe we should go right home instead of going to work." In a way the session itself has demonstrated the power of the tease, and I build on the good feeling that's been generated by saying something like *"You both seem very open to this. . . . I think you've been wanting to get together again and just didn't know how."*

Though many couples respond positively to my suggestion of "erotic touching," others are not comfortable with this suggestion. They feel that they just don't have desire for their spouse, and imagining doing and receiving that kind of touching feels awkward and unnatural. Though they know intellectually that it is normal for sexual desire to decrease over time simply because of the familiarity that they have with one another, their implicit model of how sexual contact of any sort occurs is that desire must come first. When their partner suggests having sex, they rebuff the overture because they do not feel desire. They have a hard time accepting that all they need is to have the wish to have sex become part of their life with their partner, not the bodily sense of sexual arousal. I explain that for most people once they are touched and/or see that their partner is aroused, they begin to feel the desire in their body that they did not spontaneously have before they actually got started.

I have found it useful in these instances to use Iasenza's (2010) analogy of planned sex as akin to going out to dinner with one another, and say something like *"You make dates with one another for dinner, and even if you aren't that hungry, you usually get an appetite once you're in the restaurant. The items on the menu entice you even if you weren't hungry when you sat down to eat. If you think of having sex as an activity which you are likely to enjoy even if you weren't initially in the mood, you might not only feel comfortable with making a 'date' for sex, but also enjoy the anticipation."*

Getting the reluctant partner to give it a try is only the first step, however. We then discuss what each can do to make the date more interesting. *"What can make the encounter sexy even if it is planned and not arising out of spontaneous desire? Showering together? Music? What's a turn-on in terms of the way your partner could dress? High heels? Seeing him in tight jockey shorts? Tight jeans? Wearing a black t-shirt? Thongs? Costumes? Is it sexy if she slowly unbuttons your jeans? If he unbuttons your shirt? If you slowly strip in front of him? If you use oils? Incense? Have a cocktail together?"* My aim here is to trigger their imaginations and to get them to be less inhibited with one another.

Again, using Iasenza's (2010) analogy, I also talk to them about expanding the number of items on their sexual menu. As part of this expansion, in order to help them be less inhibited with one another, I raise all sorts of possibilities. For instance, I might ask, *"Do you like slow gentle sex or sex that's a little rougher or more edgy? Does s/he touch you with the rhythm and pressure that you like or would you like it to be different? Do you like your nipples sucked? Pinched? Do you like to use a vibrator? Do you use it on him too? Do you like anal touching or penetration? Do you like handcuffs or being tied up? Do you like to try out being different genders, dress like a man? A woman? Do you moan, scream, cry, laugh? Do you like him or her to talk dirty? Do you like to look in the mirror?"* Despite the initial embarrassment, often this kind of questioning leads to surprising and productive discussions about what they each might be willing to experiment with. If they are going to try something new, we discuss limits and safety and the need for checking in with one another to make sure that the other is still feeling okay about what they've agreed to try.

I also schedule individual meetings with each of them to further explore what they each like and how they can awaken their sexual self if it feels that s/he doesn't have much of a sex drive. Women, more often than men, seem to feel that their sexual self has gone into hibernation.

I suggest to them that there are things they can do to bring back their sexual self. For one, they can allow themselves to linger in looking at the sexual images that surround us in advertising. I might say, for instance, *"When you see a billboard advertising Jockey shorts, really look at it, or if you see an ad with a couple in a sexy embrace, spend a few seconds really taking in the image."* I also suggest that women put on music that makes them move in a sexy way and dance around when they are alone or in the shower. In addition, I have found Ester Perel's (2010) question "How do you turn yourself on?" (adapted from Ogden, 2008) very useful. Equally important is the corollary question she asks couples: "How do you turn yourself off?"

When people do already feel sexual, the individual meetings are used to help the person feel comfortable talking about the type of sex s/he would find most arousing. I encourage each person to think about the best sexual experiences they have had and what sexual images they have that can bring them to orgasm. I inquire about whether they are comfortable using those images while they are having sex with their partner. Many people feel that they are being disloyal or that it makes them feel they are disconnected from their spouse if they are engaged in sexual fantasies while having sex. We discuss whether that is a topic we could talk about in the couple session and whether sharing information about the *specific* fantasies would or would not be okay to do. After the individual meetings, many people are more comfortable sharing with their partner more about what sexual images are arousing. Often there is a way to incorporate each person's preference into their sex life.

If it is difficult for a person to get aroused, not just by their partner, but even with fantasies or pornography, I suggest that they consult with their physician about the possible effects of medications they may be taking or whether their hormone levels are in the normal range.

Additional Issues

Sometimes one person is unwilling to try to have sex, and none of the suggestions just described help. In an individual session, I discuss with him or her what this is about. At times a person just can't get over the cruel things that their spouse has said about his or her body—for example, your vagina is too big, your penis is too small, you have a fat rear end, your vagina smells bad—and though the relationship has improved, having sex is so associated with hurt, anger, and self-consciousness they feel that they just "can't go there." Often we have already spent some time discussing these hurtful comments, but it is clear that more work needs to be done to see if there is any way to repair the profound hurt that occurred. As discussed earlier in Chapter 9, these types of cruel statements may have been when the person has "split off" loving feelings and discussing this topic again— perhaps linking this to legacy issues—may help the hurt person not only forgive, but not see this as a "true" statement about how the spouse feels.

In the course of an individual session the person who isn't interested in having sex may reveal that s/he has an aversion to the other's body. S/he might say something like "I know it's a problem and not good for our relationship, but I just *can't* do it. I'm not attracted to him or her and, to be honest, I feel a little repulsed by his or her body." The first thing I do in response to a statement of that sort is to explore with the person what it is that s/he finds "repulsive." Some of the things that are repellent are things that are "fixable," but either s/he does not feel it is his or her place to ask that of his or her partner—for example, becoming more muscular—or s/he *has* asked and the partner was hurt, angry, and resistant to doing anything about it (for example, losing weight, drinking less, giving up smoking). When the "revulsion" is of this sort, I discuss with the person whether it is true revulsion or actually a power struggle. I'll say something like *"I can understand your frustration in this, but I'm concerned that you're caught in a vicious circle by trying to get him or her to change by withholding sex. If you let go of that struggle, could you enjoy sex?"*

But sometimes it is a true phobic reaction. For instance, Arnie, a man in his 50s said, "I know it's terrible . . . it's me. I know my wife's body is fine for a woman of 48, but I just can't stand any flabby skin at all. I've been in therapy, and I'm sure it has to do with my mother, who walked around the house busting out of her bra, but I'm still disgusted by soft skin." Or, Emily, who said, "I love Alan but I'm really turned off by how pale and sort of pasty his skin is. It's superficial of me. I know it shouldn't matter but I can't talk myself out of it. A feeling comes over me when I look at him—I guess it's disgust—I feel so guilty saying that."

In response, I'll ask them if they would like to try finding ways around this aversion, and I give them a sense of some of the things they might experiment with. *"For instance, we could discuss with your spouse, his or her wearing silky t-shirts and you would concentrate on the smooth sensuous feeling of stroking his or her body through the silky covering. Or you could put lotion on your hands and with closed eyes see how it feels to run your hands along the curves of his or her body. You could also see how it would be if you focused on the pleasurable bodily sensations you felt as your spouse touches you."* If the person is willing to try overcoming the aversion, I refer them to an individual therapist who will work with them directly on this issue.

Sometimes people do not want to have sex with their spouse because they are having an affair with someone, and not having sex with one's spouse is a way to be loyal to the third person. When I suspect that this might be the case, I do not ask the person about this suspicion because I do not want to know anything that I couldn't share with the partner. But in a meeting alone, I will suggest that the person go into individual therapy to sort out their feelings about their spouse. *"By not being willing to have sex with your spouse you are putting the brake on how much intimacy the two of you can have. Perhaps you feel that this kind of marriage is okay with you and that your spouse can accept it too. But I think this would be helpful for you to sort out in individual therapy because I sense your ambivalence about how close you want to get to your spouse."*

And lastly, some people resist the intimacy of sex not because they're having an affair, but for unconscious reasons like fear of merger, dependency, loss of autonomy, or loss of some kind of psychic strength. As I have discussed in Chapters 8 and 9, some of these issues can be worked on in couple therapy. But sometimes the issues are too much out of awareness for couple therapy to be helpful, and then, after explaining this, I make a referral for individual therapy.

COMMUNICATION SKILLS, COLLABORATIVE CONVERSATIONS, AND "BRAINSTORMING"

The ongoing work of couple therapy often involves helping a couple understand and put into action some skills that make the relationship go more smoothly and thus enhance the possibility for closeness and intimacy (Lerner, 2002; Jacobson & Christensen, 1996; Heitler, 1990). What I think of as the "how-to" aspect of the work goes hand-in-hand with the insight and emotional connecting that we have been focusing on thus far. Without "know-how," couples can readily revert to interactions that make it difficult to sustain closeness and intimacy. We will look here at some of the skills that therapists can help a couple to develop. For a fuller exposition of the wide range of behaviors that are involved in maintaining a good relationship, the reader may want to look at my self-help book for couples, *We Love Each Other, But . . .* (E. F. Wachtel, 2000).

Simply put, many couples do not know how to speak to one another. I am not talking here just about the communication of deep emotions or vulnerabilities, but rather the ability to have conversations of *all* sorts. This section focuses on the work one can do in couple therapy to help couples learn to speak in ways that not only help them avoid unnecessary conflicts, but also help them enjoy spending time with one another. Many couples do not even have an image of how to have a collaborative conversation rather than a debate. Frequently couples end up arguing when there is no real disagreement. Though it is possible, or even probable, that there are underlying psychodynamic reasons—for example, anger at one's spouse, anxiety about merger—that have perhaps led to this way of interacting, I start with a more straightforward assumption: that they are in need of some skills, and that a large part of why they may be hurt or angry is due to the way they communicate.

I want to emphasize that this is not an either/or approach. The behavioral and the psychodynamic perspectives go hand-and-hand. For instance, one woman described feeling that she was very constricted around her husband and that she knew this came about because she was anxious that he would respond scornfully. She spoke about how hurt she felt when he spoke to her that way and how insecure it made her feel. Before we could work on their learning new ways of talking to one another, we had to address this issue. I asked him if he *intended* to be scornful and said, *"If that's not your intention, do you get why Gracie [his wife] experiences it that way?"* We discussed whether he thought other people experienced him that way and if not, did he speak differently when talking to them? Not until it was clear that he actually did want to be closer to his wife, and "got it" that he responded in a way that made her feel put-down, was the couple ready to learn *how* to discuss things in a different manner.

But with another couple, the behavioral aspect of their difficulty in communicating was the starting point. The husband was a self-described "fast-talking, type-A New Yorker" who said, "I love my wife deeply, but her leisurely midwestern style can drive me out of my mind." His wife chimed in, "I can't talk to him without him barking at me 'Get to the point, get to the point,' and so I've pretty much given up trying to talk to him." As we looked into this dynamic further, it became clear that though there were some behavioral things they could do to be more in sync—for example, they could set up a specific time to talk so that he could plan for it and it wouldn't feel like an interruption; she could try to speak in shorter chunks, thus giving him space to interject more frequently; he could deal with his nervous energy by perhaps doodling as he listened—there were also other nonbehavioral concerns that were at play here. For one, Linda, the wife, often talked about her close friends, and Jared, the husband, confessed that he found this kind of conversation "boring." As we explored this issue further, it became clear that her involvement with so many people left him feeling "unimportant"; he felt that she wasn't as interested in the day-to-day aspects of his work as he wished she would be. But his impatience with having to fill in background and details when she *did* ask him about work had led her to avoid the topic. Understanding the feelings behind their conversational pattern enabled us to fine-tune some of the communication skills needed to better reflect what they both really wanted from one another.

The balance between the behavioral and the psychodynamic perspective is more a matter of what *relative* weight to give to each with a particular couple. Both aspects are always present, because people's underlying assumptions lead to behaviors that all too often, ironically, create "accomplices" who unwittingly confirm these assumptions. (P. L. Wachtel, 2014a; see also the Epilogue). So a person who believes that she will never be understood may go into so much detail that her partner turns off, loses the thread, and unfortunately confirms his wife's feeling that she won't be attended to and heard. Adding a systems perspective to the psychodynamic and cognitive-behavioral points of view utilizes this understanding to help the couple develop and mutually reinforce new behaviors that turn the pattern around.

It is important to note that working with couples on developing skills is contingent on each person feeling *motivated* to do so. For this reason I don't *initially* focus on skills. As I discussed in the chapters on the first few sessions, before we proceed further each person needs to feel deeply understood, and the pivot of the sessions needs to shift from complaints to an understanding of what each person is longing for. Once hopefulness about getting their needs met is established, the couple is much more motivated to look at the "how-to" aspect of making this happen.

Taking Positions: An Adversarial Stance

Many couples start conversations about decisions that need to be made by immediately staking out their positions. With some couples, almost no topic is exempt from this modus operandi. A conversation in which two people throw around ideas and bounce off one another's input just isn't in their repertoire. They approach each conversation with a *position* even if at heart the decision being made isn't that important to them. They start with an assumption that they are, or will be, at odds; that they want different things; and that someone will win and someone will lose.

It is easy enough to see how this attitude may be the result of underlying concerns such as anxiety about being dominated, an assumption that one's desires are of no importance to one's loved one, or the feeling that you are in danger of losing your sense of separate self if you don't forcefully assert yourself about what you like or don't like. Again, the behaviors that come out of these assumptions can ironically sometimes result in exactly what one has dreaded. When the tenor of the loving relationship is adversarial, it becomes a "confirmation" of the belief that led to the behavior in the first place—for example, that one must look after oneself and can't assume that one's partner is going to spontaneously care about your concerns. When one person behaves in an adversarial manner, the other is likely to do so in return. Here again, we see how people can make one another into "accomplices" in maintaining their problematic schemas and behaviors.

In order to help a couple change this type of interaction, the therapist needs to get them to see and understand the problem with their habitual "conversational" style. Sometimes couples really can't imagine any other way of talking. So, for instance, when I pointed out to Ethan and Loretta that they were *starting* a conversation from positions that were so strong that it would take effort and an unpleasant exchange for each of them to budge, Ethan looked puzzled. "But we have our opinions, don't we. Are we supposed to pretend that we don't?" The first order of business then is to explain to the couple what one means. In response, I might say something like *"It's the difference between coming in with a strongly advocated opinion and feeling that you will either win or lose, or starting off with an* <u>*inclination*</u> *toward some point of view, even a strong inclination, but with a sense that it might change in one direction or another depending on what your partner says, and even more important, an <u>interest</u> in what s/he has to say. A good conversation is one in which each person has the mental set of being open to influence rather than the set that one will either get one's way or will not." Or I might say, "A good conversation is one in which you both feel relatively happy with the outcome. That's possible to achieve if you do not each start out with an already iron-clad opinion about what you want. If you think about it, there probably aren't that many things that are crucially important to you or that you have thought about so much that there's no use in getting any more input about it. If you start with a 'case-closed' attitude, you are shutting your spouse out, almost like saying 'Shut up.' You may get your way at the cost of a good relationship."*

Once the couple "gets" what I mean by the difference between a "brainstorming" tone and an adversarial one, it is important for them to understand something about *why* they approach conversations with one another in this way. For instance, Paul said about his wife, Greta, "I have to be very strong with Greta or she'll end up persuading me to do something I really don't want to do. I'm a math guy—not so good with words. Greta is much more verbal and she makes such a strong case, that unless I am really strong and shut down the conversation, she'll outtalk me." In a similar vein, Heather said that she felt her husband, Brent, was used to having to be forceful all day because he was a lawyer and that he didn't know how to be different at home—"So, I have to be just as strong as he is or he'll roll right over me." Jesus said about his wife, Tricia, "She's like a dog with a bone. Once she gets an idea about something, there's no stopping her. You think you've reached some kind of compromise—and then the next day it's like the conversation never occurred, and she's back to the same issue. So the best thing is to not give an inch in the first place; it just encourages her and she's at it again. Compromises don't work."

In order for the couple to overcome this zero-sum approach to their exchanges, they each need to be reassured that what led to this style in the first place is being addressed. In this, the therapist needs to help the couple utilize their understanding of one another. So, for instance, in the case of Paul and Greta, together we came up with some ideas for how they each would behave differently. Though Greta disagreed that she could "outtalk" Paul, she accepted the perception that he felt that way. They came up with a plan that would give Paul time to think about what he wanted to say rather than answer in the moment. After Greta proposed something, *she* would suggest to Paul that he think about her idea for a little while before they talked any more about it. That would give Paul a chance to pull his thoughts together and to honestly reflect on his opinion rather than reflexively protecting himself with a strong position that automatically countered Greta's.

In the case of Jesus and Tricia, Jesus felt his wife didn't really accept compromises that he thought they had agreed upon. He was willing to start from a more flexible position if he could be assured that any decision they'd make would be respected and that Tricia would not attempt to revisit it an effort to persuade him anew. Because there was often a good deal of confusion about what actually *had* been decided, the couple agreed that at the end of a conversation, they would summarize what they had concluded and write it out. I noticed, however, that Tricia was only half-heartedly agreeing to this idea. In order to come up with a viable solution the therapist needs to make sure that both parties are really comfortable with the plan. When I commented that *"I'm sensing that you have reservations about this but are trying to be agreeable,"* Tricia said, "I guess—sometimes I think of something later—this seems too rigid." That comment then became the basis for further problem solving. Instead of the original plan, they would write down what was decided as a *tentative agreement.* She needed to make it clear that in her mind it was still unresolved and that she felt they needed to talk about the issue again. Though this could seem similar to the "dog with a bone" scenario that Jesus complained about, he thought it would feel different because "at least I'm not being blind-sided—thinking we'd reached an agreement when we hadn't." Once again, I want to alert the reader to the importance of wording. Had I said to Tricia, *"I think you're not really comfortable with this"* or *"I think you are not being completely forthright,"* she could easily feel criticized. Saying instead, *"I'm sensing that you have reservations about this but are trying to be agreeable,"* gets us to the same place without her feeling "called out" on a deception.

Discussing communication issues often leads back around to a discussion of sensitivities and legacy issues. For the sake of clarity, communication issues are being presented as a separate topic. But in practice, one might talk about them as part of the "legacy" work described in the previous chapter. And conversely, the legacy work is revisited in many different contexts and is not something that one deals with once and for all in a few sessions. Thus, for instance, Jesus's need to have issues settled quickly might be something that relates to childhood experiences in which he felt that promises were not kept, or that a sibling always got the best of him, or that a "dog with a bone" approach was his mother's way of dealing with Jesus's very controlling father. Insight into the origins of these assumptions can lead the spouse to be more empathic as well as help the person distinguish between legacy concerns and the current reality. This chapter is intended to give the reader a sense of the ongoing work of couple therapy, and here we can see that much of the work involves chipping away at problems by utilizing many different perspectives.

Being in a "debate" mode often gets in the way of a couple being able to have enjoyable conversations that have nothing to do with problem solving. Though there are some couples where both parties enjoy "debating" issues, be they politics, religion, movies, or whatever, often one person does not enjoy this sort of "conversation" and eventually closes down, resulting in the couple feeling that they have nothing to talk about when they are alone together. As much as I try to resist gender stereotyping, it does seem to me that more often than not it is the woman who feels that everything she says is challenged and that the kind of "joining" discussion she has with women friends is not something she can do with her spouse. Many men have told me that their spouse is taking this too personally and that they are silently skeptical of what almost *anyone* says. As in all the difficulties discussed thus far, the couple therapist invites them each to elaborate on what they feel and to come up with some ideas that would enable them to change this dynamic. One woman described feeling that she was failing a test, and that her husband "smirked" at what he regarded as "ignorant" and naive. Though he recognized this attitude and even apologized, he felt that his wife made no effort to learn about things that were of interest to him, and just repeated unthinkingly anything she heard. The couple had gotten into set roles and definitions of themselves that needed to be challenged. Did he *always* need to be skeptical? Did she always need to talk about *feelings*, not facts. Could they try having a different sort of conversation? The reasons for this sort of interaction differ from couple to couple, as do the solutions. But the common thread is that the "debate" style is often behind the feeling of loneliness and lack of pleasure in the relationship.

Differing Expectations Regarding Listening and Interruptions

One of the most common complaints that couples have with one another, and one that often gets enacted in sessions, is that the other *interrupts* and doesn't let him or her finish speaking. Sometimes this is clearly true. One or both may have little patience for hearing the other out and have a difficult time controlling the impulse to interject. Earlier in this book we looked at the importance of helping couples learn to listen for what they can agree with rather than what they want to rebut. Here again, we see how *communication* issues cannot always be separated out from larger couple issues like a lack of trust in the intentions or goodwill of the other, or a tendency to blame, or feel blamed too readily, or a tendency to be defensive, regardless of whether or not one is actually being blamed.

Sometimes, however, sensitivity about being interrupted can be explained more straightforwardly. It's not uncommon for people to have unrealistic expectations in regard to how long their partner ought to listen before having an opportunity to say something. I discuss with couples the need to speak in shorter paragraphs. Rather than go on and on, and then be interrupted because one's spouse is getting impatient, the speaker can stop after a paragraph or two and actively invite the other to say something so there is no need to interrupt. This can be quite difficult for some people. People who suffer from ADD have difficulty not saying everything that comes to mind, and feel frustrated when they are asked to summarize or be more concise. Other people have difficulty because they operate from an assumption that they will not be understood and feel a need to elaborate in order to make their point. When this occurs, part of the difficulty for the partner is that it can feel that the speaker isn't engaged in a real conversation, and is talking *at*, not *to*, the spouse. Thus, it can be helpful if the speaker can *acknowledge* when s/he is talking for a long time by saying something like "Can you hear me out, I'll finish up in a minute." Often there is a great deal of intensity to a person's anger at a spouse for interjecting before s/he has completed what s/he wanted to say. The tone and harshness of a person's reaction to being interrupted can seem to the therapist disproportionate to the offense. When someone is *fiercely* angry about the other's interruptions, I do not treat this as a communication skills issue. Rather, I explore with the couple the meaning of this anger. I would say something like *"Clearly, this bothers you a lot. Can you say more about this? What's it about?"* My intention here is to get at the source of the anger, and then to work with the couple to find some solutions. There are a myriad of reasons for interruptions being a source of significant anger, ranging from legacy issues, like being unheard in one's family growing up, to more current issues, like feeling that one's spouse is the "important" one in the relationship who tends to get the lion's share of respect and interest in social situations. As always, an understanding of these concerns leads to a better ability to come up with some solutions. So, for instance, if one person is perceived as dominating social occasions, s/he can make an effort to make sure that the other can more easily join in a conversation.

Even when couples have learned to accommodate to the other's style and expectations regarding interruptions, they may still find it difficult to be with one another's family, where different "rules" of conversation prevail. Here again the couple needs to think about some practical ways to help one another. Rather than saying "That's just the way they are" or "You need to be able to tolerate it better," the couple can brainstorm together to think about ways they can minimize the stress of these interactions. Should the spouse talk to his family in advance? Would it be okay with the spouse if her partner doesn't go to certain kinds of events? Could the partner take the initiative and say to the family, "Hey, everybody, please let Shaun finish what he was saying." Each couple will need to come up with solutions that work for them. The main point is for couples to have empathy for how distressing these style differences can be and to try to help one another as best they can.

Trying to Bolster One's Point by Referencing Other People

Discussions quickly take a wrong turn when, to prove the validity of some criticism, a person references other people. Comments like "Everyone sees you as too aggressive" or "Casey talked to me about being intimidated by you" or "Even your family sees you as being too dependent" inevitably backfire. Feeling shamed and ganged-up upon, the partner becomes defensive. Instead of taking in what the spouse is saying, the person on the receiving end of these sorts of comments experiences the spouse as disloyal and undermining.

The therapist needs to help the person who says these sorts of things understand how counterproductive, and even harmful, comments like this are. As always, I am careful not to make the person feel blamed or scolded. I would start by asking, *"Why are you telling your wife this? What's leading you to say these things when I think you already know that it doesn't really help?"* The answer is usually something like "Because I'm trying to get her to see—she dismisses what I say—I guess I get so frustrated that I can't get through to her." And to the wife, I might ask, *"How does it feel when your husband brings in your friends' opinions?"* She may say she feels hurt, or that she feels he's trying to "punish" her, or that she is outraged that he's talking to people behind her back.

It's easy for the therapy to lose focus at this point. After dealing with the feelings that have been expressed and "normalizing" both parties' reactions, the therapist needs to help them get back to the original issue that they were trying to discuss. But, before doing that, it's important to underline how even though referencing other people to bolster one's position might be very tempting to do, it is a temptation that needs to be resisted.

Sometimes couples will say, "Isn't it important for me to give my spouse feedback? Isn't that what being close is about?" The answer to that is "Yes, but" or "It depends." As I repeatedly say to couples, intimacy also requires tact. There may be times when your spouse can hear something that will be wounding but will in the end be helpful. But too often feedback about how others see one's partner is unnecessary and hurtful, and is being used as a hammer in an argument.

Revisiting Old Hurts

Not infrequently, one person in a couple will bring up in the session—and in arguments at home—an event that occurred years ago. This revisiting of past offenses results in frustration for both parties. The spouse will usually react with "Can't you ever let go of that?" or "Am I going to have to pay forever for a mistake I made years ago?" or "I'm sick of hearing about this.

I've had it!" And the person who has raised the topic is equally frustrated by the spouse's inability to understand *why* she has brought the topic up once again. Often the person who raises the long-ago hurt *isn't* actually still bothered about that specific incident any more. So in response to her spouse being upset—or even incensed—about her raising it again, she argues that she *has* gotten over the hurt and that she *has* let go of it. The spouse may say, "You haven't—or you wouldn't keep bringing it up . . . you hold on to things forever." This impasse can often be resolved by my helping both parties understand that in a sense they are both right; the hurt partner really isn't upset about that *particular* event any more but she *hasn't* fully gotten over it in the sense that there is something about their current interactions that feels similar. The past incident is being raised as an emblematic example—as a way to demonstrate or explain something—but it is certainly easy to understand why the other person takes this to mean that it is still an unresolved issue. For example, when Elise revisited a time that her husband assumed that an injury she had was minor, and left her alone in order not to miss a business meeting, she did so because she *still* felt that he tended to put work above all else. Or when Raymond brought up that his wife "never consulted me about anything to do with our wedding and relied exclusively on her family," he did so because he still felt that his opinions were not valued by her. Though these events had occurred many years prior to therapy, they were repeatedly raised because they seemed like good examples of a trait or way of behaving that was still present, but generally to a lesser degree.

With many couples this kind of exchange occurs repeatedly despite the fact that it is almost common knowledge that bringing up past "offenses" when talking about current concerns is not productive and rarely results in the recognition or acknowledgment that one is hoping for. Both parties need to understand not only *why* the person keeps raising the issue, but how the partner feels when forced to hear about the event once again. Often in addition to anger and hopelessness, feelings of shame are evoked. Furthermore, s/he may also feel embarrassed about being "exposed" in front of the therapist. The hope is that the person who is bringing the past up *not* because s/he is still hurt and needs to work it through, but because s/he feels it is "illustrative" of something more current that needs to be resolved, will really "get" that the point s/he is trying to make is undermined by the defensiveness that is being set off in the partner.

Complaints, Countercomplaints, and Countering Defensiveness

Many people report that when they try to discuss something that is bothering them with their spouse, the exchange inevitably goes badly. Rebecca, feeling hopeless about ever being able to raise issues with her husband, described it this way: "If I try to tell him about something he did that upset me, it turns into what *I've* done wrong and all the things *he's* frustrated about. I think he's just trying to divert the criticism and throw it back on me—he never raises these things spontaneously—only when I have something to say to him does he suddenly have complaints about me. He always manages to turn things around that way." The scenario she described is one frequently reported by couples. Voicing complaints can lead to hours of painful mutual accusations that leave each partner feeling misunderstood, hurt, and angry.

After "normalizing" this experience as an all-too-common one for couples, I explain *why* this so frequently happens and what they each can do to prevent this terribly frustrating scenario from happening in the future. *"Most people are sensitive to criticism and react defensively in a variety of ways. Of course, as we've discussed before, the key to resolving difficulties is for each of you to try hard to listen nondefensively—to listen for what has* some *validity rather than what's wrong with what the other person is saying. But there are also some other fairly simple things that you each can do when raising difficult topics that will make nondefensive listening easier."*

One important thing that the complaining spouse can do is to begin with what Gottman (1999) has called a softened—instead of a harsh—startup. A soft opening is a way of making a hard point in a way that is more likely to be heard, not just dismissed or argued with. For example, when Reina wanted to talk to her husband about how upset she was about his angry explosion at someone trying to cut in the line at an airport, I asked her to think about whether or not this was a common occurrence for him, *why* she thought it had happened, and how she thought *he* felt about losing his temper. She answered that she felt he was ashamed of what had happened because he's been trying to control his temper and these types of explosions don't happen nearly as often as they used to. "He hates flying—so I guess he was tense. But it's still unacceptable to me. I don't *care* how tense he was." Based on what she said, I modeled for her what a "soft" opening would sound like. It would go something like this: *"I know this kind of explosion doesn't happen nearly as often as it used to and that you probably feel pretty bad about it, but I'm still very upset and angry and would feel better if you'd acknowledged that it was inappropriate or at least talked more about why you think it happened."* The point here is that the therapist not only discusses and demonstrates what a soft start looks like, but explains to the couple the need to ask themselves the kind of reflective questions that enable them to start in a way that shows some empathy for the other.

In another case, Wally wanted to tell his wife about how hurt he felt that she choose to go to a social event related to business rather than cut short her trip to be with him on his birthday. He could start the discussion by saying something like "I know you have a very demanding career and contribute a lot to our family financially, and I really appreciate what a balancing act you have to do, but. . . . " Or "I know that you often do choose family commitments over work commitments . . . it's not that you never do that, but. . . . "

Another helpful lead-in is to acknowledge one's role in what happened. So, for instance, Wally might have felt embarrassed about making a "big deal" about his birthday and thus have given mixed messages to his wife about how important it was to him. If that was the case, he could start by saying something like *"I know I didn't make it clear that it was important to me to be with you, and maybe that's why you treated it casually, but I still felt bad about it and would have thought that you would 'get it' even if I wasn't clear."*

Many people experience criticism as a total rejection of themselves. They cannot hold on to the feeling that the person who is criticizing them can simultaneously love and admire them. Specific complaints can feel like a total devaluing of anything good about them or the relationship. Thus, putting the complaint in perspective can mean starting the discussion with a statement that wards off this kind of overgeneralization. So, for instance, when Michael wanted to tell his wife, Catherine, that he felt that she ignored his preferences and did just what *she* wanted, he could start off the discussion by saying something like "I know that you are a terrific mother and plan all kinds of great activities for the family, and that means a lot to me. But a lot of times I feel ignored and I'm frustrated that I can't seem to get through to you that I want. . . . " I assure the couple that though this may seem an unnatural way to start what is basically a complaint, with practice most people find that it become fairly easy to do. *"But it will only work if you each sincerely mean what you are saying when you lead with some affirming acknowledgment, and that gets back to learning the habit of noticing the things about each other that you truly do admire and respect."*

Legacy issues often account for the global generalization of criticism that makes a relatively circumscribed dissatisfaction seem like a denouncement of the whole person. When Anita would complain about being frustrated that she couldn't get her husband, Bradley, to commit to leaving work earlier so that he'd see their son before bedtime, he would respond as if Anita had said he was a worthless human being. Having grown up with a mother who made numerous suicide attempts, Bradley's insecurity about whether he had what it takes to "hold" another's love would be activated by criticism. To ward off those feelings, he would become angry and defensive. Knowing that Bradley's insecurities were easily activated, which then led him to be defensive and angry, Anita needed to preface her complaints by saying something like "I know how hard working and how ambitious you are, and I love that about you. And I know that you want so much to make us all happy, but it's frustrating to me that. . . . "

There are other factors that contribute to discussions or disagreements spiraling into drawn-out sessions of mutual escalating accusations. By focusing on the circumstances that lead to the escalation rather than to the *content* of the argument, the therapist enables the couple to think about what they could each do differently in the future. Many couples realize that conversations are much more likely to turn into arguments when one or both of them have been drinking. Another common situational factor is starting a conversation late in the evening, when the listener is tired or doesn't want to talk because it will interfere with his or her sleep. People are not at their best when exhausted, and generally have less ability to control the impulse to strike back. Often one person will say "Do we have talk about this now?" but the other insists on having the conversation.

The therapist can help them agree to a plan to deal with this scenario by examining more closely what each person's experience is at that time. So, for instance, we might discuss questions such as *"Does the person who wants to talk have difficulty delaying discussing something that's on his or her mind? What would help the person feel more comfortable delaying? Would it help to write things down? Would agreeing on a definite time to talk help? Could the 'tired' person listen if s/he knew that the conversation would be a short one? How would they keep it short?"*

Other "timing" factors may also play a role. For instance, sometimes the spouse's individual therapist might be encouraging him to speak up when something upsets him rather than hold it in and feel resentful. Though that might be appropriate in some situations, it can also lead to arguments if the circumstances are such that the "listening" spouse feels "ambushed" while in the middle of something else. Sessions can be used to jointly decide how to handle it when one person is upset about something that just happened, but the other person is not receptive to talking about it then and there. We discuss, for instance, what if anything would enable the upset person to delay talking about something without "stewing" about it and becoming more resentful. If s/he said, "I'm upset about something that just happened and want to talk about it later," would the other person be able to put the discussion on hold? The aim here is for the therapist to help the couple focus on *process*—the *how* and *when*—rather than just on the content. It turns out that these structural changes often make a big difference in whether or not conversations are productive or turn into fruitless arguments.

Often couples feel frustrated that if they have an argument, one person wants to forget about it and move on, and the other raises it again later to process it, leading to still another argument. Here too brainstorming about how to have these "after-argument" conversations can be quite helpful. One person may not want to revisit a prior argument because s/he assumes it will not clarify anything but just start the argument up again. And often that is precisely what happens. The therapist can help the couple come to some agreement about the type of arguments that they can just move on from without having to discuss them later, and which types one or both feel a need to process. And if they *are* going to revisit the argument, the session can be used to discuss *how* and *when* they will approach it and what they each need to do to put the argument behind them.

In addition to collaboratively problem solving with couples, I do, from time to time, throughout all stages of the work, offer some straightforward advice (see *We Love Each Other, But* . . . [E. F. Wachtel, 2000]). For instance, I suggest that they limit talking about things that are bothering them to just one person's complaints at a time. For instance, when Frida raised in a session that she was feeling resentful that her husband, Alfie, came home from work whenever he wanted to while she had to rush home to relieve the babysitter, he responded by saying that "if you want to start talking about things you resent, I have a lot I could complain about too—like the way you never put your things away even though you know that I hate clutter." When this kind of exchange occurs in the session, I explain that *"problems are much less likely to get resolved if after one person raises something that bothers him, the other person, says, and 'this is what bothers me.'"* I assure the person who has countered a complaint with grievances of his own, that his dissatisfactions are *important* and deserve to be focused upon, not as an *afterthought* or as part of a response to his spouse's complaints, but rather more fully, by our dedicating time and effort later in this session or in the next, to understand his feelings without having to simultaneously address his wife's dissatisfactions.

Dealing with one issue at a time is not always possible or sensible. Often what is offered to counter a criticism is in fact organically related to the initial complaint. If, for instance, in response to Frida's complaint about Alfie coming home whenever he wanted to he was to counter with *his* feeling that she didn't appreciate the difficulty of his commute, "and won't even discuss the possibility of their moving," his response is not a separate complaint but is an integral piece of the problem being raised. As I discussed earlier in the book, couple therapists need to keep the session on focus but what is *relevant* and what is a *side issue* is a judgment call that isn't always so obvious or easy to make.

Dealing with "Turn-Offs" Specific to One's Spouse

Thus far, I have been presenting some general principles that apply to most couples. But in addition to this issue, couples need to tailor their conversational style—when disagreeing about something or even when just chatting—so as to accommodate to what may bother their spouse even though it isn't necessarily something that would bother other people.

Hot Buttons

Often couples have difficulty conversing even about noncontroversial or neutral topics because they speak in ways that are a "turn-off" to one another. One might think that after years of being with one another and seeing what works and what doesn't, couples would *know* how to speak in a way that the other can hear. But often it is only when the couple therapist spells this problem out that the couple really understands what they need to *do* and *not do* to improve communication, be it when they are going out to dinner together, trying to make a joint decision, or resolving a dispute they may be having. A number of different types of communication issues fit into this category. But first the couple therapist needs to get the couple on board with the idea that even with one's spouse, one cannot just do and say what comes naturally.

Everyone alters their speech to fit the person to whom they are speaking. If they want to, most people are able to be tactful and take care not to offend. But couples often assume that they *shouldn't have* to take care when speaking to their partner—that home is a place to be *natural* and let one's guard down. Noticing moments in the session when one or both of the partners are talking in ways that show an awareness of and sensitivity to what works for the other, can help the couple achieve a more complex—and effective—sense of what it means to be "real" with each other.

We saw in Chapter 8 how people tend to use certain adjectives in describing people that have very personal connotations, whether positive or negative. Even without doing a genogram, therapists soon learn what words and phrases each person is particularly reactive to. An important skill as a therapist is communicating in a way that will not be off-putting, and conversely, using words that help a person feel understood. We are quick to read a person's reactions and, rather than persist in saying something in a way that will make the person defensive, we find another way to say what we want to communicate. In essence, a big part of our task as couple therapists is to help the *couple* develop a similar kind of sensitivity to each other.

Some couples learn to do this with one another spontaneously, listening to and taking in how the therapist communicates with each of them. But often couples persist in using buzz words that almost ensure that they will not be heard. Again, we could examine the motivation behind this, but I have found that often such explorations go nowhere, and unless one is very careful, can feel quite blaming. If, instead, the therapist approaches the problem as an extremely common phenomenon—we *all* have a tendency to keep doing things that just don't work—the couple more readily "gets it," and even if they slip or need reminders, they begin to be more open to learning new ways of talking to one another. Sometimes I create with the couple a list of the words that the other reacts to and suggest that they should try hard to eliminate these words from their vocabulary when talking with their spouse. Couples need to think through whether or not there is another way to say what they mean. If not, then like it or not, the "hot button" words must be said. So, for instance, does one person really feel the other is *abusive*? If so, it's important not to soft-pedal that feeling to make it more palatable to one's spouse. But often "abusive" (for example) is a dramatic—and counterproductive—way of pointing to behavior that *can* be described, and honestly, in other terms. And, indeed, even if that term does feel accurate to the person speaking, spelling out what one *means* by "abusive" may be a sufficient and more effective than using the term itself. So, for instance, Mariana would say, "Chuck is abusive. He takes out his moods on me. If he has a bad day at work, I'm the one who ends up paying for it. He'll pick a fight with me." Instead of dealing with the substance of what his wife was saying, Chuck would be indignant about being called "abusive." To him that meant somebody who was physically violent or terrorizing, not someone who was in a bad mood and maybe a little "picky." Having grown up in a home where he and his siblings, as well as their mother, were intimidated by his explosive, alcoholic father, Chuck simply could not tolerate being characterized that way. Mariana felt she needed to use the word "abusive" because to her, coming home with a chip on your shoulder and looking to find something to criticize, was really *wrong*. She agreed it was not the same level of "abuse" as someone who is violent and frightening, but she did need Chuck to take her being upset with this behavior seriously. They agreed in the session that she would no longer say "abusive," but would instead use phrases like "wrong of you," "not nice," and "extremely inconsiderate" if she felt a need to call attention to what she felt was unacceptable behavior. Of course, further work needed to be done in the couple therapy about this interaction, regardless of how it was named or described. But by working first on the "hot button" buzz words, that further work is often facilitated.

Though the word "abusive" is a potent word for *many* people, many "hot button" words are rather idiosyncratic, in the sense that they have a particularly negative connotation for a person even though others may not find them objectionable. For some people, for instance, saying that they seemed "anxious," "depressed," or "worried" will feel incorrect and set off a defensive reaction even if the spouse means it sympathetically. For example, one woman, trying to be supportive, would ask her husband if he was "worried" about doing a good job on the project he was working on. In response to that question he'd say with irritation, "I'm not worried, why would I be worried?" His wife was hurt by this response, and experienced her husband as emotionally closed and unwilling to be honest about his feelings. He, in turn, felt that she persisted in trying to dig up negative emotions and that she was projecting her own feelings on to him. It became clear that "worried" had a different meaning for him than it did for her. It meant *excessive* concern rather than an appropriate level of stress. Had she asked him if he was concerned about doing a particularly good job on the project or talked about the pressure on him, he might very well have expanded upon his feelings.

It's important to emphasize to the couple that they *each* have words that rub them the wrong way. But there is also *another* side to this equation; there are particular traits and characterizations that, when acknowledged, make the person feel intimately *known*, and thus *help* him or her be receptive to what is being said. These may not be the person's most obvious personality characteristics, and may not be the ones that the world at large sees. For instance, Warren, a hard-driving, aggressive lawyer, took a lot of pride in how "present" he was as a father, regardless of his very demanding job. He tried his best to go to school events, and took his children to school every morning. He felt—and his wife concurred—that he was a very accepting and accessible father. His wife, Elvira, recognized what a devoted father he was, but she rarely mentioned it aloud. Explicitly acknowledging these valued characteristics of the other is not a matter of being strategic. It goes to the heart of what makes love last in a couple. And positive feedback is even more meaningful when it is about the characteristics that the person him- or herself takes pride in. Including references to aspects of a person that s/he feels pleased with is one of the most important things couples need to learn to do.

Often when I discuss the importance of doing this more, someone will say something like "But she *knows* I think she's a very empathic person" or, "*Of course*, I know he's someone who can be counted on—he *knows* that I appreciate that." I explain that the other person may not be so sure about how much you value the trait, and that even if it's clear that you do, "*Most people like hearing it again from time to time. We all like to feel recognized and appreciated for things that are important to us.*" The wording here is important. By saying, "*We all like to feel recognized . . . ,*" I am including myself in the statement. I do this because some people feel embarrassed by the pleasure they take in being acknowledged. They may regard it as "weak" to want or need feedback. By saying "we all" want recognition, the desire is easier to accept and talk about.

Tolerance for Details

Some people find it frustrating and difficult to listen to a lot of detail. They want the other party to get to the point more quickly, and find that the other's more meandering style leaves them tense and impatient. Though there may be some slight gender differences here, they are by no means determinative. Many women want to scream "Get to the point!" just as often as men do when listening to their wives recount their conversation with a friend. Often these differences are talked about judgmentally, and each feels hurt, angry, and misunderstood. Both need to accommodate more wholeheartedly to the other's style. Impatient people need to give themselves over to the conversation more fully, and this is often possible if a conversation is planned for rather than occurring spontaneously. And the person who gives a lot of detail needs to try to "cut to the chase" more quickly. Similarly, simply acknowledging the other's experience is in itself helpful. If the person giving a lot of detail says something like "Are you following me?" or "Is this more than you want to know?," the other person may be able to more readily relax.

The Need to Stay on Point

A common complaint in couple therapy is that one partner feels that when s/he tries to talk to his or her spouse about something important, the conversation is frustrating because the spouse picks up on an irrelevant detail. Not infrequently, the person speaking concludes that it's not worth sharing things because the spouse won't "get" it, and the one speaking is left feeling annoyed and frustrated. When there is an intense reaction to the spouse being "off point," the reasons for that reaction need to be examined. What does it mean to the person that his or her partner is responding to the wrong thing? How does s/he understand why that happens? Sometimes it feels to the person that his or her spouse hasn't really been paying attention or hasn't remembered prior conversations. A spouse may feel hurt, angry, or hopeless about the other's lack of interest or involvement in what is important to him or her. When these feelings are there, we are dealing with far more than a straightforward communication issue.

There are times, however, when the question of responding to the wrong thing *can* be more usefully addressed as a more straightforward communication issue. Some people impulsively respond to some minor point rather than thinking through what the main point is. And others have an almost obsessive reaction to details and feel a strong need to correct anything that isn't quite right, thereby disrupting the flow of the narrative and missing the forest for the trees. This tendency can be exacerbated if the speaker throws in a lot of details that are not directly related to the point s/he wants to make. When this is a communication mismatch more than a reflection of deep dynamic issues in one or both partners, the couple can often come up with some ways to better handle the problem. Perhaps the speaker can start the conversation by framing it in a way that helps the listener know what's important and what's not. And, of course, the person who gets distracted by the details needs to make an effort to ask him- or herself, "What's the main point, what's important, what's the forest not the trees?" It can be surprising to the individual therapist who begins to work with couples how much can be accomplished by this "tweaking" of their behavior with one another, and how much genuine change in feeling can ensue without intensive focus on individual dynamics. This is not always the case, of course, but having the tools to try these more "surface" efforts first can be a great service to the couple.

Reactivity to Imprecision or Exaggeration

Some people have a very strong reaction to their partner using language that they regard as not sufficiently precise. With such people, phrases like "You never . . . ," or "You always . . . ," "He hates . . . ," or "It's been years since . . . " will invariably lead to a correction or denial of what has been asserted. In some instances, this is a defensive way to not respond to the essence of what is being said. At other times, however, the listener is generally a "stickler" for accuracy regardless of who is speaking or what is being discussed. In these situations, a balance needs to be reached between one person being more mindful of the other's need for accuracy and the reactive person developing a greater tolerance for minor inaccuracies.

Earlier, I discussed teaching couples to listen with the mental set of *"What can I agree with, what's basically right about what's being said?,"* rather than what's wrong and needs to be rebutted and challenged. With the "stickler-for-accuracy" person, the therapist may need to work particularly hard to positively reinforce those moments in the session when the person is listening in that way. Most often there is an obsessive–compulsive quality to this style, and it will take a good deal of effort for the person to respond to what was *meant* even if it was not presented with complete accuracy. I might say, *"What do you think your wife is actually trying to say? Maybe 'hate' is too strong a word for what you feel, but is she basically right, is she in the right ball park?"* And as always, when the person seems to be even a bit more able to pay attention to the content and not just the less-than-precise detail of what's being said, I will underline it and help the person take pride in developing that skill (see P. L. Wachtel, 2011a).

There are numerous other *specific* things people may have idiosyncratic reactions to—for example, speed of talking, voice volume, "obsessing" out loud, or picking at one's nails while speaking. Generally, the approach is to try to understand the reaction and then first see if it can be modified in some specific behavioral way that can facilitate better conversation. So, for instance, one man complained that his wife "always turned a conversation back to herself." He gave the following example: "One night I came home after a terrible day and I told her how 'everybody wanted something from me and I ended up losing my temper at my assistant.' The next thing I know she's telling me about a time she yelled at someone in a store and felt terrible about it." His wife was stunned and hurt by this example. "I was just trying to show him that I understood how bad he felt." She went on to explain that when she gets together with her women friends, one story leads to another and she just didn't understand how he could see that as "self-absorbed."

This man experienced his mother as always being the center of attention, and for this reason as well as many others, he "shut down" when he was in her presence. So, when his wife responded to something that he felt was changing the subject so that it was about *her*, he just let her talk and made no effort to continue his story. Of course, this coping mechanism led to a self-fulfilling prophesy, because then, indeed, the conversation *did* became about his wife's experiences rather than his. Understanding his sensitivity to this problem, his wife made a strong effort to find other ways of joining than referring to something similar that had happened to her. But equally important, her husband needed to resist the temptation to close down and instead to bring the conversation back to what he wanted to talk about.

There are countless numbers of specific things that can bother one person or another. Though both parties need to try to accommodate to what annoys the other, it is also important that each make an effort to be less focused on the habits and conversational style that they find irritating.

Tone of Voice

Perhaps the biggest impediment to closeness for couples is the issues they have regarding their perception of each other's tone of voice. In sessions, one person will explain his or her comment as a reaction to the other's hostile or disdainful way of talking. Over and over again I hear statements like these: "On the way here, I asked him a simple question while he was looking at a text, and the way he said 'What?' was incredibly nasty, like I was doing something terrible to interrupt him." Or "She says she asked me nicely to put my stuff away, but she was actually seething. I wish she could hear her tone of voice. It's as if she were saying, 'You idiot, can't you do anything right'—the fact that she said *please* doesn't mean anything." Or "When I try to talk with him about something I learned in my continuing ed class, he always responds with an inflection that's like—That's *new* to you? You didn't know *that*?"

Often one person feels the other talks about him- or herself with a tone of implied superiority to his or her partner. So, for instance, sentences like "I know my son, he's *not* into basketball, he's just humoring you" or "I deal with businesspeople every day, I'll handle it" can be experienced as denigrating the other. Many arguments start because one person heard something different than the other claims s/he said. Frequently, one person is referring to the tone while the other is referring to the literal words. So, when Charlotte says, "You didn't invite me to the dinner where other people were bringing their partners," Roger responds, "Didn't I say wives are invited, you can come if you want to?" But Charlotte is picking up an inflection that implies, "I could care less if you come" rather than "I want you to come," and thus in Charlotte's mind Roger didn't actually invite her.

The first thing I try when I encounter this kind of impasse is to ask the person who is being accused of having a hostile tone whether or not s/he knows what his or her spouse means. *"Can you see how your wife experienced what you said in that way?"* Sometimes the person says one of many versions of "Yes, but . . . "; "Yes, but that's because I've asked him dozens of times to stop bringing food into the bedroom—or at least clean it up if he does—and I keep finding bowls with dried-up food on the floor near the bed!"; or "Yes, but look who's talking—he's always sarcastic with me!"; or "Yes, but she takes it too personally—I was a little irritated and distracted in the morning because of a meeting I was going to have with my boss— what's the big deal if I said 'What'?" We then go on to discuss these issues and problem-solve in the ways I've discussed throughout this book—for example, if one person is "oversensitive," can the other accommodate to that or say something that helps the other not take it personally? Or if they are both talking to each other with a harsh tone, what is behind this way of being with one another and what could they each do to bring out the softer aspects of the other?

Often, the spouse doesn't think there's any problem with his or her tone, and essentially says it's a complete projection on the part of the spouse. When this happens, I ask the other spouse to imitate the tone s/he heard and then to talk about what it felt like to hear it that way.

Rather than getting into a debate with the person who might not want to admit that the tone imitated by his or her spouse does sound familiar, I suggest that s/he just give some thought to this, since, whether or not his wife or her husband is "right," it is the way s/he experiences it and perhaps s/he can do something to help change that. I also suggest that they give some thought to whether or not they would use the same tone in talking to their spouse if the conversation were occurring in the presence of someone in their life from whom they wanted respect. *"Just give it some thought. For example, if one of your students was a fly on the wall, or your boss, or your grandfather, would you be comfortable with them hearing you speak in that tone of voice? No need to answer or share your thoughts—just honestly ask yourself that question. Maybe your answer would be sure, why not? But maybe it would help you to see how you could modify your tone so your wife [or husband] would experience it differently."*

HELPING COUPLES LEARN
TO RESOLVE DIFFERENCES

Many couples bring to sessions issues that they feel "stuck" about. They describe being unable to reach a resolution about some serious issues on which they disagree, such as where to live, how money should be handled between them, where the children should go to school, whether or not to adopt a child, and so on. Sometimes the impasse is not only on large issues, but also on many of the mundane decisions that couples need to make. Some couples will leave their home mostly unfurnished because they can't agree on a style of furnishing. And much of the pleasure of vacations or evenings out can be diminished because the process of trying to come to an agreement feels like a tug of war. The communication skills and attention to tone discussed earlier are, of course, crucial ingredients in resolving these differences. So too is having a "brainstorming" rather than an adversarial mind-set. But in addition to focusing on general communication skills, there are some specific strategies that couples can learn that help resolve conflicts.

For one, I encourage each person to elaborate more on *why* something appeals to them. It may seem odd that one would need to suggest to couples that they do this because it seems like an obvious thing to do. Yet very often couples don't fill in enough about what they're thinking and feeling, and, when encouraged to do so in a session, it often has a transformative effect on the conversation. Couples often wrongly assume that their partner knows all the aspects of why they prefer one thing over another. By spelling it out in more detail, one partner is increasing the chances that something will grab the imagination of the other. So, for example, when Sherrie said that even though living in the suburbs would involve a commute, her vision was that it would enable them to spend more time together—"For one thing, we'd both be better at setting boundaries about work because we would *have* to if we were going to make the train, but also on weekends we'd be together more because so much of what people do in the suburbs are activities that involve the whole family"—this was very clarifying to her husband, Domingo. Of course, this was not entirely new to Domingo, but hearing his wife talk about her own issues with boundaries and about wanting them all to spend more time together did soften him a bit on the idea. And when he spoke about his wish to stay in the city as not just about commuting time, but also about not wanting to disconnect from his inner-city origins—though the neighborhood they lived in was becoming increasingly gentrified—his wife said she had a greater understanding of "where he was coming from." Again, it's not that she had never heard that before, but his emphasis had been on the commute, and additionally she thought she had addressed his identity concerns by choosing a multiethnic suburb. The slight shift in emphasis led to increased empathy on both their parts and the ability to generate some new ideas that might make each more comfortable with the other's preference. I suggest to couples that they need to learn to say to one another things like "Tell me more" or "How do you see it?" or "What else enters in to your wanting that?" Not only do these questions encourage greater elaboration, but the very act of actively trying to learn more coun-teracts the impulse to debate.

Another skill that couples can learn is to notice when there *has* been some agreement. Often I will "rescue" a discussion that is beginning to go badly by stopping the couple and pointing out that they just *agreed* on some-thing. Surprisingly often couples are so sure that they want different things that they don't even notice areas of agreement. Being able to notice when what they want overlaps can help them come up with some third alternative that might satisfy both of them. So, for instance, when Elena elaborated on how she envisioned it if they moved near her family in Argentina for the next school year and put their two young daughters in a local school so they would learn Spanish while they were still very young, her husband responded, "I could see that—it would be great for them to become fluent in Spanish—but I think it's too late to plan something like that—we'd need more time." I interrupted their conversation, which was heading toward a debate, to say, *"I'm struck by something here. You are both on board with doing this for a year. That's great. It's a big thing to do and you're both say-ing, 'Yes, let's do it!' The only issue is timing, and I think if you throw some ideas out around that you'll come up with a plan."*

Another crucial aspect of "brainstorming" conversations is for each person to throw out some ideas without feeling that s/he is committing him- or herself to anything. I'll say to them, *"Use tentative phrases and be explicit that it's just a <u>thought</u> and you're not sure you yourself are comfortable with it even if you are the one who is offering up the idea."* In this spirit, Russell, who was opposed to his wife's wish to send their son to a private school, said "I don't know. Maybe I'd be okay with it if it were a school that had a campus and took sports seriously. But I have to think more about that." It's important for the other person to acknowledge that s/he understands it's a *tentative* thought.

Not infrequently, when talking about an issue in the session, the couple resolve their differences and come to a decision. Quite often, however, it turns out that they each understood what was agreed to somewhat differently and after the session they may end up debating whose interpretation was correct. When the misunderstanding is discussed in the next session it often is the case that one person thought s/he had voiced an objection and believed that the other had understood and agreed to the modification of the plan. This is an indication that in the future the couple has to work hard to make sure they are actually on the same page, so I suggest to them that they put in writing what they agreed upon to make sure there that there is in fact no misunderstand-ing. But even when the couple understands the agreement in the same way, I encourage them to take a little time to give it some more thought. I do this because the cooperative stance people have in the session may have led them to agree to something that they actually are not comfortable with.

A Word about Solutions

There are a number of different ways for couples to resolve differences when they have "brainstorming" conversation. One way resolutions are achieved is that one partner changes his or her mind as a result of the conversation, and thus there is no longer a difference in preferences. Another way is that the couple *compromise*, in the sense that each goes along with what the other wants some of the time even though it isn't their preference, and the partner does the same an equal amount of time. The third possibility is that they find a third alternative that is agreeable to both parties. Taking turns can work for things that are relatively unimportant in the sense that they do not have an enduring impact on the other's life, like where to go on vacation, or whether and where to have a holiday party. But for more significant decisions taking turns doesn't work very well. "I went along with your wish to move to the suburbs, so now I should get to decide how the house is furnished" may feel *fair* in some ways, but it can leave the other (or *both* of them) feeling unhappy. For decisions that are important ones, it is far better for the couple to try to find a *mutually* desirable alternative. Usually this will be something that has *some* of the features one wants and some of what the other wants. But there is an exception to this that I have called "the little pig's wise solution" (see E. F. Wachtel, 2000). The idea comes from a children's book (Preston & Bennet, 1976) in which a pig having a temper tantrum says about a pie that's being divided, "I should get the most because I love it the most." The pig's logic for why she should get the largest piece struck me as eminently sensible. The idea here is that something may be *much more important* to one person than to the other, and that on that basis the other could be gracious and generous and let his or her spouse make the decision. So, for instance, after discussing an issue, one person could say to the other, "I see this means a lot more to you than to me, so you can make the decision" (e.g., the person who loves gardening could make the choice about the landscaping of a new house, or the person who cares more about music will get his or her say about the location of speakers.)

When couples learn how to listen to one another and brainstorm, they often come up with solutions to problems that previously seemed unsolvable. But, of course, not *all* differences can be resolved. There are issues about which no compromise seems possible, and where no matter how well it is discussed, one person cannot change the other's mind. One such issue is, of course, whether or not to have a child. When the couple reaches an impasse of this sort, they will each have to do some soul searching about what they can or cannot accept. One way a therapist can help is to explore with them whether there is anything the other could do that might help make acceptance more possible. For example, Julie didn't know if she could stay married to Aaron, who remained firm in his feeling that he did not want to have a child. "I know I might lose Julie over this, and I'd feel terrible if that's what she decides, but I just don't want a child," said Aaron. "She always *knew* I didn't want more children, and until a year ago, she seemed fine with that. I understand more about her feelings and why she changed her mind—and I hope she understands why for me, at my age, and having two grown kids, it's just not something I want to do. I thought about doing it for her, because I know it's so important to her, but I just can't." In answer to my question *"Is there anything that might make it easier for Julie to accept your decision?,"* Aaron said, "I know being close to nieces and nephews isn't the same as being a mom, but if Julie wanted to, I'd relocate to L.A. so we'd be near her sisters and their kids."

Another way therapists can help couples who, despite having a productive, nonadversarial conversation about something, still remain on different sides of the issue, is to highlight the way they each really tried to be open to the other's preference. Hopefully, having had good, open-minded conversations about the topic will mitigate the feelings of anger and resentment that so often occur when one partner's wishes come up against the brick wall of the other's *no*. If the couple feels that they each were really heard by the other, and *tried* to find a way to make the other happy, they may still feel frustrated, and perhaps sad, but also less angry at their partner. For example, when Toni, who had a very good job in the city, just couldn't get herself comfortable with the idea of commuting each day and being far from the children and their school, her husband, Ike, was accepting of her decision because he believed that she had honestly considered his point of view and had willingly looked at some houses with him. The fact that she had even gotten excited about a couple of the houses told him that she wasn't just being stubborn and narrow-minded. Feeling bad that Ike was going to be deprived of a lifestyle he really wanted, Toni volunteered that though she doubted she'd fine a job in the suburbs that she would want, she was open to it and would put feelers out to "headhunters" just in case something came their way. Again, though not all issues will be resolved, a change in the process from an adversarial one to a brainstorming approach is highly beneficial in itself and often transforms anger and bitterness into simple sadness that they genuinely want different things and will have some difficult choices to make.

COMMUNICATION SKILLS FOR THERAPISTS

Many of the communication skills just discussed are the same ones that the couple therapist himself needs to employ. We know, for example, that many people reflexively argue with statements that seem too authoritative. Therapists need to start with a lead-in that's collaborative, saying something like, *"I've had some thoughts about what might be going on that I want to share with you and get your input on."* I do this not only to minimize the chance of resistance, but as a way of inviting the couple to join with me in the exploration of their dynamics. I put out ideas in a way that invites the couple to correct and refine what I am saying so that it is more accurate. So after throwing out an idea—for example, perhaps you're feeling concerned that if you let your guard down you'll be disappointed again or maybe it feels easier to live with something that bothers you than to risk his being angry—I'll ask, *"Does that make sense to you, or not really? Does it resonate at all or am I off-base here? Is there a better way to put it?"*

I am quick to back off if I've inadvertently used a word that someone is having a strong negative reaction to. Even though we take care to avoid hot button words, and to use the language that each person can best relate to, there are times when therapists are surprised by a person's reaction to a word s/he has used. When this happens, I clarify with the person *why* that particular word doesn't seem correct and then accept the better word s/he offers. This models for the couple a nondefensive attitude that avoids power struggles. So, for instance, when a man I was working with objected to my saying, *"It sounds like you're feeling stuck,"* I responded by saying, *"So stuck isn't quite it—what would be a better word to describe it?"*

Just as we work with couples to teach them to accommodate when possible to the other's style, we too need to be attuned to specific communication issues and, as best we can, to modify our approach so as not to "turn off" a person. For example, apropos an earlier discussion, if someone is a stickler for accuracy, we need to be careful not to overstate something or be too global. Thus, in describing differences a couple might have in coping with an argument, I would be careful to say something like, *"Usually you are the one who wants to just move on, whereas your wife usually wants to talk about it."* By accommodating to the person's need for accuracy by saying *usually*, I am making it easier for him or her to agree.

Similarly, some people are very reactive to repetitiveness and may experience the therapist as belaboring a point that s/he has made. When the therapist senses this reaction, s/he needs to be careful to speak in a more succinct manner. Nonetheless, there are times when underlining and revisiting a point made earlier in the session feels important to do, and accommodating to one person's impatience would undermine the effectiveness of the work. It can help in those instances to acknowledge that you are repeating something said earlier and that the person may feel that s/he has already "got" it. So, for instance, I might say something like *"I'm repeating what I said earlier in the session, and I know you probably already have gotten the point, but if you can bear with me for a few minutes, I just want to put out there the implications of what we discussed earlier."* Note that this way of putting it does not blame or criticize the person or even call into question whether or not s/he has actually "gotten" it. I don't say, for instance, *"I know you feel that you 'got' it, or that you think you 'got' it."* Rather, it joins with the person by saying *"You probably already have gotten the point."*

In my first session with a couple I explain that I will be periodically interrupting them, and that I hope they can bear with me on that. Even though forewarned, some people have particular trouble with keeping statements short and with my interrupting them. If possible, I try to accommodate this problem and let him or her talk for longer chunks of time. But, when this long-windedness is interfering with the effectiveness of our work, I preface my interruption with an acknowledgment and explanation. For instance, I might say something like *"I'm sorry to be interrupting you, but I know you want these meetings to be productive, and part of my job is to help move the conversation along so that you will feel you've accomplished something by the end of the meeting."* If this is difficult for someone to do, I suggest scheduling extra time or even having individual sessions with each of them so they have time to expand on what they want to say.

Just as couples need to acknowledge the positives in speaking to each other as a preface to saying something that is hard for the other to hear, so does the therapist need to couch negative feedback in a way that acknowledges strengths, and even, where appropriate, as an *exception* to the person's usual way of acting. So, for instance, if the therapist wants to point out to someone that s/he is having a hard time listening nondefensively, s/he might say something like *"This topic seems to be a particularly difficult one. When we talked about . . . I was impressed with how open you could be . . . and in general, I think you've been trying really hard to give serious thought to what your husband/wife is saying—but today, you seem to be having a hard time doing that. You seem to be waiting to respond so you can rebut what's being said, rather than listening with an open mind as you've done before."*

And just as couples need to help one another feel good about themselves, whenever possible I give the couple credit for ideas they have that contributed to a good discussion. With that in mind, I might start a session by saying, *"I thought about how apt your description was last time,"* or *"I want to go back to something you said a little while ago in the session—I thought you described yourself in a way that helped me 'get you,' "* or *"The modification on my idea that the two of you came up with was really interesting. I might suggest that to other couples if that's okay with you?"*

I also try to model openness and nondefensiveness. For instance, if a couple wasn't able to follow through on a suggestion I made, I might say, *"I'm not sure that was a realistic suggestion"* or *"I think I was off-base there . . . Let's put our heads together and see if we can come up with a better idea."* If I'm genuinely puzzled about something that goes on between them, I might say, *"I don't think I'm really understanding this dynamic yet. Could you describe it to me a little more? I'm not there yet."*

I try my best not to say anything that is a "put-down" or accusatory (P. L. Wachtel, 2011a). When I can't find a tactful way to say something, I might say, *"I'm having a hard time finding the right word to describe what I mean."* Often then the person will provide the harsher, more critical word, giving me a chance to say something that modifies it. So, for instance, when I was feeling that Dominick was being a little grandiose in his certainty about always knowing the best way something should be done, I said, *"I'm not quite sure how to describe how you come across. There's a strength to how you say things—something that feels a little too much."* "Do you mean I'm being grandiose?," Dominick replied. In response I would say, *"I'm not sure if that's quite it, but maybe something along that dimension. You can come across as certain that your way is best—I guess a little grandiose does fit."*

There are times, however, when the therapist must be absolutely direct and not beat around the bush in any way. Even then, there are ways to buffer the negative input and maintain the sense of fairness that is so crucial to the therapeutic alliance. So, for instance, when Charles insisted that his wife, Miranda, who was a physician, was being controlling and bossy by what he described as "pulling her doctor card," and that he should have equal input about whether to call the pediatrician or take their daughter to the emergency room, I said, *"I don't agree. Miranda has knowledge that you—or I, for that matter—just don't have. Even though I agree there are often power issues between the two of you, I really don't see her as being concerned with that in those moments. It looks to me like she's worried and knows more about what symptoms need to be attended to than you and I would know."* (Note that I am joining with him at the same time that I am directly contradicting him.)

Relatedly, when Emmy asserted that she was "always able to tell when someone is lying, and nothing her husband could say would change her mind," I challenged her certainty by saying, *"I'm sure you are very sensitive to facial cues and nuances, but I think you're too certain of your judgment. You could be right, but I think you do yourself a disservice by not allowing for any doubt. I'm struck by this, because in so many areas you're very able to acknowledge self-doubt. My guess is that you're being excessive in your certainty because you are so afraid of being terribly hurt once again."*

Good clinicians know that tact and timing are crucial elements of being therapeutic, and this is even more true in working with couples, where one person can use an inadvertently "accusatory" interpretation" against the other, and where maintaining a therapeutic alliance with both parties is a continuing balancing act. The communication skills just described help therapists steer an even course in waters that are often quite turbulent.

The Therapist's Use of Self

There are times in a session when I experience one or both of the couple as speaking in a hostile, competitive, dismissive, or "lecturing-from-on-high" tone. A therapist can be very tempted to give direct feedback to that person about how s/he is coming across to you, and on rare occasions such feedback may be helpful. But one must take great care in giving feedback of that sort. The person can readily feel ganged up on or humiliated. S/he may experience you as not understanding his or her point of view. Additionally, there's the very real danger that the spouse, feeling validated, can hold it over the person and during arguments say, "Even the couple therapist agrees with me." For all these reasons, if I am feeling that the person would benefit from knowing how *I* experience him or her, I schedule individual sessions with each partner so that I can give feedback to each of them without being concerned that they will feel exposed or embarrassed in front of their spouse or that my feedback will add fuel to the fire of an already contentious relationship.

There may be times when it feels that the best time to explain about the tone and undercurrents of the person's way of speaking is to do so while it is happening. But I resist doing so unless I have an exceptionally strong relationship with the person and can put negative feedback in a context that counters the risks of it disrupting the therapeutic alliance and the person's trust in my neutrality. If I do give negative feedback in the joint session, then wherever it is possible and to the degree that it can feel neither false nor contrived, I underline and attribute to the person some positive motive that will make the negative feedback easier to accept. So, for example, I might say something like *"I think you may have a bit of a blind spot here. You know that I think you've been working very hard in these sessions, but I think somehow with <u>this</u>, it's hard for you to quite see yourself. Of course, my experience is subjective too, and you can dismiss it for that reason. But I think it's important for me to share with you what I experience."* With one couple I worked with, the husband would often speak to his wife in the sessions in a manner I experienced as extremely angry and cold. He felt that he had every right to be angry because of "the way she puts me down." I said to him, *"Yes, of course, you have a right to express your anger and frustration, but I don't think you have a sense of how intense and fierce your expression is. Though your words are polite, it comes across to me as if you were saying 'You're a worthless person.' I know you don't really feel that way about her, and in fact you've been doing a lot to make this marriage better."*

People often are taken aback by my giving this kind of feedback, and will argue with me about it. "I don't agree. I'm angry and I have a *right* to be. I don't see what's so extreme in what I'm saying." In response I'll say, again, *"It's the tone, not the words."* But because I don't want to get into an argument with the person, I'll add, *"But of course, as I said earlier, this is a subjective judgment. I think we've hit it off quite well, and I know you're working hard on the relationship. I'm hoping you'll give some thought to what I've said."* Though this feedback might be initially rejected, it is my experience that nonetheless it will have a big impact and the person is apt to work harder at monitoring his or her tone.

Feedback of this sort is useful for more subtle issues too. Finding a way to tactfully let someone know that there's a tone of "I know what's right" or "I'm better than you" requires all the clinical skill that we have been discussing throughout the book. Again, if at all possible, I give this feedback in an individual meeting with the person. Attributional statements are particularly useful when giving feedback that can easily be experienced as critical. I might say, for instance, *"I do experience you as sometimes getting into the mode of 'teacher' and I have a feeling I'm not telling you something that you don't already know about yourself but aren't always aware of when it's happening."* I also try to start with an acknowledgment of a person's effort. *"I think you've been making a lot of effort not to get into power struggles, and have really been good at mastering the impulse to 'win,' but I think in subtle ways there's still a tone of superiority that your husband responds to."* I then follow this general comment up with a specific example. *"For instance, when you said, 'Jimmy comes to me with problems because I spend hours working with him at night,' it felt to me like an implied comparison in which you were asserting that you're more devoted to the children than your husband is."*

There are times when I will share not only my perception but the *reaction* I am having to a person. For instance, one woman came across as always "knowing" what was right. There was something in her tone of certainty and lack of acknowledgment that there might be other ways to view a situation that stirred in me a desire to argue with her. Again, when the timing was right, and when I could honestly convey positive feelings about her, I was able to say, *"There's a way you're talking about this topic that stirs a wish in me to argue with you. I think it's a tone that doesn't allow for any uncertainty or acknowledgment of the subjectivity of your judgment. Of course, it's possible that it's mainly just touching something in me, but I don't generally feel an urge to debate people. So, for instance, in the session last week with your husband, when you said something about how he wastes his time reading sci-fi novels, I found myself wanting to get into a debate with you about their value. And that's particularly strange because I don't even read them. I think it has something to do with what comes across as absolute certainty about your opinion being right. My point in sharing this with you is that if there's something about your tone that stirs this in me—even though it's clear that I like you a lot—it's something that if you could work on would perhaps help your husband not be as argumentative with you."*

A REMINDER ABOUT FOCUSING ON STRENGTHS

In Chapter 3 I discussed the importance of motivating the couple by noticing steps in the right direction and giving positive feedback. Carefully choosing what to respond to enables one to convert complaints to wishes and build on strengths that the couple may take for granted. But as the work proceeds, it is all too easy for therapists to focus excessively on the couple's problems and to forget to notice their strengths or the ways they are changing and "becoming." For instance, if a couple is beginning to be more comfortable talking to one another about sexual preferences—laughing and kidding around as they do so—the therapist could interject a comment about how they really seem to know how to banter and seem to get a real kick out of one another. Similarly, when the focus is on enabling the couple to have an emotional experience in the session, the therapist could interject encouraging statements, such as *"I see you are both trying hard to put aside your wariness about opening up, and I get a glimpse of the trust in each other that you described having when you first met"* or *"It's important to notice how you are talking about what you feel without <u>blaming</u> the other."* Similarly, it is useful to call attention to *"the way you deescalated the tension of a difficult conversation by smiling at each other,"* or *"how you let yourself respond with empathy to his or her hurt even though s/he's angry at you,"* or *"I'm struck by how you used last week's conversation to open up with each other at home too."*

Statements with a similar kind of structure can, of course, also be made when the focus is a conversation, or problem-solving skills, or any of the other dimensions we have discussed. The point here is not tied to the specifics of what is said, but rather that the therapist, from the first session to the last, should always be on the look out for where s/he can highlight or build upon some change in the right direction, refer back to things that remind the couple of a good experiences they once had, expand each person's sense of self, and help them both become aware of positives not just about themselves as individuals but also about the quality of their relationship.

11

❦

Troubleshooting
Common Challenges

*T*his final chapter addresses the most common concerns expressed by beginning couple therapists as well as the seasoned clinicians who consult with me about their work with couples. It covers a wide range of topics, starting from some of the specific challenges of working with couples where there has been an affair, to the moral and ethical questions that couple therapists may face, like thinking about whether the therapy is doing more harm than good, or relatedly, whether one or both partners might actually be better off if they separated. It also addresses some of the emotional challenges that couple therapists face, as well as the countertransference issues that are stimulated by the therapist's exposure to a particular couple's dynamics.

SLOW PROGRESS WHEN WORKING
WITH COUPLES AROUND AFFAIRS

Working with a couple who is seeking therapy because of the discovery of an affair can be quite challenging. Therapists are faced with situations that can leave them feeling "stuck," frustrated, and at times even annoyed, because they, like the spouse, have been deceived by being told that an affair has been broken off when it has, in fact, continued. Here are some of the common situations therapists encounter:

- Even after months of therapy, the hurt person is preoccupied with what happened, and continues to search for more information about which she constantly interrogates her spouse.
- The person who had the affair gives a superficial explanation about what happened and why, and it doesn't make sense to the spouse.
- The betrayed partner discovers his spouse is still in contact with the person she had been involved with, even though she had agreed to cut off all contact.
- The spouse who had the affair wants to put it behind her and move on, and is frustrated by her partner's continuing focus on what happened.
- The betrayed spouse is unwilling to examine the dynamics in the relationship that existed before the affair because it seems like "sharing the blame."
- The betrayed person wants more details, and her spouse refuses to give more information.
- When more detail *is* offered, it leads to another round of hurt and anger, and seems like a setback.
- The injured person wants some tangible proof that her partner is committed to her—for example, that he change jobs if the affair was with a coworker, or that he sign over property (e.g., title to their home).
- The injured party wants the partner to do something hurtful to the lover as proof that he is less important than the spouse.

The first thing to remember when working with couples around the hurt, mistrust, and anger about an affair is that the work is usually *slow*, and the therapist needs to help the couple have realistic expectations about how long it will take to recover. Sometimes it takes many weeks for the hurt person to even decide whether s/he wants to work on the relationship at all. The person who has betrayed his partner may get impatient with how slow the process is and feel that s/he'll never be out of the "doghouse," so to speak. It's important to be clear with that person that s/he needs to have patience, and that, of course, if s/he'll forever be the "guilty" one, the relationship indeed won't work. I often say something like this: "*In my experience, if you are scrupulously honest in the future, about big things and small, if you work on your tendency to avoid conflict by being evasive or telling small lies, if you show your partner deep love and commitment, and, very importantly, if you both work on understanding and changing the relationship issues that were the context in which the affair occurred, the 'guilty and untrustworthy' label will eventually fade away. That's a tall order, and it will take a lot of effort and time, but it can be done. I've seen many couples emerge from affairs closer than ever.*" Note that I am joining with both parties here—the person who doesn't want to always be "guilty" and the hurt one who needs the spouse to make a big effort. But I am also reiterating that the hurt spouse must also make an effort to understand and change whatever dynamics in the relationship contributed to the affair happening.

Second, though what "works" to help couples get over an affair differs greatly from couple to couple, the methods used in therapeutic work are the same as those that have been described throughout this book. For example, the therapist might comment on the injured person's as-yet-unarticulated wish to let go of anger (an attributional interpretation), or comment on a person's effort to be nondefensive, or highlight the unfaithful person's growing ability to express feelings, or underline the couple's shared values in wanting to protect their children from knowing what happened, or focus on the ability of the hurt person to be angry without "villainizing" the spouse.

Often, the person who has been betrayed feels that ever since finding out about the affair she has changed—become a different sort of person—in ways she doesn't like. Frequently people say things like "I've never been like this before and I can't stand being so suspicious. I'm angry that he's put me in this position—he's taken away my trust." Many people become consumed by jealousy (Sheinkman & Werneck, 2010) and are preoccupied with trying to uncover yet more untruths—for example, scouring old telephone records, credit card bills, and emails—and now believing that they have been naively trusting spend countless hours trying to reconstruct events from years past when their spouse supposedly went on business trips or traveled with friends. Helping patients free themselves from the grip of obsessions is difficult, be it in individual therapy or couple therapy (Sheinberg, 1988). I usually normalize the person's obsession with questioning everything she thought she knew, and normalize too how difficult it is to free oneself from this kind of preoccupation. We explore together whether there are any specific things the partner who has had the affair could do to help the hurt person get over her need to keep searching for more evidence of prior betrayals. The answer given by Serena, the wife in a couple I had been working with for many months, typifies the "stuck" feeling that couple therapists can feel when dealing with this issue. She had discovered that her husband, whose work frequently involved travel to Asia, had been in a relationship with someone in Bangkok for the previous 5 years. She questioned whether her perception that she and her husband, Martin, had been happily married for 18 years had been accurate, and couldn't stop searching for proof that this was not the first instance of his infidelity. When I asked her what would help her trust that her husband was telling her the truth, she said, "He needs to come clean." Martin repeatedly replied to this accusation by saying, "I can't come clean about something I didn't do. Do you want me to lie and tell you I had affairs when I didn't?"

In response to this, I said, *"You are so hurt, I can understand why you might be afraid to let your guard down now. I think you might be more able to trust in what you husband is saying if you had a better understanding of 'why' he started an affair 5 years ago but not before. What was going on for him personally in his life at that time that contributed to his opening himself up to an affair then, but not previously?"* I also encouraged them to look at what might have been going on in their *relationship* at that time that made him more susceptible to having an affair than he had previously been.

Often the explanation given by the person who had the affair doesn't make sense to the partner, and that is why he is having trouble moving on. The therapist who thinks there is more to the story than is being revealed needs to make a decision about whether to encourage more disclosure. Knowing more details and the whole truth does not always make coming together again easier. Indeed, sometimes it can make it more difficult. Instead of pursuing the "the facts," I prefer to focus on what would make the injured person feel loved. I might ask, *"What would make you feel that even if you don't fully understand what happened, you know she truly loves you? Are there moments, even if fleeting, when you believe in her love for you?"* And to the spouse I say something like *"It takes a long time for trust to develop, but over time it can gradually be reestablished if your partner really feels the love you have for him. What thoughts do you have about how to show that?"*

Frequently, there are serious setbacks to the work, because the spouse, searching for more information by investigating or interrogating his or her partner, finds out s/he has not been told the whole truth. She may also discover that the partner has continued to have some contact with the third person despite promises that s/he will break it off entirely. My stance when that happens is to highlight that they each have a decision to make. Perhaps the "betrayer" hasn't really decided s/he wants to keep his or her marriage partner more than the person with whom s/he has had the affair. I suggest s/he would benefit from sorting that issue out in individual therapy. The person who has been lied to yet again needs to decide if s/he is willing to give the process more time. The reality the hurt person is faced with is that it often is difficult to break off a relationship, even if one has decided to do so. And even if there is no more communication of any sort, the offending spouse may still think about and miss the person with whom s/he had become emotionally involved. Unfortunately, I can't give assurances that in time the betraying spouse will fully get over the romantic feelings s/he had for someone else. I can say, however, that the chances of really getting over a romantic attachment are much greater if both partners commit to working to make their own relationship truly gratifying to them both.

Often the person who had the affair really doesn't seem to have an in depth understanding of why s/he did it, or why s/he let it continue, or how s/he could risk so much by getting involved with someone else. This lack of clarity contributes to the spouse's insecurity about the future. Though in the sessions with the couple I explore with them *both* the individual and the systemic dynamics, a separate meeting alone with me can help the person who has been unfaithful explore in more depth the various components that led to the affair. Sometimes the causes may be more related to individual issues than problems in the relationship. Being infatuated with someone is an emotional "high" and a temporary lift from the doldrums. Frequently, excessive use of alcohol is involved. Regardless of what individual issues were factors in the person choosing to have an affair, there are inevitably relationship dynamics that also contributed to the person's decision to be unfaithful. Helping the person who had the affair articulate those issues is often easier to do in an individual session when s/he does not have to be concerned about his or her hurt spouse feeling s/he is "blaming the victim." The individual sessions are part of the couple therapy, and thus I discuss with the person the need for us to incorporate into the couple work his or her thoughts about the relationship disappointments and frustrations that might have contributed to his or her decision to get involved with someone else.

The therapist may have strong personal reactions to the intensity of the emotions expressed when working with couples around affairs. S/he may react to the hurt person vilifying the betrayer. S/he may react to the betrayer's continuing lies. S/he may react to the one who has been betrayed exacting a "price" as a sign of love or commitment. And s/he may be troubled by the spouse's wish for revenge or desire to hurt the third person. If you are having strong personal reactions, it is helpful to talk with a trusted colleague, supervisor, or fellow therapist to get another perspective and to sort out how your own issues are influencing your perceptions and feelings. Sometimes the therapist is not reacting out of personal emotions but rather out of strong moral feelings about what is right and wrong. If the feelings remain after talking them through, it is important to be open and transparent with the couple about your position on something. So, for instance, when Leslie wanted her husband, Jorge, to show that he was willing to break his ties with the woman whom she sarcastically called "his floozy" by informing the woman's boss as well as her husband about the affair, I said, *"I can't really help you with that. Not only do I think it will ultimately lead to bad feelings between you and Jorge even if he agrees to it now, but I'm not 'good' with revenge or an 'eye-for-an-eye' approach. Of course, the two of you are free to do whatever makes sense to both of you, but I hope you'll give it some more thought and perhaps talk to someone you respect about it, before acting on that impulse."*

WHEN THE THERAPIST
IS HAVING TROUBLE STAYING NEUTRAL

As we have seen, working with couples often stirs intense feelings in therapists in a way that they rarely feel when doing individual therapy. Here's a sampling of some of the types of reactions that are not at all uncommon when working with couples:

- The relationship seems so dysfunctional that the therapist doesn't understand *why* the couple wants to stay together.
- One person seems so much more the source of the difficulties than the other that it is hard to work systemically.
- The therapist can't understand what one person sees in the other.
- The therapist is troubled by one person's acceptance of how s/he is treated.
- The therapist is troubled by the disdain one person expresses toward the other.
- The therapist feels one person is in denial about the seriousness of the other's problems (e.g., drugs and alcohol, serious psychiatric problems, or personality disorders).

It is disturbing when therapists, used to feeling empathy, instead experience negative feelings toward someone they're working with. Additionally it is also worrisome, because working with couples is a big responsibility. Though our role is not to give our opinion about whether a couple should stay together, we undoubtedly *do* have a significant impact on their decision. We influence their decision not so much explicitly, but rather in the myriad of ways discussed throughout this book: what we choose to focus on, what *motives* we ascribe to actions, whether we focus on psychopathology or on health, whether we regard something as "fixable" or an immutable personality trait that requires acceptance and accommodation.

Because we *do* have an impact on the direction they decide to pursue, having doubts about why they are trying to stay together, or what they see in one another, or having concerns that one person is getting "short-changed" in the relationship, or that one of them is far more emotionally stable than the other, can subtly infiltrate our work and have serious consequences for the couple's future.

But lest we get too overwhelmed by the effects our doubts may have, we need to remind ourselves that although we seriously contribute to the couple's decisions, we by no means *determine* the course they will take. The therapist who is wittingly or unwittingly attempting to take the couple in a direction they are not comfortable with will feel a "pushback."

It is not uncommon, for instance, for the therapist to be set to follow up on a prior session in which the couple seemed to be seriously talking about separating, only to find that they come in next time with a new topic in hand as if the previous week's conversation had never happened. This is a sign to me that, although ambivalent, the couple doesn't really want to consider the separation option. Practical considerations, as well as concern and empathy for their children who would be pained by their separation, may loom large in the couple's decision not to go down that road. But additionally, what couples *get* from one another, and the various emotional factors that bind them and make them feel that despite the negatives, they *love* one another, is intangible, complex, and not readily put into words.

The therapist's influence, of course, goes both ways. By noticing strengths and positives in the way the couple are with one another, we encourage the couple to work on the relationship rather than separate. Having an impact in *that* direction is as momentous a responsibility as the converse. Might they be happier in the long run if they separated? Are we doing them a disservice by working with them to "fix" a relationship that has so many problems? These questions are particularly haunting when one believes, as I do, that people do not *inevitably* choose the same kind of person again or reenact the same patterns in their next intimate relationship. We each bring out particular aspects of the other's personality, and as Paul has described, often unwittingly create "accomplices" who themselves need and create "accomplices" who (themselves unwittingly) aid and abet us in— and further lock us into—enacting patterns that can plague us (P. L. Wachtel, 2014a). Different personalities are more or less suited to bring out the best or the worst in us, and thus who our partner is can make a great deal of difference in what aspects of our personality are activated. To be sure, as we have seen, couples can learn to deal with and deactivate transference and legacy issues. But, nonetheless, some relationships require more *work* on these issues than others, and realistically, even with insight and effort, some couples' individual issues will clash more than others, and thus some relationships will be an uphill battle in enabling either or both partners to thrive and be their happiest selves.

These types of considerations gave me pause when working with Joanna and James, who were both soon to turn 30. They had lived together on and off since they had met in their sophomore year of college. They reported that they had broken up with each "at least four times," but after living apart for some months would end up deciding that they still loved one another and were sure that, given how much they missed each other, they would now be able to make their relationship work. But within a month or two of resuming their relationship the same issues that made them separate would reemerge. James experienced Joanna as cold and withholding. "She says she misses me when we're separated, but I don't see it—she's not a warm per-son—she's so wound up in herself and *her* stress that when she comes home from work all she can talk about is the stuff that makes her mad at work. She really doesn't seem interested in what's going on in *my* life. Somehow every place she works is filled with idiots, and only on those rare occasions when she's in a good mood does she 'deign' to pay some attention to me. When we're apart she doesn't take me for granted and actually asks about my day sometimes!" In response, Joanna said, "Yes, he can be very warm and caring, but most of the time he's *angry* and sees himself as a *victim*. He has no idea what it's like to work in marketing. Instead of empathy and support, he just complains that I'm preoccupied with work." Despite these complaints, they both said that they wanted to work on their relationship. They had tried couple therapy before, but believed that the therapist wasn't particularly good and wanted to try it again with someone else.

When I encounter a situation like this, I am conflicted about how hard they (and I) should try to make the relationship work. Joanna and James were young and had no children—an important factor in my thoughts about how much "work" they should put into trying to get what they want from one another. I asked myself, should they have to put so much effort into getting along? Wouldn't they each be better off with someone who is bet-ter suited to them? When I probed for positives, I got a sense that they had a strong sexual attraction to one another, and Joanna said, "We were a great couple when we were in college—everyone envied us—we laughed all the time. We were part of a terrific crowd—they're still our closest friends, though only a few of them live anywhere near us. We all partied a lot, and even though we were hungover half the time, we managed to study and do okay."

I made a mental note that their bond was forged during a time in life when they were surrounded by close friends, thus didn't need as much from one another, and when they *were* alone and intimate they often were drink-ing or using marijuana. Their attachment seemed more like "imprinting" than a bond characterized by true intimacy. I believe that many couples hold on to a memory of a time when "the stars lined up," so to speak, and they had an intense connection, sometimes for just months, or even weeks. That memory resides deep inside their mind and heart and it is this recollection of a brief, magical period that, despite disappointment, frustrations, and even serious disillusionment, is what people mean when they say they still "love" each other.

I remind myself, however, that it is not for *me* to decide how much they actually love one another. Perhaps I am being too cynical to think of their attachment as "imprinting," not love. Regardless of whether or not they stay together, they will learn a lot about themselves and each other by spending some time working on their relationship.

As with all couples, I regard my job not only as helping them find solutions to their difficulties, but as making sure that they see each other more clearly, have a realistic understanding of what each of them wants from the other, and understand the ease or difficulty of their each changing in the ways the other is hoping for. But, because of my "take" on them, combined with the fact that they are young and childless, I modified my approach just a bit. Thus, though I still tried to help them get what they wanted from one another—for James, more attention and less preoccupation with work, and for Joanna, more empathy and nurturance—I didn't work quite as hard as I might otherwise do to find positives. I did this because I was concerned that by underlining positives I might be encouraging them to keep trying to make their relationship work and I just didn't know if that was really in their best interest. Similarly, I was more inclined to follow up and examine some of the negative statements that they each made about one another. So, for example, I would follow up on James's sarcastic statement about Joanna that "somehow, every place she works is filled with idiots." I did this so that they both could evaluate and not sweep under the rug a possibly serious concern. Does James really feel that Joanna is prone to be negative? And if so, how does Joanna feel about being perceived that way by James? I was not as concerned about where this line of questioning might lead and what it might stir up as I would be if I was less doubtful about the relationship. If they choose to be together, James needed to let himself really know how he sees Joanna and she in turn needed to be clear about how she is perceived by James. Perhaps she too sees herself as prone to be negative and wants to work on this issue herself. Or perhaps she has similarly negative perceptions of James, and sees him as "too passive, too placating and letting people step all over him" or "not very ambitious." I asked them each to think about whether they could accept the other's personality traits and values or whether they were hoping that the other would in time change? In subsequent sessions they talked together more seriously about whether, though they still loved one another, it just wouldn't work out in the long run. They both agreed that though it would be terribly painful to finally break up for good, it would be much worse if they went ahead, had kids, and ended up finding their differences so frustrating that they would divorce down the road.

After much discussion, James and Joanna decided they wanted to continue to work on their relationship despite the serious differences between them that the sessions had highlighted. Like many couples who have a volatile relationship, their bond remained extremely strong. Knowing that I had helped them be clear-eyed about each other's traits and values, I was comfortable doing my best to help them make their relationship more stable and gratifying. As I do with all couples I work with, I helped them untangle the maladaptive patterns that they had gotten into for dealing with the things about the other that they were now committed to trying to accept. Together we looked at the role of legacy issues and tried to find ways that they could better meet each other's needs despite their very real differences.

I use variations on this same approach—helping people see each other as clearly as possible so that they really know what they are signing onto, so to speak—for other instances that give me pause about the appropriateness of trying to help the couple stay together. A particularly difficult dilemma arises when one person clearly has more serious mental health issues than the other. As a couple therapist, I have an allegiance and responsibility to *both* members of the couple. Though the "healthier" individual might be better off being with a less emotionally needy or volatile person, the more troubled person benefits from being with someone who is emotionally stable. As with the situation of Joanna and James, I work to help them each see themselves and each other accurately. So, for instance, with a couple in which one person exhibits the symptoms of borderline personality disorder, I would be clear that the volatility is an individual issue and is not something the partner can really prevent just by doing things differently. Of course, as in all of the work I am describing in this book, I *would* try to help them find responses to the volatility that, at least to some degree, would limit the *escalation* that occurs when each partner pushes the other's buttons. Though I do not use diagnostic names, I describe the phenomenon, and would say, for instance, things like *"I think you have a hard time regulating your moods,"* or *"It's hard for you to hold on to a good feeling about yourself—you can feel fine and then you can feel worthless pretty quickly,"* or *"When you feel that a person you depend on isn't available, you can be filled with rage at the person and forget the good feeling you had toward that person just a short time ago."* I reiterate that although there are some things their spouse could do to help a bit, mostly this is a psychological state that needs to be addressed in individual therapy. If the "healthier" spouse expresses frustration that the other hasn't benefited from therapy in the past, I would acknowledge that these types of psychological difficulties are hard to change and require a big commitment on the part of the patient.

When the more troubled person resists getting the treatment s/he needs, whether for anxiety, depression, mood disorders, or personality disorders, I do my best to persuade that person of the importance of getting help, both for him- or herself and because an individual's psychological problems can have a great effect on the relationship. I take a firm stand that though the partner can be of some help and can handle the problems differently, the basic issues in the marriage won't change unless the individual works on his or her own emotional difficulties. Similarly, when I feel that a large factor in the couple's difficulties is the excessive drug or alcohol use of one or both of them, I regard my role as laying out the facts and breaking though the denial that one or both may be using.

Another disturbing feeling for therapists is when they find themselves *not liking* one of the individuals in the couple and think to themselves, *"What could the spouse possibly find appealing about this person?"* When the couple therapist feels this way, s/he might well be having a personal, idiosyncratic reaction to the person. Therapists, like everyone else, have their transferences, tastes, and "hot buttons," and in couple therapy we often see quite directly the way a person hurts or negatively impacts another, and thus our particular sensitivities and attitudes can more readily be triggered. Of course, it is helpful to be as aware as possible of one's biases and emotional inclinations in this regard, and both individual therapy and consultations with colleagues can be helpful. But often even after exploring our reactions and trying to distinguish between the actual individual in front of us and the personal emotional resonances that person has for us, we may still be "stuck" with our negative feelings. One thing I have found that is quite helpful in these situations is to have one or two individual sessions with each of the individuals in the couple. Almost always, when I spend some time alone with the person that I'm having negative feelings about, I come to like him or her much better. The person tends to be less defensive and shows me a side of him- or herself that I have not seen before. Not only does this help me *like* the person better, but I can also use this experience to see if s/he can be helped to express that aspect of him- or herself *with the spouse.*

CAN YOU DO INDIVIDUAL THERAPY WITH ONE MEMBER OF A COUPLE WHILE ALSO WORKING WITH THEM AS A COUPLE?

As implied in the foregoing discussion, it frequently becomes clear when working with a couple that one of them would benefit from going into individual therapy. When making this suggestion, I of course discuss the issues that I think would be good to work on. Generally, not only do I know about these difficulties from the couple work, but because I have had one or two individual meetings with each or them, I am able to elaborate on what, why, and how individual therapy could be useful. I spell out for the couple the types of issues that, although we can continue to work on in couple therapy, could be more focally addressed in individual therapy. I am thinking here of issues like severe anxiety, depression, trouble with anger, interpersonal problems with coworkers, social anxiety, and so on. As we have seen in Chapters 8 and 9, the couple work often includes looking at how the spouse can help with some of these problems, but usually the person also needs to get individual help with these issues. When talking with the couple about the need to address these problems in individual therapy, it is very important to also underline the person's strengths, particularly those characteristics that will be beneficial in getting the most out of individual therapy. So, for instance, I might say something like *"I think your anxiety is getting in the way of you living the way you really would like to and of having the kind of marriage you would like. I've seen how hard you work in here and how open you've become to feedback. And you really have been trying to follow through on some of the new ways of being together that we've come up with, but anxiety is still getting in the way. But those characteristics—being open to feedback, being willing to try new things, and, additionally, actually finding understanding the complexity of the dynamics in your relationship quite <u>interesting</u> are what makes me feel that you are the kind of person who would use your own therapy very well and would get a lot out of it."*

If a person is ambivalent about going to individual therapy, I try to highlight the part of the ambivalence that does *want* to do so, and if possible use attributional statements to reinforce that side of the ambivalence. So, for instance, I might say, *"I sense that you have been wanting to resolve some of these issues, but that feeling that your spouse sees you as 'the problem' has held you back. But now that we're working on the issues in the relationship that are not just <u>your</u> issues, I get a sense that you're beginning to feel it's okay to acknowledge and work on your own issues."*

Frequently, when I suggest a referral for individual therapy, one or both of the couple members asks if instead seeing me alone in addition to the couple therapy would be possible. Many people are threatened when their spouse goes into individual therapy. They fear that the therapist will believe every negative thing the person says about them, and that in the account their partner gives to his individual therapist, he will minimize his own problems and highlight his spouse's. Often the spouse to be referred would also prefer to see me. They trust me, and already feel known. It can be tempting to therapists to take on this dual role. After all, we too often feel that we've managed to make a good connection with someone who isn't so easy to connect to and who, with us, has overcome his or her skepticism about therapy. But although each situation is unique, and thus there are *some* exceptions to the rule—for example, the person is too distrustful and won't follow through on a referral to someone else—in general, we should resist our inclination to give that arrangement a try. First, it is often difficult to keep couple issues out of the individual sessions, and it is much harder for the person, and the therapist as well, to stay focused on the individual issues that most need work. Second, individual work with one person in the couple tends to lead to a stronger alliance with that person, and thus affects the work with the couple. Even when the spouse has a lot of trust in the therapist's neutrality, over time s/he may feel uncomfortable with the dual role the therapist is playing. Many couples who come to see me had previously worked with a couple therapist who ended up doing individual therapy with one of them instead of couple therapy, and even if that seemed like a good idea at the time, one or both of the partners, in retrospect, lost trust in the therapist and regretted that therapy evolved in such a way.

To address concern about the individual therapist getting a distorted view of the problems, or the individual not being able to describe well his or her difficulties, I reassure the couple that I will be available to talk with the therapist from time to time and also explain my view that individual therapy can include an occasional "cast of characters" meeting in which the spouse has an opportunity to give input (see E. F. Wachtel & P. L. Wachtel, 1986). I also make clear that although I am, of course, going to refer the person to someone I think well of, there also has to be the right personal chemistry, and that isn't always easy to predict. For that reason, it's important to state that if for any reason the person *doesn't* seem like a good fit, I'll find someone else. I usually don't, however, give more than one name at a time because I want both the patient and the therapist to start with the assumption that it is likely to work out. Therapists get tense when they know the person is shopping around, and patients may be so involved in "evaluating" the therapist that they don't really give individual therapy a chance.

Even when the couple therapy is coming to a conclusion, I am reluctant to do individual therapy with one of the people in the couple. I want couples to know that they can come back for a "booster" session or two if either of them feels that the progress they made is "slipping." Thus, the question of having an alliance that would interfere with my neutrality can still be an issue. Again, there are times when I feel that, all in all, my ability to be of help to an individual is so enhanced by my having worked with him and her in couple therapy that the positives far outweigh potential alliance difficulties at some hypothetical later point. This is particularly the case when the couple and I agree that they have made very significant changes in their relationship, and that the changes are solid and likely to last. That is not to say that they won't *ever* have problems, or won't feel a need to come in together occasionally. But given the strength of my connection to *both* of them, and the likelihood that my individual work will further strengthen the progress they've already made, I may sometimes conclude that my ability to be helpful to them in a joint session from time to time will not be impeded.

KNOWING WHEN IT'S TIME TO STOP

One way I know a couple is ready to cut back or stop is that they begin to come to sessions with nothing particular they want to talk about. The sense of urgency is gone. If they need to cancel a session, they are comfortable missing it and don't feel a need to try to reschedule as soon as possible. And although they, and I, can raise topics that are useful to discuss, there may be a feeling that we are working to figure out how to productively use the time. This is not to say every issue has been completely resolved. The couple may be getting along much better and even enjoying just being with each other, yet still not have a physically intimate relationship; or, again, despite overall getting along much better, they may still occasionally have rather bad arguments; or find that they still sometimes get into hurtful conversations about each other's family. But the fact that they no longer feel a need to discuss these topics in sessions indicates the problems that still exist are occurring in the context of a relationship that, *overall*, is going well.

Of course, one must also consider that the sessions may be feeling a bit flat because the couple has begun to avoid some difficult topics that are still unresolved and, one might say, next on the agenda. But as I have presented throughout this book, I don't *start* with assumptions of pathology or resistance, though I obviously attend to and consider both. At this point in the therapy, the therapist has to walk a fine line, on the one hand, between raising topics to see if one person is concerned about something that s/he is hesitant to raise and, on the other hand, taking care not to undo or destabilize real progress that has been made. Certain topics that the therapist is especially concerned about must not be avoided even if the couple is content to let them be—for example, the seriousness of excessive drinking, untreated depression, or anger that turns physical.

There are times too when I believe the couple is disengaging from couple therapy not because their relationship has significantly improved, but for other reasons that they have not been explicit about. Perhaps the couple might be less engaged because they are feeling discouraged about progress in a certain area. Or perhaps one person in the therapy is having a reaction to the meetings—for example, feeling that I am taking the other's side, or feeling his or her spouse is taking up too much of the focus—and is withdrawing rather than being honest about what s/he is experiencing.

When I have serious questions or reservations about the couple's stopping because I don't think they've made sufficient progress or really engaged their issues, I raise with the couple (in a tone of curiosity and concern, *not* criticism) my observation that they've been missing sessions, coming late, or not seeming so involved, and ask them what might be going on. Sometimes the answer will be simply that they've been busy and that things have settled down between them. Sometimes one of them will explain what his or her spouse has not felt comfortable voicing—for example, that s/he is feeling frustrated with the sessions, or that s/he sees me as taking the spouse's side, or that the sessions are stirring too many negative feelings, or that the other partner dominates the discussions. Once the spouse voices such a concern, the other will often elaborate on or correct the other's description of what s/he has been feeling. When I get feedback of this sort I take it very seriously and start with the assumption that there is probably some truth to what the person is feeling. I respond as nondefensively as I possibly can and communicate to them that I take to heart their "complaints." I talk with them about how we together could make changes in the session to address their concerns. So, for instance, if one person feels she is not getting enough time to speak and explain her point of view, perhaps it would be useful to have longer sessions, or to meet with her alone for a session. Or, if someone feels I am asking more of him than of his spouse, I would suggest that not only should he raise this issue when that feeling occurs, but also assure him that even if he doesn't raise it, I will periodically check in with him to see if he is still feeling that way.

When a couple has made considerable progress, I often try to raise the possibility of cutting back, and eventually stopping, before they do. I believe that *my* raising the topic powerfully highlights, and gives them credit for, the progress they've made. If it happens that one of them actually beats me to it, I would say, *"I'm glad you've raised this issue. I've been thinking too that you've made quite a bit of progress, and meeting less frequently might make sense at this point."* Sometimes one of the partners in the couple expresses anxiety about cutting back, and as we talk about his or her concern, problems that s/he had been hesitant to bring up emerge. When that happens, in addition to recommitting to working on those difficulties, we discuss why the person had been hesitant to raise issues that were still bothering him or her and try to work on making that easier in the future.

When a decision is made to end couple therapy, the final session is spent summarizing what has changed, how that came about, and what each of them has been doing differently. I also let them know the ways they have *let* me be of help to them. With some couples, I also work with them to articulate negative patterns and issues that could readily be reactivated, and we discuss what they each can do to prevent that from happening. I suggest that they might want to come in from time to time for a "booster" session to keep them on track. And I urge them not to hesitate to call me to arrange for a session or two if either of them feels that they are slipping back a little. I emphasize that coming in occasionally does not mean that they need to start over or that the couple therapy has failed.

There are times when I raise the issue of stopping therapy not because the couple has made considerable progress, but because I'm concerned that the couple work is actually doing more harm than good. Sometimes one person is too unstable or emotionally fragile to tolerate even the gentlest of feedback. S/he may respond as if s/he is being attacked, and no matter how hard the therapist tries to be reassuring, positive, and supportive, s/he may experience the therapist as taking the spouse's side.

Or one or both people in the couple may be so volatile that none of the methods I described in Chapter 6 help the couple use the sessions productively. Instead, meetings become a forum for attack, counterattack, and escalating rage. And for some couples, the opening up about concerns and dissatisfactions—even when great care has been taken to focus on resolving, not merely uncovering, problems—seems to have made things worse, not better.

There are also occasions when one person uses the opportunity to be "honest" in a cruel way. S/he might say extremely hurtful things that would be very difficult for his or her spouse to get over—for example, his penis is too small or I knew when I met her that she wasn't very intelligent. Sometimes it is hard to know whether the person *intends* to be cruel, or whether s/he may be so lacking in emotional intelligence, or even possibly be "on the autism spectrum," that s/he is simply being too literal in response to my questions.

With some couples, even if the discussion in the session was calm, it leads to intense arguments at home. When there is a history of physical abuse, one must be particularly careful that couple therapy is safe (Stith et al., 2011; Goldner, 1998). If things said in the session spark violent arguments, then couple therapy is not an appropriate modality for working on the relationship.

When I tell a couple that I don't believe couple therapy is the correct course for them right now, I also make suggestions about what I think would be more helpful and what I think might make couple therapy more useful at a later point. So, for example, if the couple is too emotionally volatile, I would strongly suggest that they explore meditation and specific help for managing anger. And with the "emotionally fragile" person who needs a lot of support, I would suggest that s/he pursue her own therapy with a therapist who would be open to having an occasional session that included his or her spouse.

If a couple really wants to continue in couple therapy despite these difficulties, I am sometimes open to changing the format. For instance, with some couples, I find it useful to meet with each of them individually and then, every few weeks, meet with them together. But another option is to explain to them that every couple therapist works differently and I'd be happy to refer them to a therapist whose way of working might be a better fit for them.

SOME FINAL WORDS

I've tried in this book to give you an up-close look at what I actually *do* with couples. In addition to the specific methods I've described, my intention was also to convey a nonpathologizing way of thinking and working whose aim is both to enable the couple to heal from the hurts they've inflicted on one another and to help them change their way of interacting so that they can come closer to having the kind of relationship they've each been wanting. As in individual therapy, so much of what makes the therapy work well is that the couple forms a strong bond with the therapist. Much of being a good couple therapist is being someone the couple trusts—trusts to be fair, to value them, to treat them as unique, to not have cookie-cutter solutions, and perhaps, most importantly of all, to continually examine his or her own personal reactions and preferences so s/he can minimize his or her intrusion into the work.

As I hope I have conveyed, in a session, though I am clearly the "authority," demonstrating my expertise in a myriad of ways—for example, by keeping the sessions on focus, making choices about what is productive to work on, and keeping the sessions calm—I also convey the message that the three of us in the room are a team, brainstorming and collaborating to find solutions. Part of what I hope you have learned from this book is that doing effective work as a couple therapist entails empowering and motivating the couple. Thus, I present my thoughts and suggestions to the couple in a way that invites them to correct and refine my suggestions and to come up with their own solutions that make sense to them. The tone I normally take with couples is exploratory, open, equal—for example, *"Here's what I'm thinking about what's going on."*; or *"Does that make sense to you?"*; or *"Is there a better way to describe it?"*; or *"What do you think might help?"* In short, I'm careful not to talk from *"on high."*

From time to time, I step out of my role as therapist and say things like, *"I'm going to tell you something really simple—not something you need to have PhD to say. I know I might be sounding like a minister or rabbi, but . . . "* These are generally things that out of context might sound hokey or superficial, but because of the trust that has developed out of the effort to develop a strong therapeutic alliance, the couple usually experience these statements as helpful "words of wisdom," rather than as preachy. I have in mind here things like *"We love people who make us feel good about ourselves,"* or *"Criticism erodes love,"* or even something as potentially cliché-sounding as *"Life is too precious to waste days in an argument—ask yourself, is it worth having a fight over?"* Offered in the context of the work we have done together, the couple usually hears these statements as a shorthand way of saying something that is actually both substantial and deeply important. I am also attentive to ensuring that the couple understands that actually making any of these principles a part of their life together requires a lot of practice, reflection, and serious consideration. These statements are thus not final pronouncements, but often a valuable starting point for further exploration of the complexities of when and how to actually put them into practice.

The challenges of being a couple therapist are great, but so too are the rewards. Being a couple therapist allows you an inside view of how each person is contributing to the couple's dynamics and how the roles and patterns they have developed can result in both parties feeling hurt, frustrated, and often profoundly unhappy. It can as well open a valuable window into what works *well* with couples, what each partner does (or at least *can* do) to bring them closer and to make the other feel better and more loved. This privileged position can serve as a lens through which we can see more clearly some of *our own* relationships. As we listen to both partners' point of view on issues that in some way echo our own, we can develop greater empathy for the feelings of those who are near and dear to us. So too are we better able to recognize *our* part in problematic interactions. By witnessing it in the couples we work with, we become more aware of instances of our own defensiveness, or the futility of criticism, or the hurt we might be unwittingly inflicting. In truth, the homey wisdom that I sometimes impart has been acquired through years of exposure to the pain and frustration experienced by the couples with whom I've worked—and through the process of living through life's complexities that is a part of all our lives.

It has been enormously gratifying to help couples free themselves from self-constraining roles and ungratifying ways of being with one another. It is my hope that this book has given the reader the tools to get the same gratification—both personal and professional—out of the work that I have had, and that, like me, you will learn something new with every couple you work with.

Epilogue

ᛒ

Principles of Change in Individual and Couple Therapy

Paul L. Wachtel

*T*urnabout is fair play. Ellen wrote a chapter for my book *Thera-peutic Communication* (P. L. Wachtel, 2011a), illustrating how the ideas presented in that book—which were directed toward work with individuals—could be extended to work with couples. So it is only appropriate that now, in her book on working with couples, I should discuss how her work is rooted in a range of principles that provide the foundation for sound therapeutic work of all sorts, individual or couple.

Of course, Ellen discusses these principles throughout this book, often quite explicitly. But in this chapter I intend to place them in the context of the larger body of theory and research that underlies the practice of psychotherapy in general. To be sure, as Ellen conveys so beautifully in this

Paul L. Wachtel, PhD, is CUNY Distinguished Professor in the doctoral program in clinical psychology at City College and the Graduate Center of the City University of New York. He is a Fellow of Divisions 12, 29, and 39 of the American Psychological Association (APA) and is a recipient of the Hans H. Strupp Award for Psychoanalytic Writing, Teaching, and Research; the Distinguished Psychologist Award from Division 29 (Psychotherapy) of the APA; and the Scholarship and Research Award from Division 39 (Psychoanalysis) of the APA. He is past president of the Society for the Exploration of Psychotherapy integration.

book, there are many ways in which couple therapy requires still additional conceptual tools and perspectives and an even greater measure of delicacy, skill, tact, and clinical sensitivity than is already very copiously required in good individual work. As enormously variable as the possibilities are for how any individual patient or client may respond to our comments and interventions, those possibilities are still further multiplied when working with couples. One of the exquisite torments of couple work is offering what feels like almost the perfect response—smart, empathic, perfectly attuned— and then having it sabotaged right before one's eyes by a response from one of the partners that is perfectly designed to wave a red flag in the face of the other. Whatever one can say about couple work, it is—for better or worse—almost never boring! These differences notwithstanding, however, the work described in this book is largely rooted in the same set of underlying principles that provide the foundation for good therapeutic work of all sorts. And as Ellen demonstrates so amply, these principles can be *taught*.

Psychotherapy, whether with individuals or couples (or, of course, families or groups), needs to be grounded in sound evidence. Arbitrary assertions by the therapist that amount simply to "trust me" are appropriately met with skepticism. But equal skepticism must be applied toward the ways in which the call for "evidence-based" practice has become a faddish and largely rhetorical slogan that is not really very clearly or carefully articulated by many of its proponents. *Evidence* is not like a stone, solid and unchanging over millions of years. Evidence is, inevitably, *constructed* and *interpreted*. One important reason for the continuing existence of different "schools" of therapy is that each has its own version of evidence, its own way of gathering, interpreting, even *noticing* the data on which its vision and clinical approach is grounded. We have been plagued in recent years with a kind of mechanical thinking about evidence and evidence-based practice that has as often impeded progress in our field as it has promoted it (P. L. Wachtel, 2010a).

In contextualizing Ellen's couple work in this chapter, my comments significantly draw upon the findings of contemporary psychotherapy research; but I will draw upon the evidence (and the principles to which it points) in a fashion that I hope is less mechanical and less overweeningly certain than is common among many who champion "evidence-based" practice or "empirically supported" treatments. To be genuinely evidence-based is to be aware of the very significant *limits* of the evidence we presently have available. All too often these days, in order to meet a set of criteria that have become far more prominent in the politics of our field than they deserve to be (P. L. Wachtel, 2010a), evidence is gathered (and the very nature of what is and is not evidence is defined) in ways that have little to do with offering the best treatment for the majority of people actually seen in our clinics (Westen, Novotny, & Thompson-Brenner, 2004). The criteria for calling an approach "evidence-based" or "empirically supported" are cherry-picked to meet ideological or economic agendas. They are then presented to the profession as if they were "the" requirement for scientific legitimacy—often in a way that mocks the very spirit and nature of science (P. L. Wachtel, 2010a) and that has as its real agenda the promotion of particular "brands" of therapy that are competing in the marketplace (Ablon, Levy, & Katzenstein, 2006; Rosen & Davison, 2003).

The way evidence will be considered and addressed in this chapter—as it is, in fact, at least implicitly, throughout this entire book—eschews this marketing-oriented approach to evidence that aims to demonstrate that one's favorite brand is "empirically supported" and, often not so subtly, to suggest that competing brands are not.[1] In reading much of this literature, I am reminded of the famous line from *Saturday Night Live*, in which the comedian Chevy Chase introduces his pseudonews show with the words "I'm Chevy Chase . . . *and you're not.*" In contrast, my approach to understanding the implications of the available evidence is much the same as in Castonguay and Beutler's (2003) important effort to delineate an empirically responsible alternative to what Beutler elsewhere wittily described as "the pervasive tendency to pit one treatment model against another, or to pit treatment model against relationship, in a dogma-eat-dogma competition" (Beutler, 2004, p. 229). Castonguay and Beutler's emphasis is on empirically supported *principles* of therapeutic change rather than on competing brands. One of the most well documented of those principles is that the therapeutic relationship and the therapeutic alliance are among the most important considerations in whether a therapeutic effort is effective (see, e.g., Norcross, 2002, 2010; Duncan, Miller, Wampold, & Hubble, 2010; Lambert & Barley, 2001). Establishing an effective therapeutic relationship cannot be done mechanically. Good relationships (whether between partners in a couple or between therapist and patient) cannot be established in cookbook fashion. But at the same time, as Ellen illustrates so thoroughly in this book, neither are they arbitrary.

Underlying *principles* are central, but they are principles that must be applied with sensitivity to the specifics of each person, of each relationship, and, indeed, of each *moment*. Doing today what worked yesterday, without attending to *why* it worked yesterday and why something different may be required today, is to fall into the kind of deadening mechanical trap that characterizes "manualized" treatments at their worst. I do not simply dismiss out-of-hand all efforts at manualization. I am familiar with a variety of manualized treatments whose developers and practitioners I greatly respect; but I do believe that the rationale for manuals as a requirement

---

[1] Here the important contribution of Shedler (2010) provides a powerful challenge to this motivated misrepresentation.

for establishing that a therapeutic approach is grounded in evidence has been riddled with confusion and double-think (Wachtel, 2010a). And I am especially concerned with the tendency that has entered our field recently in which—by a muddled logic that compounds and extends the confusions that problematically led manualization to be thought of as a requirement for meaningful psychotherapy *research*—therapists in training are more and more being required to learn manualized approaches to their *clinical* work. Perhaps for the less educated (and therefore less expensive) therapists that insurance companies are attempting to make the norm for our profession, a "manual" may be a useful supplement to their minimal training. But anyone who has ever been put repeatedly on hold while a poorly trained computer technician keeps checking his manual knows the great relief that comes on those rare occasions when you have a sense you are talking to someone who "knows it in his bones."

I think of this book as a manual for therapists who are wary of manuals. It offers the same kind of detail about just how to proceed and what to say that most purported manuals do, and it provides the same kind of clearly articulated theoretical rationale to guide the therapist through the various choice points encountered in the course of clinical work. But for readers who are concerned about the potentially mechanizing, deskilling impact of manualization, it has surely been evident that this book—which *is* ultimately a book, and not a "manual"—is grounded in respect both for the complexities of clinical work and for the need for the therapist to bring not only her intelligence and knowledge to bear in the work, but her humanity and empathic attunement. Despite the current emphasis in our field on branded treatment packages promoted as superior to competing products much like brands of toothpaste or detergent (Ablon et al., 2006; Rosen & Davison, 2003; Beutler, 2004), there is plenty of strong evidence that the skills of the therapist and his or her capacity to relate to and communicate with the client account at least as much for whether or not change occurs as what "brand" of therapy the therapist employs (Duncan et al., 2010; Norcross, 2002, 2010; Wampold, 2015; Anderson, Ogles, Patterson, Lambert, & Vermeersch, 2009). The aim of this book is to help the reader further develop those skills.

A PRINCIPLES-ORIENTED APPROACH

Good couple therapy is not achieved by following the right manual but by establishing the right relationship and by proceeding in a way that builds upon the basic processes of change that have been shown in countless studies—not just in psychotherapy outcome research but in basic research in personality and social psychology—to be the foundations of change in the way people act, feel, and perceive themselves and others. By building skillfully upon those processes and principles, the therapist, whatever her style or identi-fied orientation, can enhance her effectiveness as a clinician. In that sense, this book is addressed equally to couple therapists who identify their basic orientation as cognitive-behavioral, psychodynamic, systemic, or experien-tial. The fundamental foundations are not "owned" by any orientation, and can be applied in multiple ways and multiple styles (Castonguay & Beutler, 2006; P. L. Wachtel, 1997, 2011a; Castonguay, Goldfried, Wiser, Raue, & Hayes, 1996; Ablon & Jones, 1998, 2002; Jones & Pulos, 1993).

EXPOSURE

One of the most studied and best validated of the principles that under-lie therapeutic effectiveness, regardless of official orientation, is *exposure*. Exposure is frequently thought of as a specifically behavioral or cognitive-behavioral intervention, but careful attention to what actually transpires in therapy sessions makes it clear that in fact exposure is an important characteristic of successful therapy regardless of the orientation with which the therapist identifies (see, e.g., P. L. Wachtel, 1997, 2008, 2011a). Psy-chodynamic therapists, for example, promote exposure when they make effective "interpretations," because essential to any truly helpful interpreta-tion is that it does more than intellectually call attention to an unconscious thought or feeling, but rather brings the person *into contact with* the feeling and promotes directly *experiencing* the previously avoided inclination or affect—that is, it promotes *exposure* to it. Similarly, it is of the very essence of the various experiential and emotion-focused approaches to therapy that, again, they emphasize directly *experiencing* the previously unacknowledged emotional response or—again—*exposure* to it. Each of the various orienta-tions goes about promoting exposure in different ways, and each tends to emphasize exposure to a different set of experiences (though those expe-riences overlap more than is commonly recognized—see, e.g., Weitzman, 1967). This is one more reason why a more comprehensive and integrative therapeutic approach has advantages over one rooted exclusively in only one of our field's several major theoretical orientations (P. L. Wachtel, 1997; Norcross & Goldfried, 2005).

It is certainly the case that it was the behavioral orientation in which the value of exposure was first strongly emphasized (though see Dollard & Miller, 1950, for an early account, rooted both in Hullian learning theory and psychoanalysis, of how unreinforced exposure to experiences that have felt threatening, and hence been avoided, is at the heart of psychoanalytic therapy too). It is also important to acknowledge that exposure has received much more explicit and prominent attention from behavioral and cognitive-behavioral therapists than from therapists of other orientations, and often it is employed by them in a more focused and systematic way. That is one of the strengths of behavioral treatment, and I have learned much from the proponents of exposure in the behavioral tradition. But these practitioners and theorists do not "own" exposure or have an exclusive franchise on its use. When they are not clear about this fact, they not only misunderstand and caricature other orientations but generate research studies that are embarrassingly tendentious and poorly conceived.

Edna Foa, for example, has been an enormously productive and generative thinker about the processes that underlie therapeutic change, and much of her writing on the sources of psychological maladaptation and the principles that can help to resolve it has been among the most illuminating in the entire therapeutic literature (e.g., Foa, 2011; Foa & Kozak, 1986; Foa, Huppert, & Cahill, 2006). But when trying to appropriate for her particular approach the exclusive franchise for exposure, she and her colleagues lapse into absurdity. In a study supposedly comparing her version of prolonged exposure with psychodynamic therapy in the treatment of posttraumatic stress disorder (Gilboa-Schectman et al., 2010), the study protocol called for the psychodynamic therapists in the study to *not mention* the traumatic event, and if the patient did spontaneously bring up details of the trauma, to somehow "refer to the meaning of the event in the context of the central issue, without further encouragement to discuss the memory" (p. 1037). I am not completely sure what their fantasy is of what exploring "meaning" is apart from—or totally separate from—exposure, but in the bid for purity of factors (promoting their brand?) they create an absurdity. The version of "psychodynamic therapy" they compare their approach to is one that no competent psychodynamic therapist would recognize and that indeed, if practiced in the fashion their study requires, would create great worry in a training program whether that therapist has the requisite skills or talent (or even common sense) to continue in his or her training.

The ubiquity—and importance—of exposure in almost all therapeutic efforts is important to bear in mind as one reads this book, especially from the vantage point I am emphasizing here: focusing one's understanding of what is transpiring in the therapeutic work primarily on the underlying *principles* of change rather than on the differences between discrete manualized packages that utilize those underlying principles in a particular acronym-branded way. Ellen does not prominently frame her discussion of how she works in terms of exposure, but any perceptive reader will see clearly that much of what she does can be understood as promoting the experiencing and assimilation of feelings and inclinations that one or both members of the couple have learned to fear and avoid, and as enabling them to discover, in a direct experiential fashion, that it is safe to reintegrate those feelings into their individual sense of self and their ways of seeing and interacting with each other.

BUILDING ON POSITIVES

One of the reasons it is easy to miss the significance of exposure in the work described in this book is that many of the experiences Ellen works to make room for or reintegrate are not the obviously forbidden or frightening experiences that are usually the focus of exposure, but rather what might ordinarily be thought of as quite *positive* experiences—most notably feelings of love, of trust, of being able to count on or depend on the other. Promoting such experiences may seem to be an obvious focus of couple therapy, and of course it is the ultimate aim of almost all couple work. But, continuous with the general field of psychotherapy, it is often the *problem* patterns that are the central focus of the work, with the return of access to loving feelings essentially treated as a secondary consequence of confronting the negative tendencies. At times, certainly, this is the case (indeed, even in Ellen's work). Attention to and building upon the positive does not mean that sessions are a vacation in "La-La Land." When people are suffering or alienated or angry, these feelings must be addressed and little good comes of pretending that they are not there.

It will be clear to the reader that Ellen's emphasis on building on positives in no way means avoiding or glossing over the painful or negative. But it does mean (1) being more attentive to the positive than is common among therapists—this is perhaps the central "art" that the book teaches and that she teaches in the seminars and workshops she conducts; and (2) that one can approach the negative *through* the positive, reversing the lens of the observing instrument but looking at the same phenomenon. Thus, one can address the ways in which one or both members of a couple bicker and find fault by pointing this out or highlighting it (in a way that many therapists view as simply confronting "the truth"); *or* one can address the very same pattern by waiting until they are being a little *less* this way and noting, "You seem to be more able today to hear the validity in each other's viewpoint rather than fault-finding as you've been tempted to do in the past." This latter approach to the pattern is equally attentive to what has gone wrong in the past—and indeed, equally (if not more) likely to help the couple be aware of it. But instead of grounding the observation in a potentially accusatory or discouraging emphasis on how problematic their way of interacting is (cf. P. L. Wachtel, 2011a; Wile, 1984, 1985), it makes the point in a way that also highlights the couple's ability to be *different*—and in doing so it also *enhances* that ability to be different.

There is a passage from Leston Havens that I have been fond of quoting in my own writing because it captures in a wonderfully pithy way the quality in all-too-much therapeutic work—with couples as well as individuals—that Ellen so deftly avoids. In Havens's words, "In the current interpretive climate of much psychotherapeutic work, patients sit waiting for the next insight with their fists clenched. Small wonder, for it is rarely good news"

(1986, p. 78). Ellen's work with couples offers them plenty of good news, news about how to capture the lost potential in their relationship, how to regain their own individual vitality, and how to expand their sense of self and way of being. But this good news comes not at the *expense* of insight but as the most effective way of promoting it. As in the crafting of therapeutic communications more generally (P. L. Wachtel, 2011a), the approach of building on positives is a way of addressing the negatives—the pain, the compromises, the problematic patterns of behavior—but in a way that aims to go beyond merely naming them or calling attention to them. If the person is to *truly* see them, to see them in a way that goes beyond words to genuine acceptance, and, eventually, to genuine change, they must be conveyed in a way that points to new more adaptive ways of being and experiencing even as it enables clearer appreciation of what has indeed been problematic. Throughout this book, the reader will find ample illustrations of how this can be done.

ATTRIBUTIONAL COMMENTS AND INTERPRETATIONS

Another way to understand what is entailed in what I have thus far discussed in terms of building on positives is that Ellen makes use of what I have elsewhere (P. L. Wachtel, 2011a) called *attributional* comments and interpretations. These therapeutic framings point to new directions that may be only incipient at the moment, but in the very process of being discussed in an attributional fashion, their fuller manifestation is made more likely. I use the term "attributional" because many of these comments *attribute* to the patient, client, or couple inclinations that may not yet be clearly evident or visible. They *give the person credit*, in essence, for having already achieved a valuable new perspective or way of interacting, and in the process of doing so, they make it more likely that it will happen. There is a suggestive element in these comments (see P. L. Wachtel, 2011a, for a fuller discussion of this dimension and its complexities), but the suggestion is not something covertly foisted upon the individual, trying insidiously to coax him or her in a direction s/he does not want to go. Rather, the suggestion essentially magnifies and encourages a still-budding inclination that the person has *already* showed signs of to at least some degree but that is still fragile, tentative, or in danger of being submerged in more familiar, if problematic, ways of behaving or seeing things. The aim is to support and encourage a tendency that, without that support, would very possibly go back underground or even disappear.

Attributional comments are rooted in an essentially *constructivist* epistemology that is shared by a growing number of both psychoanalytic and cognitive therapists (see, e.g., Hoffman, 1998; Mitchell, 1988; Stern, 1997; Aron, 1996; Mahoney, 1995, 2003; Niemeyer, 2009; Feixas & Botella, 2004; Guidano, 1991).[2] At their heart is the implicit assumption that there is not just one thing that the person wants but rather that there are multiple ways that the person's desires and interests can be understood or constructed, and that each choice or each focus can lead in a potentially different direction. If there is assumed to be *only one* true understanding, then any effort to describe it differently, and especially to influence the direction in which the person moves, will be regarded as untoward influence. Both Rogerian and classical psychoanalytic therapists shared the (essentially nonconstructivist) assumption of there being an already structured underlying meaning or feeling that could be discovered and articulated (cf. Stern, 1997) and that must be respected as the person's true feeling; hence both perspectives shared a strong aversion to the therapist's *influence* as an assault on the patient's or client's autonomy (see Mitchell, 1997, for an interesting and complex consideration of these issues). From a constructivist vantage point, however, if the therapist highlights one aspect of the individual's manifest or potential experience, she is neither making something up nor denying the reality or validity of other potential ways that the person's experience may be structured. Rather, she is calling attention to (and potentially helping to strengthen) an inclination or experience that is already genuinely the patient's or the couple's but has had difficulty emerging more fully.

The tone of an attributional statement generally conveys an assumption that the trend or inclination the therapist is referring to has already been noticed by the patient. Instead of calling attention to itself as an "interpretation" (and, importantly, instead of calling attention to *the therapist* as the one who has insight into what the patient is not yet able to see), an attributional framing *gives away* the insight, credits it to the patient. Often it states things in an almost incidental way, so that instead of eliciting resistance or a defensive reaction to what might feel an alien presence or a challenge to the patient's familiar ways of seeing things, it comes across as an *acknowledgment* of what the person *already* knows. Thus, in its simplest form, an attributional comment may be framed as "As you've already conveyed to

---

[2] Here is another place where the assumptions and conceptual structures that guide clinical work from nominally different theoretical orientations overlap far more than is generally acknowledged or understood. This is not to say that there are no significant differences between the approaches of (even constructivist) psychodynamic therapists and cognitive-behavioral therapists; if there were not such differences, the general agenda of *integrating* their complementary strengths and perspectives would offer little advantage over using either of them separately. It is the complex amalgam of difference and reconcilability that makes the project of combining them of value. But appreciation of the degree to which they do converge is hampered by antagonisms and misunderstandings whose properties resemble those of *ethnic* conflict far more than genuine intellectual or scientific differences (see P. L. Wachtel, 2011b).

me," or "As I know you already know," or "If I'm understanding what you are telling me. . . . " But the way the therapist says what she "hears" the patient having said may take the patient's way of seeing things or experiencing things a good deal further than it had yet been articulated.

In an attributional framing, the therapist might say something like "I can see that you're tired of the pattern of pulling away every time Jill ruffles your feathers and would like to be able to really talk it through with her and then be able to come together, with the issue resolved and both of you feeling closer and more known. But that still feels too dangerous and it's still hard to see just how to do it." In such a framing, the therapist, to begin with, *attributes* to the patient being *tired of* pulling away. Thus, instead of the therapist's directly suggesting or recommending that the husband change his behavior, she conveys the understanding that *he himself* wants to do so, that he himself is tired of it and ready to change it. If, of course, he is *not* tired of doing this, is *not* at all inclined to stop or change it, then the comment will have little therapeutic value or little likelihood of being accepted or initiating change. As in all aspects of therapeutic work, being effective requires being perceptive. If the therapist doesn't "get it," she will have little impact. But it is also worth reminding ourselves that the flip side of this is that the therapist is unlikely to be a secret Svengali, manipulating people to act in ways that are against their interests or genuine inclinations. If the comment doesn't resonate—if it is not the leading edge of a tendency already seeking to emerge, even if as yet still fragile or conflicted—it will likely simply be a dud.

The sample attributional comment just described has other elements besides the attributing of "being tired of it" to the husband. It also implicitly conveys what would be helpful to the relationship in his responding differently to his wife, but it does so not as a lesson imparted to the patient by the all-knowing (or at least more knowledgeable) therapist but, again, as something the husband *already knows*, something that the therapist is not *instructing* him about but simply *acknowledging*. It thus inhabits a therapeutically propitious realm of ambiguity: the therapist *is* offering input, *is* conveying her expertise regarding what works in relationships and what could be a potentially salutary change in their interaction. But she is doing so in a way that shares credit for that knowledge with the patient and, again, in a way that will only "take" if in fact it does resonate with something that the husband already senses, if only in a very preliminary and incomplete way.

Finally, the last part of the comment—*But that still feels too dangerous and it's still hard to see just how to do it*—contains several important further dimensions that do heavy therapeutic lifting. To begin with, acknowledging that it feels dangerous (and, implicitly, that being hesitant to pursue this change is not simply the husband being "resistant," but reflects his perception that it really might not be such a good idea) is likely to make it easier for him to receive and listen seriously to what the therapist is saying. It makes the therapist's comment not an assault on his perceptions, denying any validity to how he has been seeing things so far, but rather a statement that *validates even as it points toward change*.[3] Moreover, in stating it as "it's still hard to see" just how to do it, it implicitly underscores the *desirability* of doing so even in the very acknowledgment of the difficulty, and it implies as well that *there is* a way to do it and that the therapist is willing to help him find that way.

Attributional comments, like many facets of the therapist's repertoire, have the potential to convey complex and subtle messages even when (or perhaps especially when) seeming very simple and straightforward. A range of emotionally significant surplus meanings are often subtly packed into just a sentence or two. The more one understands and reflects upon the overtones and connotations of what one says as a therapist—I have elsewhere discussed them as metamessages that complement the focal message of which both patient and therapist may be more aware (P. L. Wachtel, 2011a)—the more likely it will be that the communication will have a therapeutic effect. The reader will find many examples in this book of the ways in which the subtle overtones of the therapist's communications can be harnessed to enhance the therapeutic effort and find a path through potential resistances, and will see how the skillful use of attributional comments can help couples to overcome tangles capable of ensnaring a more straight-ahead approach to the work.

It may be useful in further understanding the attributional dimension to bear in mind a closely related concept that Ellen has introduced in discussing therapeutic work with children and their parents. In a very important paper (E. F. Wachtel, 2001) she discusses what she calls *the language of becoming*. This is a mode of therapeutic communication that is not designed exclusively for the therapist's use; she also often teaches parents to use it with their children at home in order to promote and amplify change. Examples of the language of becoming might include saying to a child who has been fearful and hesitant to take on challenges, "I see you're becoming the kind of kid who can do new things even if you're feeling scared" or to a child who has been embroiled in constant arguments and problematic rivalry with a sibling, "I've noticed you're becoming good at being supportive of your little sister and that the two of you are having more fun together."

---

[3]Here again we may point to an understanding that is increasingly shared by therapists of a wide range of orientations. Both Linehan (1993, 1997), in the fundamental premises of dialectical behavior therapy, and Bromberg (1998b), writing from a relational psychoanalytic perspective, highlight the importance of validating the patient's currently existing perceptions and actions as a crucial element in helping the patient to *change* those very perceptions and actions. See also Schechter (2007) and P. L. Wachtel (2011a).

The style and linguistic forms employed in the language of becoming are often simpler and have a more "naive" quality than is the case in what I have been referring to as attributional comments, as befits their being directed toward children. But the basic communicational and relational structure is very similar: the person, whether adult or child, is given credit now, in essence, for what s/he is capable of being in the future (and for the *preliminary versions* of that future that can already be pointed to). In that sense, there is an intriguing parallel between the "credit" that the therapist offers the patient in these kinds of comments and the seemingly very different kind of credit offered to a business by a bank: the bank lends the business money that at this very moment it does not have the resources to pay back; but in the very extending of the credit, the bank enables the business to *develop* those resources and, eventually, not just pay the money back but do so with interest. Similarly, when, via an attributional interpretation or the language of becoming, we give people credit for already understanding something or already beginning to initiate change, it enables them to develop resources and move in directions that they might not have been able to do without the extension of that credit—thereby justifying the credit given to them as an accurate assessment of their potential. Pursuing a little further this whimsical, but yet potentially illuminating, analogy, one can say that both bankers and therapists are in the business not just of assessing the present but of predicting (and influencing) the future.

Fortunately, we may note, the consequences are usually less severe when our predictions are erroneous than when a banker's are. No one loses money or goes bankrupt; we simply take two steps back, reassess where we took a wrong step, and pick up the thread. Often, indeed, if we are able to own up to them and work with them, our mistakes can be a productive (perhaps even essential) part of the therapeutic process itself. Important research conducted by Safran, Muran, and their colleagues suggests that a process of rupture and repair in the therapeutic alliance can be a key element in therapeutic progress (Safran & Muran, 2000; Safran, Muran, & Proskurov, 2009; Ruiz-Cordell & Safran, 2007).

BUILDING ON POSITIVES, ATTRIBUTIONAL COMMENTS, AND THE PERSPECTIVE OF REINFORCEMENT AND SHAPING

In further elaborating on the surprising and often unacknowledged convergences between therapeutic orientations that are often treated as radically separate and opposed, we may also note that the clinical strategies and perspectives I have just been describing have interesting parallels with the concepts and methods that are described from a very different theoretical vantage point as "reinforcement" and "shaping." For many therapists of other orientations, especially those with a psychoanalytic or humanistic point of view, thinking in terms of reinforcement may appear soulless or mechanistic. And these days many academics and researchers too are critical of the behavioristic foundations that underlie much discussion of these concepts. From Chomsky's (1959) review of Skinner's book on verbal behavior (Skinner, 1957) to contemporary proponents of cognitive psychology and cognitive neuroscience, the behavioristic assumptions that guided Skinner's seminal explorations of the role of reinforcement and shaping—assumptions that once were the dominant conceptual framework in American psychology—have increasingly seemed anachronistic. Today, in that pure form, they remain compelling only to a relatively small cadre of committed proponents. But it is important to appreciate that however one views the explicit philosophical and methodological assumptions of the behaviorist worldview, the *observations* generated by decades of research on reinforcement and shaping and the methods of intervention that derived from them remain of considerable value.

Most contemporary psychological theorists and researchers would conceptualize the foundations of those observations in a different way from Skinner, but nonetheless the analyses of the differing consequences of different schedules of reinforcement and of the ways that new behaviors can be shaped from the elements of earlier simpler ones seem to me potentially valuable clinical tools, especially if one is simultaneously attentive to the ethical challenges that can be associated with some ways of attempting to utilize reinforcement contingencies to change behavior (see P. L. Wachtel, 1997, especially Chs. 11 and 12). The important contributions of Kohlenberg and Tsai (e.g., 1991, 1994; Kanter, Tsai, & Kohlenberg, 2010), for example, seem to me to be examples of how the principles of reinforcement can offer a perspective that is usefully complementary to those of relational and humanistic writers in pointing to how the therapeutic relationship can most effectively be harnessed to promote therapeutic change. Closer still to the focus of this book, Gurman, Waltz, and Follette (2010) have discussed ways in which Kohlenberg and Tsai's approach can be useful in work with couples.

The principles of reinforcement can be useful not only as a guideline for understanding what is happening in the session and how to ensure that the exchanges between patient and therapist or therapist and couple serve therapeutic ends; it can also very usefully remind us of factors to be attentive to *outside* the session. The central conceptualization of relational psychoanalysis, that all of our motives, thoughts, and emotions must be understood in relation to the relational matrix that is their context, can be understood as well—in a linguistic turn unlikely to be seen very often in the relational literature—as pointing to the ways in which all facets of our lives are lived in relation to a *reinforcement* matrix. We are continuous sources of positive and negative reinforcement for each other, and our individual experiences of self and—especially important in the context of this book, our experience of and behavior toward our spouse or partner—reflect that mutual shaping and reinforcement in significant ways. It will be apparent to the reader of this book that Ellen is keenly attentive to these mutual reinforcement patterns. One cannot get very far as a therapist unless one is attentive to the ways in which behaviors that are rewarded become more likely to occur and those not rewarded tend to drop out.

To be sure, sophisticated application of this principle requires keener understanding than is often evident among proponents of the reinforcement paradigm of how what is rewarding for one person may not be rewarding for another; of how sometimes what might seem on the face of it to be quite *un*desired and *un*sought consequences may in fact be powerfully operative reinforcements; of how people can be quite *unaware* of the contingencies to which they respond and the motivations that give meaning to those contingencies. That is, in my view, it requires complementing the findings of reinforcement theorists with a healthy dose of psychodynamic understanding. But understanding clearly how reinforcement contingencies operate in our lives remains nonetheless quite critical.

Of particular importance to the therapeutic effort, whether with individuals or couples, is a concept without which the understanding of reinforcement contingencies alone would provide only limited illumination—namely, *shaping*. One of the key insights of Skinner and other early behaviorists was that to explain behavior in terms of reinforcement contingencies one must go beyond showing how behaviors already in the repertoire are strengthened or weakened according to their consequences. That much even the average schoolboy or schoolgirl already largely understands, at least implicitly.[4] The more subtle and original insights involved the understanding of how *new* behaviors evolved. By gradually changing the requirements for obtaining reinforcement, Skinner and his colleagues and followers found, new behaviors could be brought about that were not originally in the individual's repertoire (although obviously the *potential* for such behaviors must be in the repertoire—the reason pigs can't fly). Over time, building on the elements of what already existed prior, wholly new behaviors evolve. The process is akin to that of natural selection over the scale of evolutionary time. How do primitive organisms give rise to vertebrates, vertebrates to mammals, mammals to primates, or primates to human beings? Each change is small and gradual, built on the foundations of what already exists, and yet, over time,

---

[4]The role of what Skinner called different *schedules* of reinforcement, in contrast—the differing consequences, for example, of continuous reinforcement and intermittent reinforcement—was far less obvious and remains an intellectual triumph of the behaviorist era.

astounding qualitative differences arise. Human beings, hummingbirds, octopi, and sea slugs are remarkably different—in a sense, each eventually came to be something utterly new under the sun (or sea)—and yet each represents a gradual branching (a shaping by selective contingencies) from an earlier form. In that sense, the ontogeny of behavior follows a pathway similar to the phylogeny of species: small changes can, over time, yield changes that are not only bigger but, eventually, seem to yield something *qualitatively new*.

What is most relevant about shaping in understanding the approach to couple therapy that Ellen describes in this book is that shaping is essentially a process of building on positives. It is the small initial movements in the desired direction that spawn the later, more elaborated and sustainable versions that constitute what could be viewed, from one vantage point, as a couple's learning to create a mutually reinforcing pattern of loving and satisfying interactions. The approach described in this book is especially marked by its emphasis on finding and building on positives (though always, as Ellen makes abundantly clear, with a clear-eyed attentiveness to the problematic features of each partner's behavior and the interactions between them). Ellen is remarkably good at finding those initial kernels of new or positive behavior that can be nurtured and encouraged to help build increasingly positive interactions.

The perspective on this process that derives from the literature on reinforcement and shaping points to one more way in which the way of working described in this book is in fact evidence-based, if that term is understood not just as attending to the results of randomized controlled trials (RCTs) of manualized treatment packages, but also as making use of *principles* and *processes* that have been supported by a broad foundation of basic and applied research. The rhetorical depiction of RCTs as constituting a "gold standard" has introduced much confusion. RCTs most definitely offer certain kinds of assurances about causality that other investigative strategies do not as fully; but as they are generally conducted, especially in the realm of psychotherapy (where a double-blind design is virtually impossible), they bring their own limitations to a sufficient degree that without complementary evidence from multiple kinds of basic and applied studies, they constitute a shaky foundation for constructing an evidence base for clinical practice. Elevating one kind of study to a "gold standard," and thereby downplaying the equally essential complementary studies and research strategies needed for an approach to practice that is truly based on a solid foundation of evidence, is an exercise in obfuscation.

For some therapists, I am aware, my highlighting of the elements of shaping and reinforcement in the approach Ellen describes in this book may create concerns about possible *manipulation* of clients or problematic efforts on the therapist's part to shape the couple's behavior and interactions to conform with her own vision of healthy behavior rather than the couple's. There are legitimate concerns that can be raised about therapists aiming to shape others' behavior (I discuss the complex ethical and conceptual questions this perspective raises in P. L. Wachtel, 1997, especially Chs. 11 and 12). But it is worth noting as well that the perspective of shaping can be understood and employed in ways that come closer to a rather different social and ethical framework, that of taking the person "where he's at," of aiming to create change not on the basis of some ideal that treats as "lesser" the way the person presently behaves but, quite the opposite, as seeing the path to more satisfying behavior as starting with *how the person already is* and with encouraging movement in directions in which he has struggled, but often unsuccessfully, to take further.

It is very much in this spirit that Ellen proceeds. As she puts it in Chapter 5, "A key goal for the couple therapist is to encourage couples to try new ways of being with one another. When behavioral change feels like a natural manifestation of evolving feelings rather than something that the couple has *contracted* to do differently, the new ways of interacting are more likely to be sustained. They will feel like authentic expressions of feelings that were already present but not displayed because the couple had gotten into negative cycles of interaction." This emphasis on creating conditions that enable the spontaneous expression of feelings to evolve and be maintained, rather than attempting to negotiate an explicit quid pro quo behavioral contract (which means addressing behavior that is already in the couple's repertoire), seems to me not only to be consistent with the enormous body of empirical research on reinforcement and shaping but also to reflect a more sophisticated reading and application of that research.

COUPLE THERAPY AND RELATIONAL PSYCHOANALYSIS

Further reflecting the broadly integrative nature of Ellen's approach to couple work, we may see as well a number of important convergences between the work she describes and the perspective of relational psychoanalysis, a significant evolution in the world of psychodynamic thought and practice with which, unfortunately, many therapists of other orientations seem only dimly aware (Westen, 1998). Relational theory is a version of psychoanalytic thought that is especially suited for couple work (Goldner, 2104; P. L. Wachtel, 2014b) because it understands personality dynamics not in terms of what Mitchell (1995) has called "a view of mind as monadic, a separable, individual entity," but rather via "a view of mind as dyadic, emerging from and inevitably embedded within a relational field" (p. 65; see also Stolorow & Atwood, 1994).

I have already mentioned the constructivist foundations of attributional comments that Ellen liberally employs in her work, and have noted how central a constructivist epistemology is to the relational point of view. Relevant as well to our understanding both of attributional comments and of Ellen's overall approach is the concept of multiple self-states, which has similarly become a central conceptual tool in the relational literature (e.g., Bromberg, 1998a; Davies, 1996; Harris, 1996; Mitchell, 1993; Pizer, 1996; Slavin, 1996). One of the aims of attributional comments is to address how qualities that people often experience as "just the way I am" (or "just the way s/he is") can mask other potentials and other ways of behaving or experiencing that are already part of the person's repertoire, even if as yet only to a limited (and perhaps even barely noticeable) degree. Attributional comments, in aiming to support and amplify emergent tendencies that have not yet been assimilated into the person's conscious sense of self, rely on a perspective that conceives of these alternative ways of being as part of a *multiplicity* of ways of being that characterize the person, or, in the language of relational psychoanalysis, a multiplicity of self-states.

Older psychoanalytic conceptualizations, in which "beneath the surface" the person's way of thinking, feeling, and perceiving was seen as reflecting a particular "developmental level" at which the person is fixated or arrested or as characterizing his or her "personality organization" are largely replaced in the relational literature with a more commodious understanding of personality dynamics, in which *multiple* ways of being are understood to be significant elements in the person's overall makeup (P. L. Wachtel, 2008, 2014a). This viewpoint is a key conceptual foundation for the utilization of attributional comments, which often highlight aspects of the self that have not been included in the person's more usual way of seeing him- or herself. It is also a foundation of the way that Ellen, even more broadly than just in the use of attributional comments, aims to build on positives in her work with couples.

The relational conceptualization usually calls particular attention to the ways that different self-states can be *dissociated* from each other, with access to one often blocked by the very emergence of another. These dissociative phenomena are of great importance in understanding various kinds of difficulties people can have, especially at the more severe end of the spectrum. But the insights about multiplicity do not require that all variant ways of being be dissociated from each other. More fundamental, I would suggest, is the understanding that personality is not organized in a strictly hierarchical fashion, with certain features "underlying" others and therefore more fundamental (see, e.g., P. L. Wachtel, 2008, 2014a). This latter, broader understanding of multiplicity can help the therapist be less pathologizing: attention to multiple self-states points the therapist toward noticing *variations* in the person's functioning and way of being and can thus be a foundation for transcending the way that pathocentric understandings of people exert a problematic gravitational pull for many psychotherapists. By enabling attention to be paid equally to how the person acts and feels in *other* states of mind, the therapist is enabled to view these alternative ways of being as not simply "defensive" covering over of the "real" or "core" pathology, but rather as *one more way the person can be.*

Another key relational concept implicit in much that Ellen describes in this book is that of *unformulated experience,* Stern's (1997) salutary contribution to the reconceptualization of what is more commonly referred to as "the unconscious" or "unconscious processes." In Stern's reconceptualization, the tendencies and experiences we have more commonly called unconscious are understood, essentially, as *incipient* processes or experiences, *potentials* for action or experience that have not yet taken a final form, often for defensive reasons because the direction toward which they might otherwise build is a potential source of anxiety. Rather than the unconscious consisting of already fully formed memories, desires, or fantasies, located in some separate zone of the psyche to which they are banished and from which they energetically try to escape, Stern's realm of unformulated experience is rooted in an understanding of mind, behavior, and personality as always in process, always dynamically shifting, taking shape in real time as a product of multiple influences and inputs. The outcome of this dynamic process includes very significantly how the person has *previously* learned to express or give shape to experience and how s/he has encountered comfort or discomfort in doing so. It will be evident to the reader that a similar vision guides Ellen's work with couples.

THE RELEVANCE OF CYCLICAL PSYCHODYNAMICS

One version of relational thought in particular is especially reflected in Ellen's discussions in this book—that of cyclical psychodynamics (P. L. Wachtel, 2014a). This is perhaps not surprising, since Ellen shares a bedroom with the developer of this point of view. (If print versions of books shared with online communications the opportunities for inserting emoticons, a smiley face would be welcome here. But more prosaically, the point that couples, if they are getting on well, tend to share many ideas and values while at the same time having room to develop them in their individual manner will be evident throughout this book.)

Cyclical psychodynamics is a framework especially suited for thinking about couples because it is centrally rooted in the vicious circles in which people can get caught, both individually and collectively. It highlights the reality that the key to understanding how people can persist in ways of living that over and over create great pain and frustration lies in noticing that they *get help* in persisting in this improbable task. The unwitting and generally unconscious recruiting of others as "accomplices" (P. L. Wachtel, 2014a) in maintaining problematic patterns is at the heart of the problems people bring to psychotherapists, whether as individuals or as couples. From this vantage point, couple work may be seen as seeking to untangle the interlocking ways in which each partner serves as an accomplice to the other in maintaining a way of being with each other that ultimately leads to pain and dissatisfaction for both—a tangle in which they are so thoroughly caught that each step in the dance seems to lead almost inexorably to the next.

The art of untangling the ironies of this state of affairs—so well illustrated in the work Ellen describes here—very largely consists of paying due attention to the maladaptive aspects of the pattern without that attention leading to a pathologizing view of the couple. If we are to help the couple to change, we need to see in clear-eyed fashion all that is wrong, but not equate what is wrong with *who the members of the couple are* or what their relationship ultimately entails. At times this is not easy. As one gets good at seeing how they reciprocally serve as accomplices in the very behaviors and attitudes of the other that hurt them or drive them apart, there is likely to be a strong inclination to place this pattern front and center. And, of course, in some ways it is essential to do so. But a central component of the skills Ellen demonstrates so powerfully in this book includes being able to do this in a way that also keeps clearly in mind the couple's strengths. As she describes, the good couple therapist, while attuned to all that has gone wrong, is also attuned to the ways in which the two partners *also* call out in each other (even if less frequently and consistently) many of the same behaviors and feelings that brought them together in the first place, or, to put it differently, is attuned to noticing where they still are able to enjoy and support each other. Accomplices, we may say, can be recruited for both good and ill, and almost all of us, in varying degrees, have a significant capacity for both kinds of recruitment.

From a related vantage point, cyclical psychodynamics is a natural framework for understanding couples because it is essentially a *contextual* perspective on personality. It shares with other relational perspectives an emphasis on the relational matrix as the context for personality phenomena that were once seen as strictly "internal." But it tends to go further than most other relational viewpoints in highlighting the actual behaviors and interactions of daily life as the way that patterns established early in life are maintained over many decades (P. L. Wachtel, 2008, 2014a). Relatedly, though sharing with other relational approaches a strong emphasis on understanding the impact of the bidirectional relational events in the consulting room in generating therapeutic change, it also highlights the importance of the cyclical (two-person or multiperson) patterns that characterize the person's daily life *outside* the therapist's office. It is thus a version of relational thought particularly suited for tracking the ways that the partners interact with each other in their daily life and, at the same time, the ways that the deeper subjective meanings of those interactions to each partner derive in good measure from experiences that have evolved over the course of their lifetimes, both before and after they got together. Individual subjectivity, *inter*subjectivity, and systemic patterns are not separate realms but overlapping perspectives on lived experience that must all be taken into account by the therapist, as Ellen beautifully illustrates throughout this book.

THE THERAPIST'S CHOICE OF LANGUAGE

Very closely associated with the evolution of the cyclical psychodynamic point of view has been a concern with the ways that subtle differences in how therapists speak to patients can make a big difference in the emotional and relational meaning that is conveyed. Slightly different ways of saying what might seem to be the "same thing" can have very different therapeutic implications (P. L. Wachtel, 2011a). Such concerns, of course, are not limited to the cyclical psychodynamic point of view, but cyclical psychodynamic thought and attention to the details of therapists' language have evolved so closely hand-in-hand that there is a special link between the two.

Ellen's discussion in this book is by no means exclusively limited to a cyclical psychodynamic point of view. Although cyclical psychodynamics itself is a systemic perspective as well as a psychodynamic one, Ellen employs a wide range of other systemic viewpoints as well. Likewise, although many of the guidelines presented in *Therapeutic Communication* (P. L. Wachtel, 2011a) for how therapists can most fruitfully talk with their patients are shared by Ellen, she takes them in new directions and adds her own distinctive contribution in the couple work described in this book.

THE ROLE OF ATTACHMENT

In recent years, the dynamics of couples and the difficulties they can encounter have been increasingly understood in terms of attachment and attachment injuries (e.g., Davila, 2003; Greenberg & Goldman, 2008; Johnson & Whiffen, 2003; Makinen & Johnson, 2006; Johnson et al., 2001). This trend parallels one in the larger realm of psychotherapy, where, after many years of being marginalized by the psychoanalytic establishment, attachment theory has assumed great prominence both in the world of psychoanalysis and psychodynamic therapy and in a still broader range of therapeutic orientations (e.g., P. L. Wachtel, 2010b; Fonagy, 2001; Fosha, 2000;

Leahy, 2005; Johnson & Greenberg, 1995; Renn, 2012, 2017; Slade, 2008; Wallin, 2007; Davila, 2003). This is an enormously salutary development, offering valuable bridges between careful empirical research on psychological development and the practices of psychotherapists.

In particular, the contributions of attachment theory and research have introduced a greater emphasis on understanding the consequences of the *actual experiences* of the growing child and his or her interactions with others. Part of the initial antagonism toward Bowlby in large parts of the psychoanalytic establishment, especially in his native Britain, derived from an inclination in the psychoanalytic theorizing of the time to view as more fundamental and more rigorously in accord with the deepest truths about human experience accounts that depicted psychological inclinations as emerging from *within*, as the innate unfolding of a genetically programmed and almost inexorable internally driven sequence. As part of this theoretical line, explanations of behavior or experience that were attentive to what is actually happening in the person's life and in his interactions with others were derided as mere [*sic*] "social" psychology—and hence as "superficial" (see in this regard Greenberg & Mitchell, 1983). In the Kleinian vision, which exerted a powerful influence on psychoanalysis in England (Bowlby's home country), as well as in many other parts of the world, what was "deep" was the drives and the supposedly innate "phantasies" they generated. Because Bowlby's theory highlighted *what actually happened* between mother and infant, and in essence treated the phantasies of Kleinian theory as secondary factors that were a consequence of the particularities of the actual mother–infant interaction, it was for several decades extruded from the mainstream of psychoanalytic thought.

Today, much has changed. To begin with, it is increasingly understood that the form of biological and genetic determinism embodied in the earlier psychoanalytic models, despite analysts' self-congratulatory understanding of themselves as more "hard-headed" and acknowledging of our animal nature, was significantly in error. We now understand that the operation of genes is not a fixed, autonomously run-off sequence but that, rather, the expression of the genetic program is a profoundly *contextual* process; what the expression of the gene leads to can be dramatically different depending on the context in which that expression occurs, and a host of variables code-termine the meaning and implication of the gene itself (see, e.g., Bronfenbrenner & Ceci, 1994; Kendler & Eaves, 1986; Lerner, 1991; Shanahan & Hofer, 2005). No longer is an emphasis on the direct expression of a purely endogenous, biologically programmed destiny a hallmark of hard-headed realism, contrasting with the theoretical comfort food that views people as malleable and adaptable to social circumstances. Today, the demythologizing light of science points toward explanations of a quite different sort—contextual accounts that attend to the staggering complexity of biological and psychological development and the reciprocal feedback processes that lead to emergent phenomena that are poorly understood by simple linear story lines.

The increasing influence of attachment theory in understanding the difficulties both individuals and couples experience has clearly been a very salutary development. But the contribution of the attachment perspective has also been limited by an excessive emphasis on attachment *categories* (secure, avoidant, resistant, etc.) as the primary focus of theory and research (P. L. Wachtel, 2010b). The findings demonstrating correlations between early measured attachment categories and future psychological qualities and outcomes have certainly been generative, and the sheer quantity of this research is impressive; clearly, it is a paradigm that lends itself well to the methods researchers presently most commonly employ. But it is essential to complement the study of attachment *categories* with an understanding of attachment in terms of *process* and *dynamics*. Attachment is not just a convenient sorting device for making statistical predictions; it is as well a critically important lens for understanding how people *interact* with each other and for understanding both the motivations and the consequences of those interactions. And although the categorical assessment of individuals' attachment status has been a useful tool in a number of ways, and Bowlby's concept of internal working models provides a helpful picture of how people come to anticipate future interactions based on past ones and of how they organize their relational and experiential world, it is essential to bear in mind that attachment is not a phenomenon residing solely inside the head of one person but is in many respects an almost quintessentially two-person phenomenon (P. L. Wachtel, 2010b). This understanding of attachment is especially relevant for addressing attachment in the context of couple therapy.

When we move beyond singular (and often static) descriptions of attachment *status* to accounts of attachment *processes*—and especially as we expand our lens to a two-person perspective that looks at the mutual and reciprocal contributions of the caretaker and the cared-for—we encounter a framework better suited for work with couples. (Of course, with couples the role of caretaker and cared-for keeps shifting; indeed, if it does not, that in itself is a sign of a problem that needs to be addressed.) When we move beyond thinking of one or the other partner as simply securely or insecurely attached, and consider *when* either feels secure or insecure in the attachment, *when* their anxieties are quelled by turning to the other and when they are exacerbated—and when we realize that even in the most well-attached and well-functioning couple, both kinds of events will inevitably happen (though obviously in different proportions)—then we can begin to be clearer as well about *what is happening* when greater or lesser security is evoked. Such a dynamic (rather than simply categorical) understanding of attachment still builds on the research that illuminates the features of secure, ambivalent, avoidant, and disorganized attachment. But it acknowledges as well—much as in theorizing about multiple self-states—that each of us can be quite variable even if we have a central tendency that can roughly characterize us; and it points to how we can relate that variability to the context in which we are participating (and, in the case of couples especially, to the ways that people become the context for *each other* and, through their actions and experiences, maintain either a continuity or a change in that bidirectional context).

All of this dynamic variability—and all of the ways that attention to this variability provides the couple therapist with the tools to bring out submerged potentials in the couple and in the individuals who comprise it—will be evident to the reader who follows Ellen's account of how she works. But the attachment dimension in her thinking and her work may not be as immediately apparent as it might be because in recent years attention to attachment phenomena has often been associated with particular kinds of intense emotionality in the session. Breakthroughs often seem to derive from *breaking through*—from breaking through defenses, breaking through emotional walls, breaking through denials or distancing. Tolerance for intense emotion, to be sure, is an important requirement for good therapeutic work. But that does not mean drama is the same as progress. Videos with lots of tears and moments of heightened emotion make great viewing, but they do not necessarily represent the apex of therapeutic effectiveness.

One of the interesting things about Ellen's approach, distinguishing it at times from some other approaches that describe themselves very explicitly and centrally as attachment-centered, is that, as the reader has likely noted, she does not usually aim to produce "Hollywood moments" in the session. Often, of course, there is crying or deep feelings of pain that come up in the sessions—and the book describes how she skillfully deals with these strong emotional responses—but she does not particularly *aim* to produce them. And yet, the aim *is* to lead to profound experiences of closeness and attachment; it is just that the most important arena for this is in the couple's *life together* more than in the session per se. In the framework implicit in the work described here, attachment injuries are understood as persisting because of what transpires in the couple's daily interactions more than because of something from the past, though of course the past is taken into account.

AN INTEGRATIVE APPROACH
TO COUPLE THERAPY

I have touched on but a sample of the conceptual themes that are found in this book. In describing an approach marked by a very broadly integrative sensibility, Ellen draws upon psychodynamic, cognitive-behavioral, systemic, and experiential models. She approaches the couple as a system, but she attends as well to the qualities, characteristics, and vulnerabilities of each individual. She focuses on what is happening in the present, how the couple live and how they perpetuate their difficulties (as well as how they manifest already the kernels of different ways of being); but she does not ignore the past. She observes what happens in the room, but she also listens carefully to what happens outside it. She attends to them as lovers and sexual beings but also as parents, wage-earners, and members of the community. The complexity of human behavior and experience—and the ways that that complexity is even further multiplied in trying to address the issues presented by couples—means that we need to bring to bear every conceptual tool we possibly can.

Most readers will find in this book both viewpoints that are familiar and rooted in a framework that overlaps substantially with their own and perspectives that feel new, perhaps at first even alien. The integrative framework that informs the work and the thinking described provides the sinews and ligaments to hold together these disparate perspectives. As one absorbs it in reading the various chapters, it enables viewpoints that were portrayed in one's training as beyond the bounds of acceptable thought or discourse to be seamlessly assimilated into one's thinking. Each reader brings different training experiences and identifications to his or her work and to the experience of reading this book. Consequently, each will learn something slightly different from the book, and—very importantly—each will have something useful *to add* to what Ellen has described, some additional perspective to bring to bear. It is my hope that by offering perspectives that speak simultaneously (but inevitably with different resonances) to the different communities and constituencies that constitute our field, this book will spark dialogue among clinicians of different initial outlooks. If, via emails or other modes of exchange, or during workshops or seminars that Ellen offers, new questions, new challenges, and new convergences become apparent, that will be the surest sign of the book's success.

stonguay, L. G., Goldfried, M. R., Wiser, S., Raue, P. J., & Hayes, A. M. (1996). Predicting the effect of cognitive therapy for depression: A study of unique and common factors. *Journal of Consulting and Clinical Psychology, 64*, 497–504.

omsky, A. N. (1959). A review of Skinner's *Verbal Behavior. Language (LSA), 35*(1), 26–58.

vies, J. M. (1996). Linking the "pre-analytic" with the postclassical: Integration, dissociation, and the multiplicity of unconscious processes. *Contemporary Psychoanalysis, 32*(4), 553–576.

vila, J. (2003). Attachment processes in couple therapy: Informing behavioral models. In S. M. Johnson & V. E. Whiffen (Eds.), *Attachment processes in couple and family therapy* (pp. 124–143). New York: Guilford Press.

herty, W. J. (2001). *Take back your marriage: Sticking together in a world that pulls us apart.* New York: Guilford Press.

llard, J., & Miller, N. E. (1950). *Personality and psychotherapy.* New York: McGraw-Hill.

ncan, B. L., Miller, S. D., Wampold, B. E., & Hubble, M. A. (Eds.). (2010). *The heart and soul of change: Delivering what works in therapy* (2nd ed.). Washington, DC: American Psychological Association.

xas, G., & Botella, L. (2004). Psychotherapy integration: Reflections and contributions from a constructivist epistemology. *Journal of Psychotherapy Integration, 14*(2), 192–222.

dman, L. B. (1992). *Integrating individual and family therapy.* New York: Brunner/Mazel.

hbane, M. D. (2001). Relational narratives of the self. *Family Process, 40*, 273–291.

hbane, M. D. (2013). *Loving with the brain in mind: Neurobiology and couple therapy.* New York: Norton.

a, E. B. (2011). Prolonged exposure therapy: Past, present, and future. *Depression and Anxiety, 28*(12), 1043–1047.

a, E. B., Huppert, J. D., & Cahill, S. P. (2006). Emotional processing theory: An update. In B. Rothbaum (Ed.), *Pathological anxiety: Emotional processing in etiology and treatment* (pp. 3–24). New York: Guilford Press.

a, E. B., & Kozak, M. J. (1986). Emotional processing of fear: Exposure to corrective information. *Psychological Bulletin, 99*, 20–35.

nagy, P. (2001). *Attachment theory and psychoanalysis.* New York: Other Press.

sha, D. (2000). *The transforming power of affect: A model for accelerated change.* New York: Basic Books.

enkel, P. (2009). The therapeutic palette: A guide to choice points in integrative couple therapy. *Clinical Social Work, 37*, 234–247.

enkel, P., & Pinsof, W. M. (2001). Teaching family therapy-centered integration: Assimilation and beyond. *Journal of Psychotherapy Integration, 11*, 59–85.

nk, J. D., & Frank, J. B. (1991). *Persuasion and healing.* Baltimore: Johns Hopkins University Press.

edman, J., & Combs, G. (1996). *Narrative therapy.* New York: Norton.

rson, M. J. (2009). *The embedded self: An integrative psychodynamic and systemic perspective on couples and family therapy* (2nd ed.). New York: Routledge.

rson, M. J. (2013). The analyst and the significant other: Two's company, three's

References

Ablon, J. S., & Jones, E. E. (1998). How expert clinicians' prototype treatment correlate with outcome in psychodynamic and cogniti therapy. *Psychotherapy Research, 8,* 71–83.

Ablon, J. S., & Jones, E. E. (2002). Validity of controlled clinical tri therapy: Findings from the NIMH Treatment of Depression Research Program. *American Journal of Psychiatry, 159,* 775–78

Ablon, S. J., Levy, R., & Katzenstein, T. (2006). Beyond brand nam therapy: Identifying empirically supported change processes. *P Theory, Research, Practice, Training, 43*(2), 216–231.

Anderson, T., Ogles, B. M., Patterson, C. L., Lambert, M. J., & Vern (2009). Therapist effects: Facilitative interpersonal skills as a pre apist success. *Journal of Clinical Psychology, 65*(7), 755–768.

Aron, L. (1996). *A meeting of minds: Mutality in psychoanalysis.* Analytic Press.

Beutler, L. E. (2004). The empirically supported treatments movemer practitioner's response. *Clinical Psychology: Science and Practice*

Beutler, L. E., Consoli, A. J., & Lane, J. (2005). Systemic treatment prescriptive psychotherapy. In J. C. Norcross & M. R. Goldfried *book of psychotherapy integration* (2nd ed., pp. 121–143). New University Press.

Bromberg, P. M. (1998a). *Standing in the spaces: Essays on clinical pr and dissociation.* Hillsdale, NJ: Analytic Press.

Bromberg, P. M. (1998b). Staying the same while changing: Reflecti judgment. *Psychoanalytic Dialogues, 8,* 225–236.

Bronfenbrenner, U., & Ceci, S. J. (1994). Nature–nurture reconceptu opmental perspective: A bioecological model. *Psychological* 568–586.

Castonguay, L. G., & Beutler, L. E. (Eds.). (2003). *Empirically suppc of therapeutic change.* New York: Oxford University Press.

a crowd: Commentary on paper by Carla Leone. *Psychoanalytic Dialogues, 23,* 340–348.

Gilboa-Schechtman, E., Foa, E. B., Shafran, N., Aderka, I. M., Powers, M. B., Rachamim, L., et al. (2010). Prolonged exposure versus dynamic therapy for adolescent PTSD: A pilot randomized controlled trial. *Journal of the American Academy of Child and Adolescent Psychiatry, 49*(10), 1034–1042.

Goldman, R., & Greenberg, L. (2013). Working with identity and self-soothing in emotion-focused therapy for couples. *Family Process, 52,* 62–82.

Goldner, V. (1998). The treatment of violence and victimization in intimate relationships. *Family Process, 37*(3), 263–286.

Goldner, V. (2014). Romantic bonds, binds, and ruptures: Couples on the brink. *Psychoanalytic Dialogues, 24,* 402–418.

Gottman, J. M. (1994). *What predicts divorce?* Hillsdale, NJ: Erlbaum.

Gottman, J. M. (1999). *The marriage clinic: A scientifically based marital therapy.* New York: Norton.

Gottman, J. M., & DeClaire, J. (2002). *The relationship cure.* New York: Harmony.

Gottman, J. M., & Silver, N. (1999). *The seven principles for making marriage work.* New York: Crown.

Greenberg, J., & Mitchell, S. A. (1983). *Object relations in psychoanalytic theory.* Cambridge, MA: Harvard University Press.

Greenberg, L. S., & Goldman, R. N. (2008). *Emotion-focused couples therapy: The dynamics of emotion, love, and power.* Washington, DC: American Psychological Association Books.

Greenberg, L. S., & Johnson, S. (1988). *Emotionally focused couple therapy.* New York: Guilford Press.

Guidano, V. E. (1991). *The self in process: Toward a post-rationalist cognitive therapy.* New York: Guilford Press

Gurman, A. S., Waltz, T. J., & Follette, W. C. (2010). FAP-enhanced couple therapy: Perspectives and possibilities. In J. W. Kanter, M. Tsai, & R. J. Kohlenberg (Eds.), *The practice of functional analytic psychotherapy* (pp. 125–147). New York: Springer.

Hardy, K. V., & Laszloffy, T. A. (1995). The cultural genogram: Key to training cultural competent family therapists. *Journal of Marital and Family Therapy, 21,* 227–237.

Harris, A. (1996). The conceptual power of multiplicity. *Contemporary Psychoanalysis, 32*(4), 537–552.

Havens, L. (1986). *Making contact: Uses of language in psychotherapy.* Cambridge, MA: Harvard University Press.

Heitler, S. M. (1990). *From conflict to resolution: Strategies for diagnosis and treatment of distressed individuals, couples, and families.* New York: Norton.

Hoffman, I. Z. (1998). *Ritual and spontaneity in psychoanalysis.* Hillsdale, NJ: Analytic Press.

Howard, K. I., Moras, K., Brill, P. L., Martinovitch, Z., & Lutz, W. (1996). The evaluation of psychotherapy: Efficacy, effectiveness, and patient progress. *American Psychologist, 51,* 1059–1064.

Iasenza, S. (2010). What is queer about sex?: Expanding sexual frames in theory and practice. *Family Process, 49,* 291–308.

Jacobson, N. S., & Christensen, A. (1996). *Integrative behavioral couple therapy.* New York: Norton.

Johnson, S. M. (1996). *The practice of emotionally focused couples therapy: Creating connections.* New York: Brunner-Routledge.

Johnson, S. M., & Greenberg, L. S. (1995). The emotionally focused approach to problems in adult attachment. In N. S. Jacobson & A. S. Gurman (Eds.), *Clinical handbook of couple therapy* (pp. 121–141). New York: Guilford Press.

Johnson, S. M., Makinen, J. A., & Millikin J. W. (2001). Attachment injuries in couple relationships: A new perspective on impasses in couples therapy. *Journal of Marital and Family Therapy, 27*(2), 145–155.

Johnson, S. M., & Whiffen, V. E. (Eds.). (2003). *Attachment processes in couple and family therapy.* New York: Guilford Press.

Jones, E. E., & Pulos, S. M. (1993). Comparing the process in psychodynamic and cognitive-behavioral therapies. *Journal of Consulting and Clinical Psychology, 61,* 306–316.

Kanter, J. W., Tsai, M., & Kohlenberg, R. J. (Eds.). (2010). *The practice of functional analytic psychotherapy.* New York: Springer.

Kaslow, F. W., & Hammerschmidt, H. (1992). Long term "good" marriages: The seemingly essential ingredients. In B. J. Brothers (Ed.), *Couples therapy, multiple perspectives: In search of universal threads* (pp. 15–38). New York: Haworth Press.

Kendler, K. S., & Eaves, L. (1986). Models for the joint effect of genotype and environment on liability to psychiatric illness. *American Journal of Psychiatry, 143,* 279–289.

Knobloch-Fedders, L. M., Pinsof, W. M., & Mann, B. J. (2007). Therapeutic alliance and treatment progress in couple psychotherapy. *Journal of Marital and Family Therapy, 33*(2), 245–257.

Kohlenberg, R. J., & Tsai, M. (1991). *Functional analytic psychotherapy: Creating intense and curative therapeutic relationships.* New York: Springer.

Kohlenberg, R. J., & Tsai, M. (1994). Functional analytic psychotherapy: A radical behavioral approach to treatment and integration. *Journal of Psychotherapy Integration, 4,* 175–201.

Lambert, M. J., & Barley, D. E. (2001). Research summary on the therapeutic relationship and psychotherapy outcome. *Psychotherapy: Theory, Research, Practice, Training, 38*(4), 357–361.

Leahy, R. L. (2005). A social-cognitive model of validation. In P. Gilbert (Ed.), *Compassion: Conceptualizations, research and use in psychotherapy* (pp. 195–217). New York: Routledge.

Lebow, J. L. (1997). The integrative revolution in couple and family therapy. *Family Process, 36*(1), 1–17.

Leone, C. (2013). The unseen spouse: Pitfalls and possibilities for the individual therapist. *Psychoanalytic Dialogues, 23,* 324–339.

Lerner, H. (2002). *The dance of connection: How to talk to someone when you're mad, hurt, scared, frustrated, insulted, betrayed.* New York: William Morrow.

Lerner, H. (2012). *Marriage rules: A manual for the married and the coupled up.* New York: Gotham.

Linehan, M. M. (1993). *Cognitive-behavioral treatment of borderline personality disorder*. New York: Guilford Press.

Linehan, M. M. (1997). Validation and psychotherapy. In A. Bohart & L. Greenberg (Eds.), *Empathy reconsidered: New directions in psychotherapy* (pp. 353–392). Washington, DC: American Psychological Association.

Mahoney, M. J. (Ed.). (1995). *Cognitive and constructive psychotherapies: Theory, research, and practice*. New York: Springer.

Mahoney, M. J. (2003). *Constructive psychotherapy: A practical guide*. New York: Guilford Press

Makinen, J. A., & Johnson, S. M. (2006). Resolving attachment injuries in couples using emotionally focused therapy: Steps toward forgiveness and reconciliation. *Journal of Consulting and Clinical Psychology, 74,* 1055–1064.

Markman, H. J. (2001). *Fighting for your marriage*. San Francisco: Jossey-Bass.

McGoldrick, M. (1999). *Genograms: Assessment and intervention*. New York: Norton.

Mitchell, S. A. (1988a). *Relational concepts in psychoanalysis*. Cambridge, MA: Harvard University Press.

Mitchell, S. A. (1988b). The intrapsychic and the interpersonal: Different theories, different domains, or historical artifacts? *Psychoanalytic Inquiry, 8,* 472–496.

Mitchell, S. A. (1993). *Hope and dread in psychoanalysis*. New York: Basic Books.

Mitchell, S. A. (1995). Interaction in the Kleinian and interpersonal traditions. *Contemporary Psychoanalysis, 31*(1), 65–91.

Mitchell, S. A. (1997). *Influence and autonomy in psychoanalysis*. Hillsdale, NJ: Analytic Press.

Neimeyer, R. A. (2009). *Constructivist psychotherapy: Distinctive features*. Washington, DC: American Psychological Association Books.

Nielsen, A. C. (2016). *A roadmap for couple therapy: Integrating systemic, psychodynamic, and behavioral approaches* (reprint ed.). New York: Routledge.

Norcross, J. C. (Ed.). (2002). *Psychotherapy relationships that work: Therapists contributions and responsiveness to patients*. New York: Oxford University Press.

Norcross, J. C. (2010). The therapeutic relationship. In B. L. Duncan, S. D. Miller, B. E. Wampold, & M. A. Hubble (Eds.), *The heart and soul of change: Delivering what works in therapy* (2nd ed., pp. 113–141). Washington, DC: American Psychological Association.

Norcross, J. N., & Goldfried, M. R. (Eds.). (2005). *Handbook of psychotherapy integration* (2nd ed.). New York: Oxford University Press.

O'Brien, T. (1990). *The things they carried*. Boston, MA: Houghton Mifflin Harcourt.

Ogden, G. (2008). *The return of desire: A guide to recovering your sexual passion*. Boston: Trumpeter.

O'Hanlon, B., & Weiner-Davis, M. (2002). *In search of solutions: A new direction in psychotherapy, revised edition*. New York: Norton.

Orbach, S. (2004). Beyond the fear of intimacy. *Psychoanalytic Dialogues, 14,* 397–404.

Parker-Pope, T. (2010). *For better: How the surprising science of happy couples can help your marriage succeed*. New York: Plume.

Perel, E. (2010). The double flame: Reconciling intimacy and sexuality, reviving desire. In S. R. Leiblum (Ed.), *Treating sexual desire disorders* (pp. 23–43). New York: Guilford Press.

Pinsof, W. M. (1995). *Integrative problem-centered therapy: A synthesis of family, individual, and biological therapies.* New York: Basic Books.

Pinsof, W. M., & Catherall, D. R. (1986). The integrative psychotherapy alliance: Family, couple and individual therapy scales. *Journal of Marital and Family Therapy, 12*(2), 137–151.

Pitta, P. (2015). *Solving modern family dilemmas: An assimilative therapy model.* New York: Routledge.

Pizer, S. A. (1996). The distributed self: Introduction to symposium on "the multiplicity of self and analytic technique." *Contemporary Psychoanalysis, 32,* 499–507.

Preston, E. M., & Bennet, R. (1976). *The temper tantrum book.* London: Puffin.

Renn, P. (2012). *The silent past and the invisible present: Memory, trauma, and representation in psychotherapy.* New York: Routledge.

Renn, P. (Ed.). (2017). Special issue on creative attachments: Clinical practice through an attachment theory lens. *Psychoanalytic Inquiry, 37*(2).

Rosen, G. R., & Davison, G. R. (2003). Psychology should list empirically supported principles of change (ESPs) and not credential trademarked therapies or other treatment packages. *Behavior Modification, 27,* 300–312.

Ruiz-Cordell, K. D., & Safran, J. D. (2007). Alliance ruptures: Theory, research, and practice. In S. G. Hofmann & J. Weinberger (Eds.), *The art and science of psychotherapy* (pp. 155–170). New York: Routledge.

Safran, J. D., & Muran, J. C. (2000). *Negotiating the therapeutic alliance: A relational treatment guide.* New York: Guilford Press.

Safran, J. D., Muran, J. C., & Proskurov, B. (2009). Alliance, negotiation, and rupture resolution. In R. A. Levy & J. S. Ablon (Eds.), *Handbook of evidence-based psychodynamic psychotherapy: Bridging the gap between science and practice* (pp. 201–225). Totowa, NJ: Humana Press.

Schechter, M. (2007). The patient's experience of validation in psychoanalytic treatment. *Journal of the American Psychoanalytic Association, 55,* 105–130.

Scheinkman, M., & Fishbane, M. (2004). The vulnerability cycle: Working with impasses in couples therapy. *Family Process, 43,* 279–299.

Scheinkman, M., & Werneck, D. (2010). Disarming jealousy in couples relationships: A multidimensional approach. *Family Process, 49,* 486–502.

Schwarz, R. (2011). *We're no fun anymore: Guiding couples to joyful relationships.* New York: Routledge.

Shanahan, M. J., & Hofer, S. M. (2005). Social context in gene–environment interactions: Retrospect and prospect. *Journals of Gerontology, 60B*(Special Issue I), 65–76.

Shedler, J. (2010). The efficacy of psychodynamic therapy. *American Psychologist, 65,* 98–109.

Sheinberg, M. (1988). Obsessions/counter-obsessions: A construction/reconstruction of meaning. *Family Process, 27,* 305–316.

Sheinberg, M., & Brewster, M. K. (2014). Thinking and working relationally: Interviewing and construction hypotheses to create compassionate understanding. *Family Process, 53,* 618–639.

Sheinberg, M., & Fraenkel, P. (2000). *The relational trauma of incest: A family-based approach to treatment*. New York: Guilford Press.

Skinner, B. F. (1957). *Verbal behavior*. Acton, MA: Copley.

Slade, A. (2008). The implications of attachment theory and research for adult psychotherapy: Research and clinical perspectives. In J. Cassidy & P. R. Shaver (Eds.), *Handbook of attachment: Theory, research, and clinical applications* (2nd ed., pp. 762–782). New York: Guilford Press.

Slavin, M. O. (1996). Is one self enough?: Multiplicity in self-organization and the capacity to negotiate relational conflict. *Contemporary Psychoanalysis, 32*(4), 615–625.

Sprenkle, D. H., Davis, S. D., & Lebow, L. (2009). *Common factors in couple and family therapy*. New York: Guilford Press.

Stern, D. B. (1997). *Unformulated experience*. Hillsdale, NJ: Analytic Press.

Stith, S. M., McCollum, E. E., & Rosen, K. H. (2011). *Couples therapy for domestic violence: Finding safe solutions*. Washington, DC: American Psychological Association.

Stolorow, R. D., & Atwood, G. E. (1994). The myth of the isolated mind. *Progress in Self Psychology, 10*, 233–250.

Wachtel, E. F. (1979). Learning family therapy: The dilemmas of an individual therapist. *Journal of Contemporary Psychotherapy, 10*, 122–135.

Wachtel, E. F. (1982). The family psyche over three generations: The genogram revisited. *Journal of Marital and Family Therapy, 8*, 335–343.

Wachtel, E. F. (1992). An integrative approach to working with troubled children and their families. *Journal of Psychotherapy Integration, 2*, 207–224.

Wachtel, E. F. (2000). *We love each other, but . . . : Simple secrets to strengthen your relationship and make love last*. New York: St. Martin's Press.

Wachtel, E. F. (2001). The language of becoming: Helping children change how they think about themselves. *Family Process, 40*, 369–384.

Wachtel, E. F. (2004). *Treating troubled children and their families*. New York: Guilford Press.

Wachtel, E. F., & Wachtel, P. L. (1986). *Family dynamics in individual therapy: A guide to clinical strategies*. New York: Guilford Press.

Wachtel, P. L. (1997). *Psychoanalysis, behavior therapy, and the relational world*. Washington, DC: American Psychological Association.

Wachtel, P. L. (2008). *Relational theory and the practice of psychotherapy*. New York: Guilford Press.

Wachtel, P. L. (2010a). Beyond "ESTs": Problematic assumptions in the pursuit of evidence-based practice. *Psychoanalytic Psychology, 27*, 251–272.

Wachtel, P. L. (2010b). One-person and two-person conceptions of attachment and their implications for psychoanalytic thought. *International Journal of Psychoanalysis, 91*, 561–581.

Wachtel, P. L. (2011a). *Therapeutic communication: Knowing what to say when* (2nd ed.). New York: Guilford Press.

Wachtel, P. L. (2011b). *Inside the session: What really happens in psychotherapy?* Washington, DC: American Psychological Association.

Wachtel, P. L. (2014a). *Cyclical psychodynamics and the contextual self: The inner world, the intimate world, and the world of culture and society.* New York: Routledge.

Wachtel, P. L. (2014b). When the context is in the room: Extending the relational paradigm. *Psychoanalytic Dialogues, 24,* 419–426.

Wallin, D. J. (2007). *Attachment in psychotherapy.* New York: Guilford Press.

Wampold, B. E. (2015). *The great psychotherapy debate* (2nd ed.). New York: Routledge.

Weitzman, B. (1967). Behavior therapy and psychotherapy. *Psychological Review, 74*(4), 300–317.

Westen, D. (1998). The scientific legacy of Sigmund Freud: Toward a psychodynamically informed psychological science. *Psychological Bulletin, 124*(3), 333–371.

Westen, D., Novotny, C. M., & Thompson-Brenner, H. (2004). The empirical status of empirically supported psychotherapies: Assumptions, findings, and reporting in controlled clinical trials. *Psychological Bulletin, 130,* 631–663.

White, M., & Epston, D. (1990). *Narrative means to therapeutic ends.* New York: Norton.

Wile, D. B. (1981). *Couples therapy: A nontraditional approach.* New York: Wiley.

Wile, D. B. (1984). Kohut, Kernberg, and accusatory interpretations. *Psychotherapy, 21*(3), 353–364.

Wile, D. B. (1985). Psychotherapy by precedent: Unexamined legacies from pre-1920 psychoanalysis. *Psychotherapy, 22,* 793–802.

Wile, D. B. (2002). Collaborative couple therapy. In A. S. Gurman & N. S. Jacobson (Eds.), *Clinical handbook of couple therapy* (3rd ed., pp. 281–307). New York: Guilford Press.

Wile, D. B. (2013). Opening the circle of pursuit and distance. *Family Process, 52,* 19–32.

Wilson, P. (1995) *Instant calm: Over 100 easy-to-use techniques for relaxing mind and body.* New York: Plume.

Index